BASIC EXPERIMENTS IN BIOTECHNOLOGY

THE AUTHORS

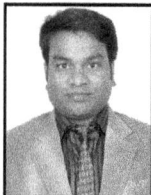

Dr. Ashok K. Rathoure shares his knowledge and experience in the field of Environment Impact Assessment with a doctoral degree in Bioremediation for M/s En-vision Group Surat. Previously he was associated with En-vision Enviro Engineers Pvt. Ltd. for EIA studies; Himachal Institute of Life Sciences Paonta and Beehive College of Ad. Studies Dehradun for teaching to Biotechnology, Microbiology, Biochemistry and other biosciences subjects. He is also associated as Editor-in-Chief for Octa Journal of Environmental Research, Managing Editor for Octa Journal of Biosciences and Executive Editor for Scientific India Magazine. His area of research is environmental biotechnology and publication includes 58 full length research papers in international and national journals of repute, 8 Course books from reputed publishers in India, 4 Research books and 6 Book chapters in Springer-verlag USA, CRC press Tayer & Francis Florida, I.K. Publishers Mumbai and Daya Publishers New Delhi, respectively. He had reviewed more than 70 research manuscript for many international journals. He is member of APCBEES (Hong Kong), IACSIT (Singapore), EFB (Spain), Society for Conservation Biology (Washington) and founder member of Scientific Planet Society (Dehradun). He has supervised 24 research scholars (UG, PG and Diploma). Dr. Rathoure was born in 1983 in village Hariharpur (UP) and completed his basic education in Hariharpur, Tandiyawan and Hardoi. He came to Kanpur for M.Sc. and was moved to Pauri for M.Tech. (G.B. Pant Engineering College) and has travelled extensively in the major cities of Northern and Western India for his education and as a teacher, trainer and taught to widen the horizon of knowledge and to sharpen his intellect. Moreover, He has also received PG Diploma in Human Resource Management (HRM) from Algappa University Karaikudi Tamilnadu.

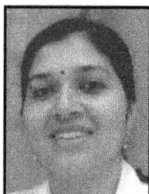

Dr. Smitha Rajesh has received her master degree in chemical engineering from SVNIT Surat in 2010 followed by doctorate degree (Doctor of Philosophy) from SVNIT Surat in Chemical Engineering. She has also received MBA degree in Operation Research (HRM) from IGNOU. Her area of research is chemical and environmental engineering. She had 12 years of industrial experience and excelled in various reputed industries in varies capacities. She had published so far 6 international technical papers along with 4 patents related to PP catalyst development. She is life member of Scientific Planet Society (Dehradun) and senior member of Indian Institute of Industrial Engineers (IIIE). She has strong command over ETP designing, Utility designing, Design of P&ID, Making of PFDs, Vendor selection, Material and heat balance, water balance, Preparation of Feasibility and Treatability Reports, Risk Analysis Report & Disaster Management. Also, she has undergone professional training on MATLAB Basics and Intellectual Property Management. She is a keen planner, strategist & implementer with demonstrated abilities in managing plant operations at commercial scale accelerating the business growth.

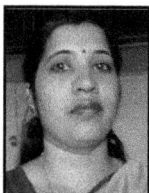

Dr. Savita Goyal Aggarwal, working as Associate Professor, Department of Chemistry, Army Cadet College IMA (Dehradun) has received his master degree from Hemwati Nandan Garhwal (Central) University, Garhwal (MSc) in Chemistry followed by doctorate degree (Doctor of Philosophy) from, FRI University, Forest Research Institute, Dehradun in 2004. She had worked as a Project Assistant in Indian Institute of Petroleum. She is an alumnus of SGRRPG College, Dehradun. She has also done her Bachelor degree in Education from Kurushetra University, Kurushetra. She is also pursuing PG in psychology. She is throughout first division. Her area of research includes environmental science, medicinal plant and natural products and research publication includes 20 full length research papers in international and national reputed journals. She has supervised more than 15 research scholars (including UG, PG and PhD). She is reviewer of many national and international journals. She is also member of many scientific societies. She has more than 12 years of teaching (at UG and PG Level) and more than 14 years of research experience. She has received national and state scholarship. She has organized many national level seminars as an organizing secretary.

BASIC EXPERIMENTS IN BIOTECHNOLOGY

Authors

Dr. Ashok K. Rathoure

Dr. Smitha Rajesh

Dr. Savita G. Aggarwal

2016

Daya Publishing House®

A Division of

Astral International Pvt. Ltd.
New Delhi - 110 002

Cataloging in Publication Data—DK
Courtesy: D.K. Agencies (P) Ltd. <docinfo@dkagencies.com>

Rathoure, Ashok K., author.
   Basic experiments in biotechnology / authors, Dr. Ashok
K. Rathoure, Dr. Smitha Rajesh, Dr. Savita G. Aggarwal.
      pages cm
   Includes bibliographical references.

   ISBN: 9789351309543 (International Edition)

   1. Biotechnology—Experiments.   I. Rajesh, Smitha,
author.   II. Aggarwal, Savita G. (Savita Goyal), author.   III.
Title.

   TP248.24.R38 2016   DDC 660.6078   23

Published by	:	**Daya Publishing House®** *A Division of* **Astral International Pvt. Ltd.** – ISO 9001:2008 Certified Company – 4760-61/23, Ansari Road, Darya Ganj New Delhi-110 002 Ph. 011-43549197, 23278134 E-mail: info@astralint.com Website: www.astralint.com
Laser Typesetting	:	**SSMG Computer Graphics,** Delhi - 110 084
Printed at	:	**Replika Press Pvt Ltd**

This Book is dedicated to

"Mrs. K.P. Rathoure"

(Meenu)

Acknowledgements

"First and foremost, we would like to thank our loving Creator for making us
a curious being who loves to explore his creation and for giving us the
opportunity to write this Book. Without him, we can do nothing."

It's our immense pleasure to thank Mrs. K.P. Rathoure for inspiring me to write
this manuscript. We express my sincere gratitude to Prof. N. Singh Dept. of
Biotechnology and Zoology, HNBGU (A Central University), Srinagar-Garhwal
(Uttarakhand); Prof. B.S. Bisht, Dept. of Zoology, HNBGU (A Central University),
SRT Campus Badshahithaul Tehri (Uttarakhand); Prof. Meena Srivastava, Head Dept
of Zoology, Prof. I.D. Singh, Ex Head, Dept of Botany, MP Govt. (PG) College, Hardoi
Uttar Pradesh (India); Prof Akhilesh Kumar, Principal, M.P. Govt. (PG) College, Hardoi
(UP); Dr. A.M. Saxena, Lucknow University Lucknow; Prof. Neelima Gupta, Dept of
Animal Science, MJP Rohelkhand University, Bareilly (Uttar Pradesh); Prof. P. Soni.
Retd. Scientist-G & Head Ecology & Environment, FRI, Dehradun; Prof. U.K. Atheya.
Ex. Head, Dept of Animal Science, G.B. Pant University of Sciences and Technology
Pantnagar (Uttarakhand); Prof. R.P. Singh, School for Environmental Sciences
Babasaheb Bhimrao Ambedkar University, Lucknow; Prof. S.C. Tiwari and Prof. J.P.
Mehta, Dept. of Microbiology and Botany, HNBGU (A Central University), Srinagar-
Garhwal (Uttarakhand); for their critical suggestions and inspirations. My special
thanks to Dr. V.D. Joshi, Ex Principal, Govt. PG College, Purola, Uttarkashi
(Uttarakhand); Prof. A. K. Chopra, Dept. of Zoology and Environmental Science,
Gurukul Kangri University Haridwar, (Uttarakhand); Dr. Harish Chandra and Dr.
Manoj Bhatt, Dept. of Biotechnology, G.B. Pant Engineering College Pauri-Garhwal;
Dr. Arun Kumar, Director Research, Dolphin Institute of Biomedical and Natural
Sciences Dehradun; Dr. A.K. Singh, Scientist E, Wadia Institute of Himalayan Geology,
Dehradun; Dr. S.P. Goyal, Scientist F and Head, Forensic Science Laboratory, Wild
Life Institute of India, Dehradun; Mr. P. Dwivedi Dept. of Biotechnology, Amity Institute
Noida; Dr. Saswat Katiyar Dept. of Biochemistry, CSJMU Kanpur (UP); Dr. Sandip
Kumar and Dr. Sandip Tripathi, NIMS University Jaipur; Dr. Ashish Thapliyal,
Scientist State Biotech Program Utterakhand; Dr. N. Rai Dept. of Biotechnology, GEU
Dehradun, Dr. Aftab Ahmad, Director Beehive College Dehradun, Dr. G. Sunil Babu,

Dept. of Enviromental Sceince. BRA University Lucknow; Dr. M.S. Khan, Dept. of Microbiology AMU Aligarh; Dr. A. K. Chopra, Dr. P.C. Joshi, Dept. of Zoology, Gurukul Kangari University Haridwar, Dr. R. Kumar, Scientist, IARI Delhi; Dr. Sanjay Gupta Dept. of Biotechnology, SBS College Dehradun; Dr Vinod K. Dhatwalia, Assistant Prof., Dept. of Chemistry, Uttaranchal University, Dehradun (Uttarakhand); Dr. Arun Bhatt, Associate Professor (Genetics and Plant Breeding), Officer Incharge Department of Crop Improvement, College of Forestry and Hill Agriculture, Ranichauri,Tehri Garhwal; Dr. Ashish Chauhan, Jr. Scientist, National Institute of Pharmaceutical Education and Research (NIPER), Sector 67, Phase 10, S.A.S Nagar, Mohali , Punjab; Dr. G. Awasthi, Assistant Prof., Dept of Biochemistry, Dolphin Institute of Natural Sciences, Dehradun (Uttarakhand); Dr. M.K. Tripathi, Senior Scientist (Biochemistry), APPD, CIAE, Bhopal; Dr. Manoj Eledath, Ecology and Biodiversity Expert and Proprietor, Ananthsree Ecocare Meghna Complex, Bhatar Char Rasta Surat Gujrat; Dr. Manoj Kumar Upadhyay, Scientist C & Quality Manager, Biotech Park Lucknow; Dr. Pankaj Chauhan, Asst. Professor, Dept of Biotechnology, Soolani University (HP); Dr. Rajib Roychowdhury, Centre for Biotechnology, Visva-Bharati Santiniketan; West Bengal; Dr. Rekha Rani, Assistant Professor, Dept. of Zoology, Navyug Kanya PG College, Rajendra Nager, Lucknow; Tejpal Dhewa, Asst. Professor, Dept of Microbiology, BCAS, Delhi University of Delhi, Sector-2, Phase-1, Dwarka, New Delhi; Dr Vishal Rajput, Assistant Prof. Dept. of Biotechnology and Biochemistry, Post Graduate Institute of Biomedical Science & Research Balawala Dehradun, (Uttarakhand) for discussions and valuable comments which have helped to improve the matter.

We also express gratitude to Dr. I. O. Agbagwa, Department of Plant Sciences and Plant Biotechnology, University of Port Hartcourt, Nigeria; Dr. Idress Hamad Attitalla, Associate Professor, Botany Department, Faculty of Science, Omar Al-Mukhtar University, Al- Bayda, Libya; Prof. Badar Alam Iqbal, Former Fulbright Visiting Professor; Claflin University; South Carolina USA; Prof. M Ekin Uddin, State University of Bangladesh, 77 Satmasjid Road, Dhanmondi, Dhaka, Bangladesh; Prof. Nelson Duran, Environmental Biotechnology and Pharmacology, Chemical Institute, UNICAMP, Campinas, SP, Brazil; Prof. Paulo Jubilut, Sao Paulo State University, UNESP Rua Quirino de Andrade, 215-Centro Sao Paulo Brazil; Prof. S. Choi, Dept. of Molecular Biology and Bioinformatics, Pusan National University, Pusan South Korea; Prof. Silas GranatoVillas-Boas, Industrial Microbiology, University of Aukland, New Zealand; Prof. Tanvir Shams Qureshi, Dept of Civil Engineering, Department of Civil Engineering, Bangladesh University, Bondorbazar, Sylhet; Prof. Nathalie Gravel, Geography Division, Université Laval, Quebec City, 2325, rue de l' Universite, Québec (Quebec) G1V 0A6 Canada; Prof. G T. P. Wong, Research Centre for Environmental Changes, Academia Sinica, Academia Rd. Nankang, Taipei, Taiwan; Prof. Welington Luiz de Araujo, Biotechnology of Microorganisms, Microbiology Institute, Universidade Estadual de Sao Paulo Brazil for encouragement and substantial support.

We thank our colleagues Dr. Pankaj Chauhan, Pankaj Dhiman, Avnish Kumar, Stephen Benjamin, Meetika Gupta, Sonal Chonde, Amar Katiyar, PV Bramhachari, Apoorva Singh and Navneet Kumar for their scientific discussions and valuable comments. We sincerely appreciate the help and support rendered by Ajay Kumar, Manvendra Kumar, Gyanendra Kumar, Atul Kumar, Abishek Kumar, Virendra N. Joshi and Jignesh Patel.

Thank you all forever!!!

Dr. Ashok K. Rathoure
Dr. Smitha Rajesh
Dr. Savita G. Aggarwal

Preface

Biotechnology is multidisciplinary science subject involving a variety of distinct subject, where various living organisms and parts of organisms are used for the human welfare. The students obviously need a book that can provide complete and comprehensive aspects of the subjects and various biotechnological procedures applied in biology. This book *Basic Experiments in Biotechnology* aims to fulfill such a need of the students and teachers as well.

One of the exciting aspects of being involved in the field of biotechnology is the accelerating rate of progress. This book has been divided into four segments. The first segment discussed about biotechnology and its emerging fields; the segment '1' has 13 basic experiments for the students who are entering into the laboratory for the first time. In this segment, they will learn about the preparation of buffer and solutions, quantitative and qualitative tests about amino acids, protein, nucleic acids, (RNA & DNA) by different methods and isolation of casein protein from the milk. In the segment '2' about animal physiology, here, the students will learn about expression of solutions in concentrations, determination of urine urea nitrogen, calculating acid number of fats, calculation of saponification number and average molecular weight of triacylglycerols, salting in, salting out and dialysis of proteins, determination of serum albumin, total cholesterol, etc., blood group analysis, ouchterlony double diffusion test and determination of haemoglobin content by haemoglobinometer. The last segment 3 has 28 experiments about biotechnology and biological techniques for microbiology, plant tissue culture, genetic engineering and industrial biotechnology. Here the students will learn about culture of bacteria on solid and liquid medium, isolation of bacteria, methods of sterilization, sterilization of nutrient media, preparation of agar plates, simple staining, Gram staining, negative staining, biochemical characterization, determination of bacterial growth by turbidimetric method, preparation of alcohol from fruit juice, sterilizing plant materials, demonstration of *in vitro* morphogenesis and totipotency of seedling, effects of hormone balance on explant growth and morphogenesis, preparation from basal salt solutions, callus formation and multiplication, establishment of suspension cultures, anther culture, culture of primary chick embryo fibroblasts (CEF), transfer of cell cultures, preservation of cultured cells by freezing, isolation of DNA from animal tissue, isolation of DNA from plant leaves (C-TAB Method), isolation of high molecular weight genomic DNA from bacteria, isolation of plasmid DNA from *E. coli* bacteria, purification of DNA, quantitative estimation of DNA by spectrophotometric method and Agarose Gel Electrophoresis (AGE) for separation of DNA. This book will extensively assist students, teachers and academicians to further extend their knowledge beyond the course work and related subject matter but onto the practical application to gain insights of what happening in the present era of applied science.

Dr. Ashok K. Rathoure
Dr. Smitha Rajesh
Dr. Savita G. Aggarwal

Contents

Segment 0
Introduction to Biotechnology and Laboratory

1. Molecular Biology

The biology begins in 1930s with the junction of various biological disciplines such as, biochemistry, genetics, microbiology and virology. With the hope of understanding life at its most fundamental level, numerous physicists and chemists also took an interest in what would become molecular biology. In its modern sense, molecular biology attempts to explain the phenomena of life starting from the macromolecular properties that generate them. Two categories of macromolecules in particular are the focus of the molecular biologist:

(i) Nucleic acids, among which the most famous is DNA, the constituent of genes.

(ii) Proteins, which are the active agents of living organisms.

One definition of the scope of molecular biology therefore is to characterize the structure, function and relationships between these two types of macromolecules. This relatively limited definition will suffice to allow us to establish a date for the so called molecular revolution or at least to establish a chronology of its most fundamental developments. In its earliest manifestations, "Molecular Biology" the name was coined by Warren Weaver of the Rockefeller Foundation in 1938, an idea of physical and chemical explanations of life, rather than a coherent discipline. Following the advent of the Mendelian-chromosome theory of heredity in the 1910s and the maturation of atomic theory and quantum mechanics in the 1920s, such explanations seemed within reach. However, in the 1930s and 1940s it was by no means clear which cross-disciplinary research would bear fruit; work in colloid chemistry, biophysics and radiation biology, crystallography and other emerging fields all seemed promising. In 1940, George Beadle and Edward Tatum demonstrated the existence of a precise relationship between genes and proteins. In the course of their experiments connecting genetics with biochemistry, they switched from the genetics mainstay *Drosophila* to a more appropriate model organism, the fungus *Neurospora*; the construction and exploitation of new model organisms would become a recurring theme in the development of molecular biology. In 1944, Oswald Avery, working at the Rockefeller Institute of New York, demonstrated that genes are made up of DNA. In 1952, Alfred Hershey and Martha Chase confirmed that the genetic material of the bacteriophage, the virus which infects bacteria, is made up of DNA. In 1953, James Watson and Francis Crick discovered the double helical structure of the DNA molecule. In 1961, Francois Jacob and Jacques Monod hypothesized the existence of an intermediary between DNA and its protein products, which they called messenger RNA. Between 1961 and 1965, the relationship between the information contained in DNA and the structure of proteins was determined: there is a code — the genetic code — which creates a correspondence between the succession of nucleotides in the DNA sequence and a series of amino acids in proteins. At the beginning of the 1960s, Monod and Jacob also demonstrated how certain specific proteins, called regulative proteins, latch onto DNA at the edges of the genes and control the transcription of these genes into messenger RNA — they direct the expression of the genes.

The successes of molecular biology derived from the exploration of that unknown world by means of the new technologies developed by chemists and physicists; X-ray diffraction, electron microscopy, ultracentrifugization and electrophoresis. These studies revealed the structure and function of the macromolecules. A milestone in that process was the work of Dr. Linus Pauling in 1949, which for the first time linked the specific genetic mutation in patients with sickle cell disease to a demonstrated change in an individual protein, the haemoglobin in the erythrocytes of heterozygous or homozygous individuals. The development of molecular biology is also the encounter of two disciplines which made considerable progress in the course of the first thirty years of the twentieth century *i.e.,* biochemistry and genetics. The first studies, structure and function of molecules which make up living things. Between 1900 and 1940, the central processes of metabolism were described: the process of digestion and the absorption of the nutritive elements derived from alimentation, such as the sugars. Every one of these processes is catalyzed by a particular enzyme. Enzymes are proteins, like the antibodies present in blood or the proteins responsible for muscular contraction. As a consequence, the study of proteins, of their structure and synthesis, became one of the principal objectives of biochemists.

The second discipline of biology is genetics. After the rediscovery of the laws of Mendel through the studies of Hugo de Vries, Carl Correns and Erich von Tschermak in 1900, this science began to take shape thanks to the adoption by Thomas Hunt Morgan, in 1910, of a model organism for genetic studies, the famous fruit fly (*Drosophila melanogaster*). Morgan showed that the genes are localized on chromosomes. Following this discovery, he continued working with Drosophila and, along with numerous other research groups, confirmed the importance of the gene in the life and development of organisms. The chemical nature of genes and their mechanisms of action remained a mystery. Molecular biologists committed themselves to the determination of the structure and the description of the complex relations between, genes and proteins. The developments of the theory of information and cybernetics in 1940s, in response to military exigencies, brought to the new biology a significant number of fertile ideas and especially metaphors. The choice of bacteria and of its virus, the bacteriophage, as models for the study of the fundamental mechanisms of life was almost natural they are the smallest living organisms known to exist and at the same time the fruit of individual choices. The study of DNA is a central part of molecular biology. Friedrich Miescher (1844–1895) discovered a substance he called nuclein in 1869. Later, he isolated a pure sample of the material now known as DNA from the sperm of salmon and in 1889 his pupil, Richard Altmann, named it nucleic acid. This substance was found to exist only in the chromosomes. In 1919, Phoebus Levene at the Rockefeller Institute identified the components and showed that the components of DNA were linked in the order phosphate-sugar-base. He called each of these units a nucleotide and suggested DNA molecule consisted of a string of nucleotide units linked together through the phosphate groups, which are the backbone of the molecule. However, Levene thought the chain was short and that the bases repeated in the same fixed order. Torbjorn Caspersson and Einar Hammersten showed that DNA was a polymer.

Discovery of Structure of DNA

In the 1950s, three groups made it their goal to determine the structure of DNA. The first group to start was at King's College London and was led by Maurice Wilkins and was later joined by Rosalind Franklin. Another group consisting of Francis Crick and James D. Watson was at Cambridge. A third group was at Caltech and was led by Linus Pauling. Crick and Watson built physical models using metal rods and balls, in which they incorporated the known chemical structures of the nucleotides, as well as the known position of the linkages joining one nucleotide to the next along the polymer. At King's College Maurice Wilkins and Rosalind Franklin examined X-ray diffraction patterns of DNA fibers. In 1948, Pauling discovered that many proteins included helical shapes. Pauling had deduced this structure from X-ray patterns and from attempts to physically model the structures. Even in the initial diffraction data from DNA by Maurice Wilkins, it was evident that the structure involved helices. But this insight was only a beginning. There remained the questions of how many strands came together, whether this number was the same for every helix, whether the bases pointed toward the helical axis or away and ultimately what were the explicit angles and coordinates of all the bonds and atoms. Such questions motivated the modeling efforts of Watson and Crick.

Complementary Nucleotides: In their modelling, Watson and Crick restricted themselves to what they saw as chemically and biologically reasonable. Still, the breadth of possibilities was very wide. A breakthrough occurred in 1952, when Erwin Chargaff visited Cambridge and inspired Crick with a description of experiments Chargaff had published in 1947. Chargaff had observed that the proportions of the four nucleotides vary between one DNA sample and the next, but that for particular pairs of nucleotides *i.e.* adenine and thymine, guanine and cytosine, the two nucleotides are always present in equal proportions.

Central Dogma

Watson and Crick's model attracted great interest immediately upon its presentation. Arriving at their conclusion on February 21, 1953, Watson and Crick made their first announcement on February 28. In an influential presentation in 1957, Crick laid out the Central Dogma, which foretold the relationship between DNA, RNA and proteins and articulated the sequence hypothesis. A critical confirmation of the replication mechanism that was implied by the double-helical structure followed in 1958 in the form of the Meselson-Stahl experiment. Work by Crick and coworkers showed that the genetic code was based on non-overlapping triplets of bases, called codons and Har Gobind Khorana and others deciphered the genetic code not long afterward (1966). These findings represent the birth of molecular biology.

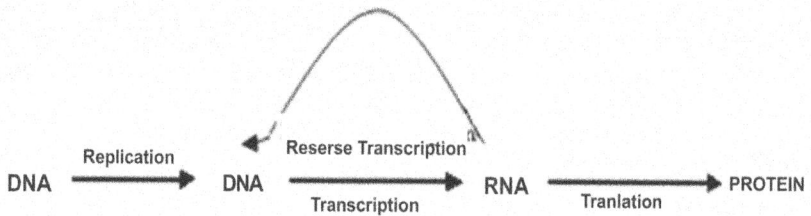

Fig. 1.1 Central Dogma of Molecular Biology

Structure of DNA

Deoxyribonucleic acid is an extremely long polymer made from units called deoxyribonucleotides which are simply called nucleotides. Deoxyribonucleic acid is a nucleic acid that contains the genetic instructions used in the development and functioning of all known living organisms with the exception of RNA viruses. The DNA segments that carry this genetic information are called genes but other DNA sequences have structural purposes or are involved in regulating the use of this genetic information. Along with RNA and proteins, DNA is one of the three major macromolecules that are essential for all known forms of life. DNA consists of two long polymers of simple units called nucleotides, with backbones made of sugars and phosphate groups joined by ester bonds. These two strands run in opposite directions to each other and are anti-parallel. Attached to each sugar is one of four types of molecules called nucleobases (bases). It is the sequence of these four nucleobases along the backbone that encodes information. This information is read using the genetic code, which specifies the sequence of the amino acids within proteins. The code is read by copying stretches of DNA into the related nucleic acid RNA in a process called transcription.

Within cells DNA is organized into long structures called chromosomes. During cell division these chromosomes are duplicated in the process of DNA replication, providing each cell its own complete set of chromosomes. Eukaryotic organisms store most of their DNA inside the cell nucleus and some of their DNA in organelles, such as mitochondria or chloroplasts. In contrast, prokaryotes (bacteria and archaea) store their DNA only in the cytoplasm. Within the chromosomes, chromatin proteins such as histones compact and organize DNA. These compact structures guide the interactions between DNA and other proteins, helping control which parts of the DNA are transcribed.

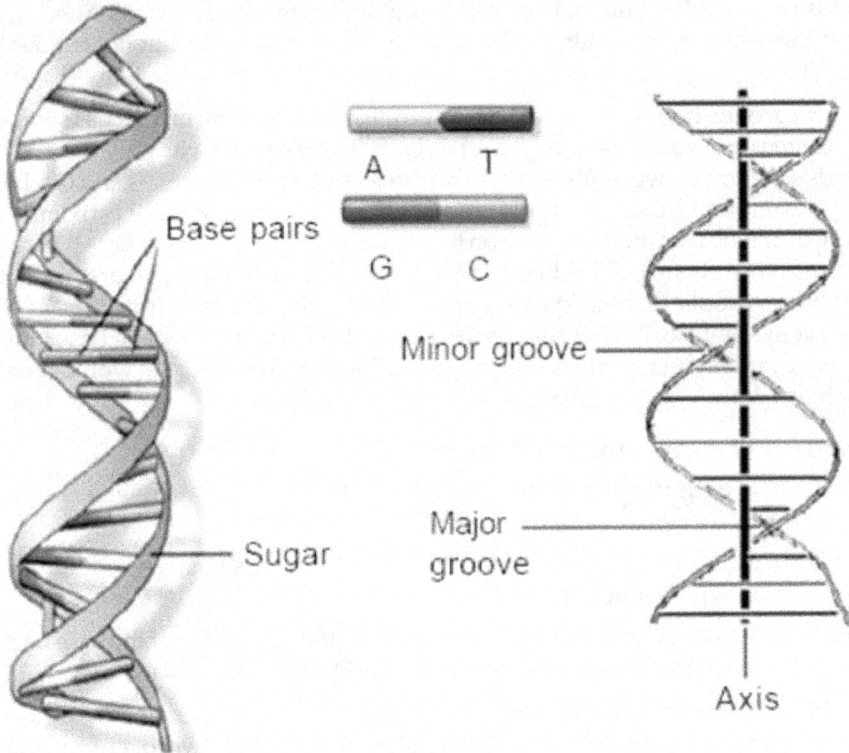

Figure 1.2 Double Helix Struture of DNA (B DNA)

Watson and Crick Model of DNA

DNA is found in cells, the smallest living units in our body or the smallest separate living organisms. DNA is the material that codes for the many physical characteristics of every living creature. The cells use different codes to determine what functions to carry out. In 1953, James Watson and Francis Crick proposed a structure for DNA that not only accounts for this pairing of bases but also explains how relatively simply the system of storing and transferring genetic information is. According to the Watson-Crick Model, a DNA molecule consists of two polynucleotide strands coiled around each other in a helical twisted ladder structure. The sugar-phosphate backbone is on the outside of the double helix and the bases are on the inside, so that a base on one strand points directly toward a base on the second strand. When using the twisted ladder analogy, think of the sugar-phosphate backbones as the two sides of the ladder and the bases in the middle as the rungs of the ladder. In effect, each strand of DNA is one-half of the double helix. The two halves come together to form the double helix structure. The two strands of the DNA double helix run in opposite directions, one in the 5' to 3' direction, the other in the 3' to 5' direction. The term that describes how the two strands relate to each other is known as antiparallel. The strands are held together by hydrogen bonds between the nitrogenous bases. In the double helix, adenine and thymine form two hydrogen bonds to each other but not to cytosine or guanine. Similarly, cytosine and guanine form three hydrogen bonds to each other in the double helix, but not to adenine or thymine.

Hydrogen bonds occur only between a Hydrogen atom on one base and either an oxygen or nitrogen atom on the other base. This explains why only two hydrogen bonds can form between A's and T's and three can form between G's and C's, because a hydrogen bond can only form where a H atom comes in close proximity to an Oxygen or Nitrogen atom of a base on the opposite strand. The every base pair contains one purine and one pyrimidine. Again, this is related to the structure of each base and how a proper fit, both in base size and chemical makeup, allows the DNA helix to exist in a physically and chemically stable structure. This type of base pairing is called complementary rather than identical. Identical base pairing would mean that A's bond with A's, G's with G's and so on.

Features of Watson-Crick base pair

(i)   The permitted hydrogen bonds are adenine with thymine (2 bonds); and cytosine with guanine (3 bonds).

(ii) The dimensions of the 2 permitted base-pairs are similar *i.e.,* C1'-C1' distance is nearly identical in both cases.

(iii) The beta-glycosidic bond is attached on the same edge of the base pair. This has implications for the structure of B-DNA, in particular.

(iv) Although some of the atoms in the purine and pyrimidine bases are involved in hydrogen bonds, there is still potential for further hydrogen bonding. This potential is particularly important for sequence specific protein binding.

(v)   The Watson-Crick base-pair is a planar structure.

(vi) The beta glycosidic bonds point in opposite directions. As a result, both chains can contain both purines and pyrimidines and the backbones of the two chains run in opposite directions.

Features of the Watson-Crick model of B-DNA

(i)   It is an antiparallel double helix.

(ii)   It is a right-handed helix.

(iii) The base-pairs are perpendicular to the axis of the helix.

(iv)   The axis of the helix passes through the centre of the base pairs.

(v)   Each base pair is rotated by 36 degrees from the adjacent base pair.

(vi)   The base-pairs are stacked 0.34 nm apart from one another.

(vii) The double helix repeats every 3.4 nm, *i.e.,* the pitch of the double helix is 3.4 nm.

(viii) B-DNA has two distinct grooves a major groove and, a minor groove.

These grooves form as a consequence of the fact that the beta-glycosidic bonds of the two bases in each base pair are attached on the same edge. However, because the axis of the helix passes through the centre of the base pairs, both grooves are similar in depth.

2. Origin of Biotechnology

The word Biotechnology is actually derived from the fusion of two simple words Biology and Technology. The Biotechnology term was used for the first time by Karl Erkey, a Hungarian Engineer, in 1919. The Biotechnology may be defined as the application of engineering and the biological science in the creativity of useful products from biological raw matter. The word 'Biotechnology' has received enormous importance and significance during last two decades, which is unprecedented. The beneficiaries from it to mankind led a greater attention towards this field. Biotechnology has touched our lives in all aspects, such as, food, health and animal life, improvement of our environment and for better healthcare, replacement of fossil fuel biofuel. Thus it has revolutionized the modern life. Biotechnology is the application of scientific and engineering principles to the processing of materials by biological agents to provide goods and services. From its inception, biotechnology has maintained a close relationship with society. Although now most often associated with the development of remarkable drugs, historically biotechnology has been principally associated with food, addressing such issues as malnutrition and famine. The history of biotechnology begins with zymotechnology, which commenced with a focus on brewing techniques for beer. By World War I, zymotechnology would expand to tackle larger industrial issues and the potential of industrial fermentation gave rise to biotechnology. Both the single-cell protein and gasohol projects failed to progress due to varying issues including public resistance, a changing economic scene and shifts in political power. The new field, genetic engineering, would soon bring biotechnology to the forefront of science in society and the intimate relationship between the scientific community, the public and the government would ensue. These debates gained exposure in 1975 at the Asilomar Conference, where Joshua Lederberg was the most outspoken supporter for this emerging field in biotechnology. By as early as 1978, with the synthesis of synthetic human insulin, Lederberg's claims would prove valid and the biotechnology industry grew rapidly. Each new scientific advance became a media event designed to capture public support and by the 1980s, biotechnology grew into a promising real industry. In 1988, only five proteins from genetically engineered cells had been approved as drugs by the United States Food and Drug Administration (FDA), but this number would skyrocket to over 125 by the end of the 1990s. The field of genetic engineering remains a heated topic of discussion in today's society with the advent of gene therapy, stem cell research, cloning and genetically-modified food. While it seems only natural nowadays to link pharmaceutical drugs as solutions to health and societal problems, this relationship of biotechnology serving social needs began centuries ago.

The origins of biotechnology culminated with the birth of genetic engineering. There were two key events that have come to be seen as scientific breakthroughs beginning the era that would unite genetics with biotechnology. One was the 1953 discovery of the structure of DNA, by Watson and Crick and the other was the 1973 discovery by Cohen and Boyer of a recombinant DNA technique by which a section of DNA was cut from the plasmid of an *E. coli* bacterium and transferred into the DNA of another. This approach could, in principle, enable bacteria to adopt the genes and produce proteins of other organisms, including humans. Popularly referred to as genetic engineering, it came to be defined as the basis of new biotechnology. Genetic engineering proved to be a topic that biotechnology into the public scene and the interaction between scientists, politicians and the public defined the work that was accomplished in this area. Technical developments during this time were revolutionary and at times frightening. In December 1967, the first heart transplant by Christian Barnard reminded the public that the physical identity of a person was becoming increasingly problematic. While poetic imagination had always seen the heart at the center of the soul, now there was the prospect of individuals being defined by other people's hearts. During the same month, Arthur Kornberg announced that he had managed to biochemically replicate a viral gene. Life had been synthesized, said the head of the National Institutes of Health. Genetic engineering was now on the scientific agenda, as it was becoming possible to identify genetic characteristics with diseases such as beta thalassemia and sickle-cell anemia.

With the discovery of recombinant DNA by Cohen and Boyer in 1973, the idea that genetic engineering would have major human and societal consequences was born. In July 1974, a group of eminent molecular biologists headed by Paul Berg wrote to *Science* suggesting that the consequences of this work were so potentially destructive that there should be a pause until its implications had been thought through. This suggestion was explored at a meeting in February 1975 at California's Monterey Peninsula, forever immortalized by the location, Asilomar. Its historic outcome was an unprecedented call for a halt in research until it could be regulated in such a way that the public need not be anxious and it led to a 16-month moratorium until National Institutes of Health (NIH) guidelines were established. Genetic engineering in biotechnology stimulated hopes for therapeutic proteins, drugs and biological organisms themselves, such as seeds, pesticides, engineered yeasts and modified human cells for treating genetic diseases. From the perspective of its commercial promoters, scientific breakthroughs, industrial commitment and official support were finally coming together and biotechnology became a normal part of business. No longer were the proponents for the economic and technological significance of biotechnology the iconoclasts. Their message had finally become accepted and incorporated into the policies of governments and industry.

By the 1980s, protein sequencing had already transformed methods of scientific classification of organisms especially cladistics but biologists soon began to use RNA and DNA sequences as characters. It expanded the significance of molecular evolution within evolutionary biology, as the results of molecular systematics could be compared with traditional evolutionary trees based on morphology. Following the pioneering ideas of Lynn Margulis on endosymbiotic theory, which holds that some of the organelles of eukaryotic cells originated from free living prokaryotic organisms through symbiotic relationships, even the overall division of the tree of life was revised. Into the 1990s, the five domains Plants, Animals, Fungi, Protists and Monerans became three i.e., Archaea, Bacteria and Eukarya based on Carl Woese's pioneering molecular systematics work with 16S rRNA sequencing. The development and popularization of the polymerase chain reaction (PCR) in mid 1980s by Kary Mullis and others at Cetus Corporation marked another watershed in the history of modern biotechnology, greatly increasing the ease and speed of genetic analysis. Coupled with the use of expressed sequence tags, PCR led to the discovery of many more genes than could be found through traditional biochemical or genetic methods and opened the possibility of sequencing entire genomes. The unity of much of the morphogenesis of organisms from fertilized egg to adult began to be unraveled after the discovery of the homeobox genes, first in fruit flies, then in other insects and animals, including humans. These developments led to advances in the field of evolutionary developmental biology towards understanding how the various body plans of the animal phyla have evolved and how they are related to one another. The Human Genome Project, the largest, most costly single biological study ever undertaken, began in 1988 under the leadership of James D. Watson, after preliminary work with genetically simpler model organisms such as *E. coli, S. cerevisiae* and *C. elegans.* Shotgun sequencing and gene discovery methods pioneered by Craig Venter and fueled by the financial promise of gene patents with Celera Genomics led to a public private sequencing competition that ended in compromise with the first draft of the human DNA sequence announced in 2000.

At the beginning of 21st century, biological sciences converged with previously differentiated new and classic disciplines like Physics into research fields like Biophysics. Advances were made in analytical chemistry and physics instrumentation including improved sensors, optics, tracers, instrumentation, signal processing, networks, robots, satellites and compute power for data collection, storage, analysis, modeling, visualization and simulations. These technology advances allowed theoretical and experimental research including internet publication of molecular biochemistry, biological systems and ecosystems science. This enabled worldwide access to better measurements, theoretical models, complex simulations, theory predictive model experimentation, analysis, worldwide internet observational data reporting, open peer-review, collaboration and internet publication. New fields of biological sciences research emerged including Bioinformatics, Theoretical biology, Computational genomics, Astrobiology and Synthetic Biology.

3. Chronological History of Biotechnology

500 B.C.: The discovery of first antibiotic, moldy soybean curds, in China.

A.D. 100: The first insecticide produced in China from powdered chrysanthemums.

1761: English Physician Edward Jenner, pioneers vaccination, inoculated a child with a viral smallpox vaccine.

1865: Gregor Mendel wrote his paper entiled Experiments on Plant Hybridization.

1869: Friedrich Miescher discovers a weak acid in the nuclei of white blood cells that today we call DNA.

1870: Development of Breeders crossbreeds cotton, developing hundreds of varieties with superior qualities.

1870: First *in vitro* corn hybrid was developed in laboratory.

1880-1890: Walther Flemming, Eduard Strasburger and Edouard van Beneden elucidate chromosome distribution during cell division.

1889: Hugo de Vries postulates that inheritance of specific traits in organisms comes in particles, naming such particles (pan) genes.

1903: Walter Sutton hypothesizes that chromosomes, which segregate in a Mendelian fashion, are hereditary units.

1905: William Bateson coins the term genetics in a letter to Adam Sedgwick and at a meeting in 1906.

1908: Hardy-Weinberg law derived.

1910: Thomas Hunt Morgan shows that genes reside on chromosomes.

1911: First cancer-causing virus was discovered by American pathologist Peyton Rous.

1913: Alfred Sturtevant makes the first genetic map of a chromosome.

1913: Gene maps show chromosomes containing linear arranged genes.

1918: Ronald Fisher publishes the Correlation between Relatives on the Supposition of Mendelian Inheritance the synthesis of genetics and evolutionary biology starts.

1928: Frederick Griffith discovers that hereditary material from dead bacteria can be incorporated into live bacteria.

1928: Alexander Fleming, Scottish scientist, discovered Penicillin.

1931: Crossing over is identified as the cause of recombination.

1933: Jean Brachet is able to show that DNA is found in chromosomes and that RNA is present in the cytoplasm of all cells.

1933: Hybrid corn was commercialized.

1941: Edward Lawrie Tatum and George Wells Beadle show that genes code for proteins.

1942: Penicillin was mass-produced in microbes for the first time.

1944: The Avery, MacLeod, McCarty experiment isolates DNA as the genetic material.

1948: Barbara McClintock discovers transposons in maize.

1950: The first synthetic antibiotic was created.

1950: Erwin Chargaff shows that the four nucleotides are not present in nucleic acids in stable proportions, but that some general rules appear to hold e.g., that the amount of adenine A, tends to be equal to that of thymine T.

1951: Artificial insemination of livestock was accomplished using frozen semen.

1952: The Hershey-Chase experiment proves the genetic information of phages to be DNA.

1953: DNA structure is resolved to be a double helix by James D. Watson and Francis Crick.

1956: Joe Hin Tjio and Albert Levan established the correct chromosome number in humans to be 46.

1958: The Meselson-Stahl experiment demonstrates that DNA is semiconservatively replicated.

1961-1967: Combined efforts of scientists crack the genetic code, including Marshall Nirenberg, Har Gobind Khorana, Sydney Brenner and Francis Crick.

1964: Howard Temin showed using RNA viruses that the direction of DNA to RNA transcription can be reversed.

1970: Restriction enzymes were discovered in studies of a bacterium, *Haemophilus influenzae*, enabling scientists to cut and paste DNA.

1972: Walter Fiers and his team at the Laboratory of Molecular Biology of the University of Ghent (Belgium) were the first to determine the sequence of a gene: the gene for bacteriophage MS2 coat protein.

1976: Walter Fiers and his team determine the complete nucleotide-sequence of bacteriophage MS2-RNA.

1977: DNA is sequenced for the first time by Fred Sanger, Walter Gilbert and Allan Maxam working independently. Sanger's lab sequence the entire genome of bacteriophage Ö-X174.

1978: Recombinant human insulin was produced for the first time.

1979: First time Human growth hormone was synthesized.

1980: Smallpox was globally eradicated after following 20-year mass vaccination.

1980: Principle of patenting organisms, which allows the Exxon oil company to patent an oil-eating microorganism, was approved by U.S. Supreme Court.

1981: The first transgenic animals by transferring genes from other animals into mice produced by Scientists at Ohio University.

1982: The first recombinant DNA vaccine for livestock was developed.

1982: Human insulin produced in genetically modified bacteria, was approved by FDA.

1983: Kary Banks Mullis discovers the polymerase chain reaction enabling the easy amplification of DNA.

1985: The Genetic markers were found for kidney disease and cystic fibrosis.

1986: The first recombinant vaccine for humans, a vaccine for hepatitis B, was approved.

1986: Interferon becomes the first anticancer compound produced through biotech.

1988: The first pest-resistant corn, Bt corn was produced.

1989: The human gene that encodes the CFTR protein was sequenced by Francis Collins and Lap-Chee Tsui. Defects in this gene cause cystic fibrosis.

1990: The first successful gene therapy was performed on a 4-year-old girl suffering from an immune disorder.

1992: Bovine somatotropin (BST) was approved by FDA for increased milk production in dairy cows.

1993: FDA approved Betaseron, the first of several biotech products that had a major impact on multiple sclerosis treatment.

1994: The first breast cancer gene was discovered.

1994: The International Commission for the Certification of Polio Eradication.

1995: The genome of *Haemophilus influenzae* is the first genome of a free living organism to be sequenced.

1995: The principles like Gene therapy, immune-system modulation and recombinantly produced antibodies enter the clinic in the war against cancer.

1996: A gene associated with Parkinson's disease was discovered.

1996: *Saccharomyces cerevisiae* is the first eukaryote genome sequence to be released.

1996: The first genetically engineered crop was commercialized.

1997: The first animal cloned from an adult cell was made in Scotland namely Dolly (sheep).

1998: The first genome sequence for a multicellular eukaryote, *Caenorhabditis elegans*, is released.

1999: The development of diagnostic test for quick identification of Bovine Spongiform Encephalopathy (BSE, also known as mad cow disease) and Creutzfeldt - Jakob disease (CJD).

2000: Virus-resistant sweet potato – the first biotech crop was tested over Kenya field.

2000: Starlink Bt corn, manufactured by Aventis Crop Science and supposedly produced only for livestock feed, is found in taco shells in the United States, to which some people claim to have had an allergic reaction. Starlink corn is subsequently discontinued, although no adverse health reactions are proven.

2001: First draft sequences of the human genome are released simultaneously by the Human Genome Project and Celera Genomics.

2002: The first transgenic rootworm-resistant corn approved by EPA.

2002: Japan's Biotechnology Strategy Council drafts the Biotechnology Strategy Guidelines, intended to guide the economic development of the life sciences in the country in the 21st century.

2002: The endangered species, banteng, cloned for the first time.

2003: First regulatory approval of a gene therapy product, Gendicine (Shenzhen SiBiono GenTech), which delivers the p. 53 gene as a therapy for squamous cell head and neck cancer.

2003 (14 April): Successful completion of Human Genome Project with 99% of the genome sequenced to a 99.99% accuracy.

On May 13, U.S. government files a challenge with the World Trade Organization stating that the European Union's anti-GM food policy violates international agreements.

On September 11, the Cartagena Protocol on Biosafety enters into force (on GMO), with the goal of protecting existing biodiversity from organisms modified through modern biotechnology.

On November 27, the Icelandic Supreme Court bars the implementation of the Icelandic Health Sector Database which contains tissue of and genetic information on Iceland's 300,000 citizens by the biotech company deCODE.

2004: Biotechnology is a complementary tool to traditional farming methods that can help poor farmers and consumers in developing nations stated UN Food and Agriculture Organization which endorsed the biotech crops.

2005: The United Nations General Assembly approves the Declaration on Human Cloning, a non-binding resolution that calls for a ban on all forms of reproductive and therapeutic cloning.

2005: The Energy Policy Act was passed and signed into law, authorizing numerous incentives for bioethanol development.

2006: The recombinant vaccine Gardasil, developed against human papillomavirus (HPV), first preventative cancer vaccine approved by FDA.

2006: Dow AgroSciences was granted the first regulatory approval for a plant-made vaccine by USDA.

2007: The first H5N1 vaccine approved for avian flu by FDA.

2007: On September 4, Celera Genomics publishes the complete human genome, consisting of a sequence of 6 billion nucleotides of the company's founder, Craig Venter.

2008: Stemagen scientists Andrew French and Samuel Wood announce that they have cloned several human embryos from adult skin cells using the somatic cell nuclear transfer technique. The embryos are later destroyed.

2009: Global biotech crop acreage reaches 330 million acres.

2009: The first genetically engineered animal for production of a recombinant form of human antithrombin approved by FDA.

2009: In March, President Obama reverses George W. Bush's policy on stem cell research, allowing hundreds of new embryonic stem cell lines to be used in federally funded research.

4. Genetic Engineering

The simple addition, deletion or manipulation of a single trait in an organism to create a desired change is called genetic engineering. Genetic engineering or genetic modification is the direct manipulation of an organism's genome using biotechnology. DNA may be inserted in the host genome by first isolating and copying the genetic material of interest using molecular cloning methods to generate a DNA sequence or by synthesizing the DNA and then inserting this construct into the host organism. Genes may be removed or knocked out, using a nuclease. Gene targeting is a different technique that uses homologous recombination to change an endogenous gene and can be used to delete a gene, remove exons, add a gene or introduce point mutations. An organism that is generated through genetic engineering is considered to be a genetically modified organism (GMO). The first GMOs were bacteria in 1973; GM mice were generated in 1974. Insulin-producing bacteria were commercialized in 1982 and genetically modified food has been sold since 1994. Glofish, the first GMO designed as a pet, was first sold in United States December in 2003. Genetic engineering alters the genetic makeup of an organism using techniques that remove heritable material or that introduces DNA prepared outside the organism either directly into the host or into a cell that is then fused or hybridized with the host. This involves using recombinant nucleic acid (DNA or RNA) techniques to form new combinations of heritable genetic material followed by the incorporation of that material either indirectly through avector system or directly through micro-injection, macro-injection and micro-encapsulation techniques. Genetic engineering does not normally include traditional animal and plant breeding, *in vitro* fertilization, induction of polyploidy, mutagenesis and cell fusion techniques that do not use recombinant nucleic acids or a genetically modified organism in the process. However, the European Commission has also defined genetic engineering broadly as including selective breeding and other means of artificial selection. Cloning and stem cell research, although not considered genetic engineering is closely related and genetic engineering can be used within them. Synthetic biology is an emerging discipline that takes genetic engineering a step further by introducing artificially synthesized genetic material from raw materials into an organism. If genetic material from another species is added to the host, the resulting organism is called transgenic. If genetic material from the same species or a species that can naturally breed with the host is used the resulting organism is called cisgenic. Genetic engineering can also be used to remove genetic material from the target organism, creating a gene knockout organism. In Europe genetic modification is synonymous with genetic engineering while within the United States of America it can also refer to conventional breeding methods. The Canadian regulatory system is based on whether a product has novel features regardless of method of origin. In other words, a product is regulated as genetically modified if it carries some trait not previously found in the species whether it was generated using traditional breeding methods *e.g.*, selective breeding, cell fusion, mutation breeding or genetic engineering. Within the scientific community, the term genetic engineering is not commonly used; more specific terms such as transgenic are preferred.

Gene Cloning

The cornerstone of most molecular biology technologies is the gene. To facilitate the study of genes, they can be isolated and amplified. One method of isolation and amplification of a gene of interest is to clone the gene by inserting it into another DNA molecule that serves as a vehicle or vector that can be replicated in living cells. When these two DNAs of different origin are combined, the result is a recombinant DNA molecule. Although genetic processes such as crossing-over technically produce recombinant DNA, the term is generally reserved for DNA molecules produced by joining segments derived from different biological sources. The recombinant DNA molecule is placed in a host cell, either prokaryotic or eukaryotic. The host cell then replicates (producing a clone) and the vector with its foreign piece of DNA also

Current cultivar   Wild relative

× Beneficial gene

Unwanted genes

Back Cross

F1 Generation

×

F2 Generation

Many Backcrosses

New Cultivar

Conventional Breeding

Unrelated organism

Beneficial gene

Unwanted genes

Current cultivar   Transfer into Plasmid in Agrobacterium

× ○ Genes required for transfer

New Cultivar

Transgenesis

Wild relative

Beneficial gene

Unwanted genes

Current cultivar   Transfer into Plasmid in Agrobacterium

× ○ Genes required for transfer

New Cultivar

Cisgenesis

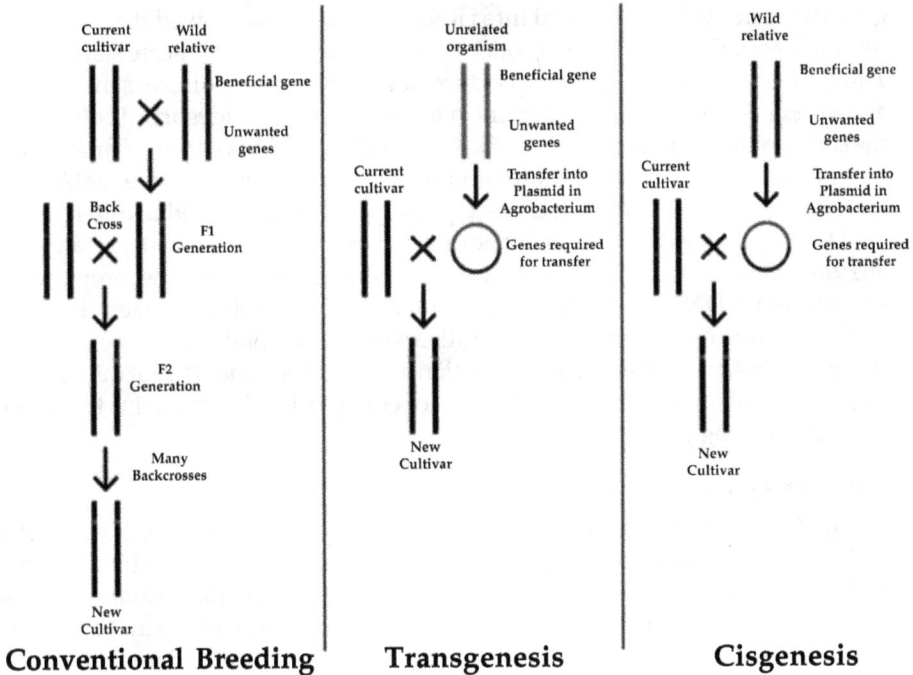

Figure 1. 3 Conventional Breeding and Transgenesis

replicates. The foreign DNA thus becomes amplified in number and following its amplification can be purified for further analysis. The process of cloning a gene involves many biotechnological techniques. Depending on what information is already availible on the gene of interest, various methods can be used to isolate and amplify it. To clone a gene means to cut it out of its original place in the host DNA and ligate it into a suitable vector where multiple copies of it can be quickly reproduced. Hamilton Smith and co-workers demonstrated unequivocally that restriction endoncleases cleave a specific DNA sequence. Later, Daniel Nathans used restriction endonucleases to map the simian virus 40 (SV40) genome and to locate the origin of replication. These major breakthroughs underscored the great potential of restriction endonucleases for DNA work. Building on their discoveries, the cloning experiments of Herbert Boyer, Stanley Cohen, Paul Berg and their colleagues in early 1970s ushered in the era of recombinant DNA technology. One of the first recombinant DNA molecules to be engineered was a hybrid of phage λ and the SV40 mammalian DNA virus genome. In 1974, the first eukaryotic gene was cloned.Amplified ribosomal RNA (rRNA) genes or ribosomal DNA (rDNA) from the South African clawed frog Xenopus laevis were digested with a restriction endonuclease and linked to a bacterial plasmid. Amplified rDNA was used as the source of eukaryotic DNA since it was well characterized at the time and could be isolated in quantity by CsCl-gradient centrifugation. Within oocytes of the frog, rDNA is selectively amplified by a rolling circle mechanism from an extrachromosomal nucleolar circle. The number of rRNA genes in the oocyte is about 100 to 1000 fold greater than within somatic cells of the same organism. To the great excitement of the scientific community, the cloned frog genes were actively transcribed into rRNA in *E. coli*. This showed that recombinant plasmids containing both eukaryotic and prokaryotic DNA replicate stably in *E. coli*. Thus, genetic engineering could produce new combinations of genes that had never appeared in the natural environment, a feat which led to widespread concern about the safety of recombinant DNA work Recombinant DNA is a form of artificial DNA that is made through the combination or insertion of one or more DNA strands, therefore combining DNA sequences as per your requirement, within different species *i.e.*, DNA sequences that would not normally occur together. Two major categories of enzymes are important tools in the isolation of DNA and the preparation of recombinant DNA; restriction endonucleases and DNA ligases. Restriction endonucleases recognize a specific, rather short, nucleotide sequence on a double stranded DNA molecule, called a restriction site and cleave the DNA at this recognition site or elsewhere, depending on the type of enzyme. DNA ligase joins two pieces of DNA by forming phosphodiester bonds.

Steps of Gene Cloning

(i) Isolation of DNA: Crude isolation of donor (foreign) DNA is accomplished by isolating cells, disrupting lipid membranes with detergents, destroying proteins with phenol or proteases, degrading RNAs with RNase and then leaving DNA at the end. If we had a little bit of DNA and knew enough of sequence to make primers we could use PCR to amplify it. If we started with RNA, then we would need to use reverse transcriptase to reverse transcribe it into DNA then PCR amplify it.

(ii) Choosing a vector: A vector is usually a piece of DNA that replicates in a bacterium. Plasmids are usually used, they are small pieces of circular DNA that are often found in bacteria which are self replicating and are maintained in the cell in a stable and characteristic number of copies. Some bacteria have very high numbers of plasmids which make them ideal cloning vectors. A gene inserted into a plasmid will be replicated many of times in single bacteria. And it is possible to grow millions of bacteria in a 1 litre flask. So this is a good way to make lots of copies of a gene of interest.

(iii) Application of restriction digestion to cut DNA: Next we use restriction enzymes to cut out the gene we want from the amplified product. We use the same enzymes to cut the vector so that the ends will be compatible. This means that if we use a sticky ends restriction enzyme, then the DNA sequences of the trailing bits will be compatible and will want to stick to each other. This makes it much easier to do. If we can't find a suitable site for a sticky end restriction enzyme then we can use a blunt ended one, which is a bit harder to make work. Once the restriction is done the piece of DNA that you want to clone needs to be separated from the parts you do not want this is done using gel electrophoresis as this will make it easier to clone. This is usually done by running the digest out on a gel and physically cutting out the fragment that you want with a scalpel.

(iv) Ligation: Once both the vector and the target DNA have been cut we mix them together and add the ligase enzyme. This enzyme ligates (connects) the phosphodiester backbone acting as a glue to stick the ends together.

(v) Transform of bacteria: This just means add the DNA back into a bacteria. There are a number of different ways of doing this, but most of them involve making the bacterial cell membrane temporarily porous so that it can take up the liquid containing the DNA mix. Then you let the cells recover and grow them up as usual.

(vi) Screening for positives: Those bacteria that have the cloned DNA in them. Sometime, the vector will just stick back to itself or stick to another vector without having any target DNA in it. Screening is often done using bacteria that makes a blue colour when fed a particular food but when a bit of target DNA is cloned into it then the gene that produces the blue colour is interrupted so they grow white. So, pick the white bacteria, grow them up and prepare the plasmid DNA from them, which contains lots of cloned gene. Now check the white one. This is done by isolating pure plasmid DNA. Then analyzing it by PCR or by use of restriction digests or by DNA sequencing to make sure your gene of interest has be cloned in. PCR products and restriction digests are analyzed by agarose gel electrophoresis.

Plasmid DNA as Vector: Plasmids are naturally occurring extra chromosomal double-stranded circular DNA molecules that carry an origin of replication and replicate autonomously within bacterial cells. The plasmid vector pBR322, constructed in 1974, was one of the first genetically engineered plasmids to be used in recombinant DNA. Plasmids are named with a system of uppercase letters and numbers, where the lowercase p stands for plasmid. In the case of pBR322, BR identifies the original constructors of the vector (Bolivar and Rodriquez) and 322 is identification number of the specific plasmid. These early vectors were often of low copy number, meaning that they replicate to yield only one or two copies in each cell. The pUC18 is a derivative of pBR322. This is a high copy number plasmid (> 500 copies per bacterial cell). Plasmid vectors are modified to contain a specific antibiotic resistance gene and a multiple cloning site, also called the polylinker region, which has a number of unique target sites for restriction endonucleases. Cutting the circular plasmid vector with one of these enzymes results in a single cut, creating a linear plasmid. A foreign DNA molecule, referred to as the insert, cut with the same enzyme, can be joined to the vector in a ligation reaction. Ligations of the insert to vector are not 100% productive, because the two ends of a plasmid vector can be readily ligated together, which is called self ligation. The degree of self ligation can be reduced by treatment of the vector with the enzyme phosphatase, which removes the terminal 5$'$-phosphate. When the 5$'$-phosphate is removed from the plasmid it cannot be recircularized by ligase, since there is nothing with which to make a phosphodiester bond. But, if the vector is joined with a foreign insert, 5$'$-phosphate is provided by foreign DNA. Another strategy involves using two different restriction endonuclease cutting sites with noncomplementary sticky ends. This inhibits self ligation and promotes annealing of the foreign DNA in the desired orientation within the vector.

DNA Ligase: The study of DNA replication and repair processes led to the discovery of the DNA joining enzyme called DNA ligase. DNA ligases catalyze formation of a phosphodiester bond between the 5$'$-phosphate of a nucleotide on one fragment of DNA and the 3$'$-hydroxyl of another. This joining of linear DNA fragments together with covalent bonds is called ligation. Unlike the type II restriction endonucleases, DNA ligase requires ATP as a cofactor. Because it can join two pieces of DNA, DNA ligase became a key enzyme in genetic engineering. If restriction digested fragments of DNA are placed together under appropriate conditions, DNA fragments from two sources can anneal to form recombinant molecules by hydrogen bonding between the complementary base pairs of the sticky ends. However, the two strands are not covalently bonded by phosphodiester bonds. DNA ligase is required to seal the gaps, covalently bonding the two strands and regenerating a circular molecule. The DNA ligase most widely used in the lab is derived from the bacteriophage T4. T4 DNA ligase will also ligate fragments with blunt ends, but the reaction is less efficient and higher concentrations of the enzyme are usually required *in vitro*. To increase the efficiency of the reaction, researchers often use the enyzme terminal deoxynucleotidyl transferase to modify the blunt ends. If a single stranded poly(dA) tail is added to DNA fragments from one source and a singlestranded poly(dT) tail is added to DNA from another source, the complementary tails can hydrogen bond. Recombinant DNA molecules can then be created by ligation.

Host Cells: A number of bacterial and yeast strains have been developed for recombinant DNA experiments. In order for a given plasmid to be replicated by a host cell, the cell must recognize its origin of replication site (*oriC*). Recombinant plasmid vectors are normally introduced into competent cells by transformation and then selected using appropriate cell culture media e.g., if the vector contains an *ampR* gene that encodes resistance to ampicillin, the culture media would include that antibiotic to ensure that only transformed cells will grow. Another method for introducing recombinant DNA molecules into host cells is electroporation. In this method, a suspension of exponentially growing host cells is mixed with a solution of recombinant DNA molecules and exposed to a high electric field for a few milliseconds. The high voltage alters the structure of the membrane so that pores are temporarily formed, allowing plasmid DNA to enter the cell. This method is fast and efficient. If bacteria are used as the host to clone eukaryotic genes, certain steps must be taken to make it possible for the bacteria to make sensible mRNA and functional proteins, since bacteria do not possess mechanisms for processing eukaryotic pre-mRNA molecules. It is necessary to isolate already processed mRNA from the donor eukaryotic cells and convert the single-stranded RNA to double stranded DNA. Reverse transcriptase from retroviruses uses RNA templates for synthesizing DNA. The resulting DNA molecules, known as cDNA (complementary DNA), can then be used for cloning in bacteria since they posses only intron free protein coding genetic information.

5. Transgenic Plants

Population of the country is rapidly increasing day by day. However, the most urgent need to the nation is to meet the food demand of the people. To remain self-dependent and to make them available with quality food, the biotechnologists have to boost up the gene revolution programmes for crop improvement so that the improved crops should have high yield, high amount of digestible and quality proteins and vitamins, disease/pest resistance and drough/herbicide/salt tolerance, etc. These can be done through the transfer of beneficial genes of a prokaryotic microorganism/eukaryotic incompatible plant in a given crop plant, alteration in metabolic pathways and making the plants resistant to invasion of pathogens/pests and herbicides/salt stress. Methods of gene transfer in a desired eucaryotic cell are: through *Agrobacterium,* through virus, co-cultivation of cells, leaf disc transformation, electroporation, etc. In recent years, plant protoplast, cell and tissue cultures have become an important tool for crop improvement, commercial production of natural compounds and many more in the development of forestry. Swaminathan (1987) emphasized the significance of biotechnological application of *in vitro* cultured plant protoplasts/cells/tissues as below:

(i) Tissue culture applications in order to capitalize upon the totipotency of cells,

(ii) Cell and protoplast cultures coupled with DNA vectors to overcome problems caused by barriers to gene transfer through sexual means,

(iii) Culture of plant cells for the production of useful compounds,

(iv) Extension and increase of efficiency of biological nitrogen fixation,

(v) Transfer of genes for nitrogen fixation ability to non-fixing species.

Due to playing with plant tissues in laboratory, this technique has been referred by some researchers as a botanical laser whose numerous uses are yet to be fully understood. In Gurgaon, the tissue culture laboratories (Euro-India Biotech Ltd. in collaboration with Haryana Agro-Industries Cooperation and Kiwi Callus (NZ) Ltd. have been set up for

(i) Micropropagation of plants,

(ii) Development and production of transgenic plants and seeds,

(iii) Development of genetically engineered plants,

(iv) Production of pure and virus free plants of rare species of high value,

Plant Improvement through Genetic Transformation

Following are some of the methods through which plants can be improved:

(i) Agrobacterium tumifaciens **mediated gene transfer:** *A. tumifaciens* can be used as a vector for transferring the desired genes into plant cells. There are several problems related to Ti-plasmid which must be overcome before using it as vector. Being large sized, it cannot be used as such because the hormones secreted by it interfere with the normal functioning of transformed cells. Therefore, T-DNA region, after removing from Ti-plasmid must be tailored so that it may join with foreign DNA. The *nos* (nopaline synthesis) gene of this plasmid which has promoter and termination signals and recognized by the host plant can be used for this purpose. Then it is allowed to join pBR322 resulting in production of tailored pBR322 T-DNA plasmid. At this stage a foreign gene of desired function is inserted into the non-essential region of T-DNA. Since the tailored plasmid does not contain *vir* genes required for transfer of T-DNA into the host genome. Therefore, the following two systems are being adopting for this purpose.

(a) Co-integrative system: In this system of gene transfer, the tailored plasmid containing foreign DNA is allowed to transform *A. tumifaciens* cells which contain a

Ti- plasmid. Consequently, *A. tumifaciens* cells have two plasmids. As a result of which there are much chances of reinserting T-DNA region to tailored plasmid into Ti-plasmid via homologous recombination at the repeated sequences.

(b) Binary vector system: It is an alternative method of previous one. In this method, *A. tumifaciens* containing Ti-plasmid, from which T-DNA has been removed, are transformed by tailored pBR322-T-DNA plasmid. Since the *vir* gene of T-DNA lacking Ti-plasmid is still effective, it integrates with foreign DNA containing tailored plasmid and transfers into plant cells. Using these techniques many more transgenic plants have been produced so far through transformed *A. tumifaciens* cells. Expression of seed storage protein of soybean in transgenic *Petunia* plants has been possible only due to successful transfer of foreign DNA into it.

(ii) **Co-cultivation (protoplast transformation) method:** In this system, the young leaves are segmented and protoplasts are isolated enzymatically by using cell wall lysing enzymes. It takes 3-10 days to protoplasts to divide and form cell walls. Protoplasts after regeneration of cell walls are mobilized to infection by *A. tumifaciens*cells containing foreign DNA. These are incubated for about 3 days. After transformation of protoplasts bacterial cells of the medium are now killed and protoplasts are cultured for 16-30 days. There develop microcalli which are plated on selective medium containing kanamycin as marker. Kan's callus grows which are then analyzed easily and recultured to develop transformed cells and finally adult plantlets within 4-6 months. In general, it is tedious and time consuming method and takes more than 4 months to develop transgenic plants, even in plants like tobacco. Moreover, it is not suitable for producing transgenic plants in calcitrant species.

(iii) **Leaf disc transformation method:** In this method leaf discs of 2 mm size are punched. The discs are co-cultivated in plates with a desired strain of *Agrobacterium* (5-10 x 10^6 cells/mL) containing the foreign DNA. Infection takes place at cut edges of leaf discs. After infection and cell transformation bacterial cells of the medium are killed. There are two methods of culturing leaf discs based on the presence of plasmids in *Agrobacterium*. If the bacterium, contains Ti-plasmid with a foreign DNA the discs are transferred onto filter paper of feeder plates for 48 hour; thereafter, the filter is transferred onto shooting medium containing kanamycin as marker. After shoots develop, these are transferred onto rooting medium. Finally, the adult plantlets are transferred in soil after hardening.

Moreover, if *Agrobacterium* contains Ri-plasmid the transformed cells are plated onto such medium which contains kanamycin and develops adventitious roots from cut edges of discs. The adventitious roots are cut and cultured on shooting medium to allow shoot formation. These are again put onto rooting medium for the development of roots. Transgenic plantlets are obtained after 4-6 weeks of incubation which later on are transferred in soil.

(iv) Virus mediated Transformation: Among plant viruses, cauliflower mosaic virus (CaMV) and Gemini viruses are being looked for potential vectors for transferring foreign DNA into plant cells. CaMV contains double stranded DNA as genetic material has increased the possibility of being used an efficient vector for genetic engineering purposes. Since its genome is tightly packed in protein coat, there remain the least chances to insert foreign DNA. Until size limitation problem is removed by using the helper virus, it cannot be used for transformation purposes. Geminiviruses e.g., curly top virus and maize streak virus are known to cause diseases on plant. They contain single stranded DNA packed in protein coat. Before using them as efficient cloning vector much is to know about the essential genes such as promoter sequence, etc.

Importance of Transgenic Plants

During the last decades, a tremendous progress has been made in the development of transgenic plants using the various techniques of genetic engineering. The plants, in which a functional foreign gene has been incorporated by any biotechnological methods that generally are not present in the plant, are called transgenic plants. As per estimates recorded in 2002, transgenic crops are cultivated worldwide on about 148 million acres (587 million hectares) land by about 5.5 million farmers. Transgenic plants have many beneficial traits like insect resistance, herbicide tolerance, delayed fruit ripening, improved oil quality, weed control etc.

Some of the commercially grown transgenic plants in developed countries are: Roundup Ready soybean, Freedom II squash, High-lauric rapeseed (canola), Flavr Savr and Endless Summer tomatoes. During 1995, full registration was granted to genetically engineered Bt gene containing insect resistant New Leaf (potato), Maximizer (corn), BollGard (cotton) in USA. Some of the traits introduced in these transgenic plants are as follows:

Stress Tolerance

Biotechnology strategies are being developed to overcome problems caused due to biotic stresses such as viral, bacterial infections, pests and weeds and abiotic stresses such as physical actors such as temperature, humidity, salinity etc.

Abiotic Stress Tolerance: The plants show their abiotic stress response reactions by the production of stress related osmolytes like sugars e.g., trehalose and fructans, sugar alcohols e.g., mannitol, amino acids e.g., proline, glycine, betaine and certain proteins e.g., antifreeze proteins. Transgenic plants have been produced which over express the genes for one or more of the above mentioned compounds. Such plants show increased tolerance to environmental stresses. Resistance to abiotic stresses includes stress induced by herbicides, temperature (heat, chilling and freezing), drought, salinity, ozone and intense light. These environmental stresses result in the destruction, deterioration of crop plants which leads to low crop productivity. Several strategies have been used and developed to build resistance in the plants against these stresses.

Herbicide Tolerance: Weeds are unwanted plants which decrease the crop yields and by competing with crop plants for light, water and nutrients. Several biotechnological strategies for weed control are being used e.g., over production of herbicide target enzyme in the plant which makes the plant insensitive to the herbicide. This is done by the introduction of a modified gene that encodes for a resistant form of the enzyme targeted by the herbicide in weeds and crop plants. Roundup Ready crop plants tolerant to herbicide-Roundup, is already being used commercially. The biological manipulations using genetic engineering to develop herbicide resistant plants are:

   (a) Over-expression of the target protein by integrating multiple copies of the gene or by using a strong promoter.

   (b) Enhancing the plant detoxification system which helps in reducing the effect of herbicide.

   (c) Detoxifying the herbicide by using a foreign gene.

   (d) Modification of the target protein by mutation.

Some of the examples are:

Glyphosate Resistance: Glyphosate is a glycine derivative and is a herbicide which is found to be effective against the 76 of the world's worst 78 weeds. It kills the plant by being the competitive inhibitor of the enzyme 5-enoyl-pyruvylshikimate 3-phosphate synthase (EPSPS) in the shikimic acid pathway. Due to its structural similarity with the substrate phosphoenol pyruvate, glyphosate binds more tightly with EPSPS and thus blocks the shikimic acid pathway. Certain strategies were used to provide glyphosate resistance to plants. It was found that EPSPS gene was overexpressed in Petunia due to gene amplification. EPSPS gene was isolated from Petunia and introduced in to the other plants. These plants could tolerate glyphosate at a dose of 2- 4 times higher than that required to kill wild type plants. A single base substitution from C to T resulted in the change of an amino acid from proline to serine in EPSPS. The modified enzyme cannot bind to glyphosate and thus provides resistance. The detoxification of glyphosate by introducing the gene, isolated from soil organism, (*Ochrobactrum anthropi*) encoding for glyphosate oxidase into crop plants. The enzyme glyphosate oxidase converts glyphosate to glyoxylate and aminomethylphosponic acid. The transgenic plants exhibited very good glyphosate ressitance in the field.

Phosphinothricin Resistance: Phosphinothricin is a broad spectrum herbicide and is effective against broad-leafed weeds. It acts as a competitive inhibitor of the enzyme glutamine synthase which results in the inhibition of the enzyme glutamine synthase and accumulation of ammonia and finally the death of the plant. The disturbace in the glutamine synthesis also inhibits the photosynthetic activity. The enzyme phosphinothricin acetyl transferase which was first observed in *Streptomyces* sp in natural detoxifying mechanism against phosphinothricin, acetylates phosphinothricin and thus inactivates the herbicide. The gene encoding for phosphinothricin acetyl transferase (bar gene) was introduced in transgenic maize and oil seed rape to provide resistance against phosphinothricin.

Other Abiotic Stresses: The abiotic stresses due to temperature, drought and salinity are collectively also known as water deficit stresses. The plants produce osmolytes or osmoprotectants to overcome the osmotic stress. The attempts are on to use genetic engineering strategies to increase the production of osmoprotectants in the plants. The biosynthetic pathways for the production of many osmoprotectants have been established and genes coding the key enzymes have been isolated e.g., Glycine betaine is a cellular osmolyte which is produced by the participation of a number of key enzymes like choline dehydrogenase, choline monooxygenase etc. The choline oxidase gene from Arthrobacter sp. was used to produce transgenic rice with high levels of glycine betaine giving tolerance against water deficit stress. Scientists also developed cold-tolerant genes (around 20) in Arabidopsis when this plant was gradually exposed to slowly declining temperature. By introducing the coordinating gene, it encodes a protein which acts as transcription factor for regulating the expression of cold tolerant genes; expression of cold tolerant genes was triggered giving protection to the plants against the cold temperatures.

Insect Resistance: A variety of insects, mites and nematodes significantly reduce the yield and quality of the crop plants. The conventional method is to use synthetic pesticides, which also have severe effects on human health and environment. The transgenic technology uses an innovative and eco-friendly method to improve pest control management. About 40 genes obtained from microorganisms of higher plants and animals have been used to provide insect resistance in crop plants. The first genes available for genetic engineering of crop plants for pest resistance were Cry genes (Bt genes) from a *bacterium Bacillus thuringiensis*. These are specific to particular group of insect pests and are not harmful to other useful insects like butter flies and silk worms. Transgenic crops with Bt genes e.g., cotton, rice, maize, potato, tomato, brinjal, cauliflower, cabbage, etc. have been developed. This has proved to be an effective way of controlling the insect pests and has reduced the pesticide use. The most notable example is Bt cotton which contains CrylAc gene *i.e.,* resistant to a notorious insect pest Bollworm *(Helicoperpa armigera).* There are certain other insect resistant genes from other microorganisms which have been used for this purpose. Isopentenyl transferase gene from *Agrobacterium tumefaciens* has been introduced into tobacco and tomato. The transgenic plants with this transgene were found to reduce the leaf consumption by tobacco hornworm and decrease the survival of peach potato aphid. Certain genes from higher plants were also found to result in the synthesis of products possessing insecticidal activity. One of the examples is the Cowpea trypsin inhibitor gene (CpTi) which was introduced into tobacco, potato and oilseed rape for develping transgenic plants. Earlier it was observed that the wild species of cowpea plants growing in Africa were resistant to attack by a wide range of insects. It was observed that the insecticidal protein was a trypsin inhibitor that was capable of destroying insects belonging to the orders Lepidoptera, orthaptera etc. Cowpea trypsin inhibitor (CpTi) has no effect on mammalian trypsin; hence it is non-toxic to mammals.

Virus Resistance: There are several strategies for engineering plants for viral resistance and these utilizes the genes from virus itself e.g., the viral coat protein gene. The virus-derived resistance has given promising results in a number of crop plants such as tobacco, tomato, potato, alfalfa and papaya. The induction of virus resistance is done by employing virus-encoded genes-virus coat proteins, movement proteins, transmission proteins, satellite RNa, antisense RNAs and ribozymes. The virus coat protein-mediated approach is the most successful one to provide virus resistance to plants. It was in 1986, transgenic tobacco plants expressing tobacco mosaic virus (TMV) coat protein gene were first developed. These plants exhibited high levels of resistance to TMV. The transgenic plant providing coat protein-mediated resistance to virus is rice, potato, peanut, sugar beet, alfalfa etc. The viruses that have been used include alfalfa mosaic virus (AIMV), cucumber mosaic virus (CMV) and potato virus X (PVX), potato virus Y (PVY) etc.

Resistance against Fungal and Bacterial infections: As a defense strategy against the invading pathogens (fungi and bacteria) the plants accumulate low molecular weight proteins which are collectively known as pathogenesis-related (PR) proteins. Several transgenic crop plants with increased resistance to fungal pathogens are being raised with genes coding for the different compounds. One of the examples is the Glucanase enzyme that degrades the cell wall of many fungi. The most widely used glucanase is beta-1,4-glucanase. The gene encoding for beta-1,4 glucanase has been isolated from barley, introduced and expressed in transgenic tobacco plants. This gene provided good protection against soil-borne fungal pathogen Rhizoctonia solani. Lysozyme degrades chitin and peptidoglycan of cell wall and in this way fungal infection can be reduced. Transgenic potato plants with lysozyme gene providing resistance to Eswinia carotovora have been developed.

Delayed Fruit Ripening: The gas hormone, ethylene regulates the ripening of fruits, therefore, ripening can be slowed down by blocking or reducing ethylene production. This can be achieved by introducing ethylene forming genes in a way that will suppress its own expression in the crop plant. Such fruits ripen very slowly, they can be ripening by ethylene application and this helps in exporting the fruits to longer distances without spoilage due to longer shelf life. The most common example is Flavr Savr transgenic tomatoes, which were commercialized in USA in 1994. The main strategy used was the antisense RNA approach. In the normal tomato plant, PG gene for the enzyme polygalacturonase encodes a normal mRNA that produces the enzyme polygalacturonase which is involved in the fruit ripening. The complimentary DNA of PG encodes for antisense mRNA, which is complimentary to normal (sense) mRNA. The hybridization between the sense and antisnse mRNAs renders the sense mRNA ineffective. Consequently, polygalacturonase is not produced causing delay in the fruit ripening. Similarly strategies have been developed to block the ethylene biosynthesis thereby reducing the fruit ripening e.g., transgenic plants with antisense gene of ACC oxidase, an enzyme involved in the biosynthetic process of ethylene, have been developed. In these plants, production of ethylene was reduced by about 97% with a significant delay in the fruit ripening. The bacterial gene encoding ACC deaminase (an enzyme that acts on ACC and removes amino group) has been transferred and expressed in tomato plants which showed 90% inhibition in the ethylene biosynthesis.

Male Sterility: The plants may inherit male sterility either from the nucleus or cytoplasm. It is possible to introduce male sterility through genetic manipulations while the female plants maintain fertility. In tobacco plants, these are created by introducing a gene coding for an enzyme e.g., barnase, which is a RNA hydrolyzing enzyme that inhibits pollen formation. This gene is expressed specifically in the tapetal cells of anther using tapetal specific promoter TA29 to restrict its activity only to the cells involved in pollen production. The restoration of male fertility is done by introducing another gene barstar that suppresses the activity of barnase at the onset of the breeding season. By using this approach, transgenic plants of tobacco, cauliflower, cotton, tomato, corn, lettuce etc., with male sterility have been developed.

Transgenic Plants as Bioreactors (Molecular Farming): Plants can be used as cheap chemical factories that require only water, minerals, sun light and carbon dioxide to produce thousands of sophisticated chemical molecules with different structures. By transferring the right genes, plants can serve as bioreactors to modified or new compounds such as amino acids, proteins, vitamins, plastics, pharmaceuticals (peptides and proteins), drugs and enzymes for food industry and so on. The transgenic plants as bioreactors have some advantages such as the cost of production is low, there is an unlimited supply, safe and environmental friendly and there is no scare of spread of animal borne diseases. Tobacco is the most preferred plant as a transgenic bioreactor because it can be easily transformed and engineered. Tobacco is an excellent biomass producer with about 40 tons of fresh leaf production as against e.g., rice with 4 tons.

Some of the uses of transgenic plants are:

Improvement of Nutrient quality: Transgenic crops with improved nutritional quality have already been produced by introducing genes involved in the metabolism of vitamins, minerals and amino acids. A transgenic *Arabidopsis thaliana* that can produce ten-fold higher vitamin E (alpha-tocopherol) than the native plant has been developed. The biochemical machinery to produce a compound close in structure to alpha-tocopherol is present in A. thaliana. A gene that can finally produce alpha-tocopherol is also present, but is not expressed. This dormant gene was activated by inserting a regulatory gene from a bacterium which resulted in an efficient production of vitamin E. Glycinin is a lysine-rich protein of soybean and the gene encoding glycinin has been introduced into rice and successfully expressed. The transgenic rice plants produced glycinin with high contents of lysine. Using genetic engineering Prof Potrykus and Dr. Peter Beyer have developed rice which is enriched in pro-vitamin A by introducing three genes involved in the biosynthetic pathway for carotenoid, the precursor for vitamin A. The aim was to help millions of people who suffer from night blindness due to Vitamin A deficiency, especially whose staple diet is rice. The presence of beta-carotene in the rice gives a characteristic yellow/orange colour, hence this pro-vitamin A enriched rice is named as Golden Rice. The genetic engineering is also being used to improve the taste of food e.g., a protein monellin isolated from an African plant (*Dioscorephyllum cumminsii*) is about 100,000 sweeter than sucrose on molar basis. Monellin gene has been introduced into tomato and lettuce plants to improve their taste.

Improvement of Seed Protein Quality: The nutritional quality of cereals and legumes has been improved by using biotechnological methods. Two genetic engineering approaches have been used to improve the seed protein quality. In the first case, a transgene e.g., gene for protein containing sulphur rich amino acids, was introduced into pea plant which is deficient in methionine and cysteine, but rich in lysine under the control of seed-specific promoter. In the second approach, the endogenous genes are modified so as to increase the essential amino acids like lysine in the seed proteins of cereals. These transgenic routes have helped to improve the essential amino acids contents in the seed storage proteins of a number of crop plants e.g., overproduction of lysine by de-regulation. The four essential amino acids namely, lysine, methionine, threonine and isoleucine are produced from a non-essential amino acid aspartic acid. The formation of lysine is regulated by feedback inhibition of the enzymes aspartokinase (AK) and dihydrodipicolinate synthase (DHDPS). The lysine feedback insensitive genes encoding the enzymes AK and DHDPS have been respectively isolated from *E. coli* and Cornynebacterium. After doing appropriate genetic manipulations, these genes were introduced into soybean and canola plants. The transgenic plants so produced had high quantities of lysine.

Artificial Seeds: Usually, we have to wait upto the end of reproductive phase for obtaining true seeds whereas artificial seeds are available within one month. The production of true seed is season bound at particular seasons of a year.The production of artificial seed is not time or seasonal bound. Life cycle of plant could be shortened in case of plant where dormancy of seed is prolonged. Artificial seeds will be applicable for large scale monoculture as well as mixed genotype plantation. It gives the protection of meiotically unstable, elite genotype. Artificial seed coating also has the potential to hold and deliver beneficial adjuvant such as growth promoting rhizobacteria, plant nutrients and growth control agents and pesticides for precase placement. Artificial seeds help to study the role of endosperm and seed coat formation.

Diagnostic and Therapeutic Proteins: Experiments are going on to use transgenic plants in diagnostics for detecting human diseases and therapeutics for curing human and animal diseases. Several metabolites and compounds are already being produced in transgenic plants e.g., monoclonal antibodies, blood plasma proteins, peptide hormones, cytokinins etc. The use of plants for commercial production of antibodies, referred to as plantbodies, is a novel approach in biotechnology. The first successful production of a functional antibody, namely a mouse immunoglobulin IgGI in plants, was reported in 1989. This was achieved by developing two transgenic tobacco plants-one synthesizing heavy chain (gamma chain) and other light (kappa) chain and crossing them to generate progeny that can produce an assembled functional antibody. In 1992, C.J. Amtzen and co-workers expressed hepatitis B surface antigen in tobacco to produce immunologically active ingredients via genetic engineering of plants. Several other therapeutic proteins have also been produced like haemoglobin and erythropoietin in tobacco plants, lactoferrin in potato, trypsin inhivitor in maize etc. The first proteins/enzymes that were produced in transgenic plants (maize) are avidin and beta-glucuronidase and are used in diagnostic kits.

Edible Vaccines: Crop plants offer cost effective bioreactors to express antigens which can be used as edible vaccines. The approach is to isolate genes encoding antigenic proteins from the pathogens and then expressing them in plants. Such transgenic plants or their tissues producing antigens can be eaten for vaccination/ immunization (edible vaccines). The expression of such antigenic proteins in crops like banana and tomato are useful for immunization of humans since banana and tomato fruits can be eaten raw. Transgenic plants (tomato, potato) have been developed for expressing antigens derived from animal viruses e.g., rabies virus, herpes virus. In 1990, the first report of the production of edible vaccine in tobacco at 0.02% of total leaf protein level was published in the form of a patent application under the International Patent Cooperation Treaty. The first clinical trials in humans, using a plant derived vaccine were conducted in 1997 and were met with limited success. This involved the ingestion of transgenic potatoes with a toxin of *E. coli* causing diarrhea. The process of making of edible vaccines involves the incorporation of a plasmid carrying the antigen gene and an antibiotic resistance gene, into the bacterial cells e.g., *Agrobacterium tumefaciens*. The small pieces of potato leaves are exposed to an antibiotic which can kill the cells that lack the new genes. The surviving cells with altered genes multiply and form a callus. This callus is allowed to grow and subsequently transferred to soil to form a complete plant. In about a few weeks, the plants bear potatoes with antigen vaccines. The bacteria *E. coli, V. cholerae* cause acute watery diarrhea by colonizing the small intestine and by producing toxins. Chloera toxin (CT) is very similar to *E. coli* toxin. The CT has two subunits, A and B. Attempt was made to produce edible vaccine by expressing heat labile enterotoxin (CT-B) in tobacco and potato. Another strategy adopted to produce a plant-based vaccine, is to infect the plants with recombinant virus carrying the desired antigen that is fused to viral coat protein. The infected plants are reported to produce the desired fusion protein in large amounts in a short duration. The technique involves either placing the gene downstream a subgenomic promoter or fusing the gene with capsid protein that coats the virus.

Advantages of Edible Vaccines: The edible vaccines produced in transgenic plants will sole the storage problems, will ensure easy delivery system by feeding and will have low cost as compared to the recombinant vaccines produced by bacterial fermentation. Vaccinating people against dreadful diseases like cholera and hepatitis B, by feeding them banana, tomato and vaccinating animals against important diseases will be an interesting development.

Biodegradable Plastics: Polythenes and plastics are one of the major environmental hazards. Efforts are on to explore the possibility of using transgenic plants for biodegradable plastics. Transgenic plants can be used as factories to produce biodegradable plastics like polyhydroxy butyrate or PHB. Genetically engineered *Arabidopisis* plants can produce PHB globules exclusively in their chloroplasts without effecting plant growth and development. The large scale production of PHB can easily be achieved in plants like *Populus*, where PHB can be extracted from leaves.

6. Record Making and Keeping

The records are very important documents for practical exercises in the laboratory. The students should prepare records very carefully. They reveal job done in laboratory. Use the following heads when preparing the documents/Practical note books.

Purpose/Introduction

In two or three sentences state exactly the purpose(s) and objective(s) of the experiment; what was done, to what, and why. Do not include as a part of this abstract familiarization with equipment or techniques, unless applicable. A short conclusion stating results/ideas may be added, if applicable.

Materials and Methods

Include here only any deviations, or additional equipment/procedures, from those stated in the laboratory manual. Otherwise, merely write, No deviations from the planned procedure were performed. However, accurate and complete cross-referencing to any references or procedures is mandatory.

Data/Results

All data generated should be recorded during the experiment. This includes recopying any tables, graphs, formulas, etc., from the laboratory manual and/or making new tables, graphs, as necessary, to represent the data accurately and neatly. Also, this section should include all calculations, averages, error analyses, and corrections of re-corded data.

Discussion and Conclusion

This section should include interpretations, conclusions, or suggestions regarding the results obtained. If applicable, include the expected results, and discuss why they were or were not achieved. State evidence for the views, including any assumptions has been made.

References

Include any that were consulted for the experiment or made in reference to the report. This is usually at least laboratory manual.

Notes

1. Be honest and concise.

2. Label all tables and graphs to indicate what they represent.

3. Do not use different colour pens or pencils in any portion of the reports.

4. Graphs should be numbered on axes in divisions that are easy to work with *i.e.*, 5, 10, 15, 20, etc.; not 2.3, 4.6, 6.9, etc.

5. Remember, this is not a personal diary and should not include any personal notations.

6. An accurate representation of them, with an intelligent explanation or hypothesis for any data obtained, is far more important.

7. If available, word processing and spreadsheet software will facilitate report writing and data analysis.

Record Keeping

1. Use a record book with permanent binding to avoid page deletions and insertions.

2. Make two copies of all notebook entries, one of which should be kept safely at a separate location.

3. Enter data and information directly into the record book promptly as generated. The students may wish to sign and date each page of the record book at the time of entry (signing is required procedure for industrial research notebooks). Do not rely on memory or informal loose sheets for entries with the intention of later putting these into the bound record book.

4. Use permanent ink, preferably black, which will reproduce well when photocopied.

5. Identify errors and mistakes and explain them.

6. Attach support records to the record book or store such records, after properly referencing and cross-indexing, in a readily retrievable manner.

7. Use standard accepted terms; avoid abbreviations, code names, or code numbers if possible.

8. Keep the record book clean; avoid spills and stains.

9. Keep a table of contents and index the record book as soon as it is filled.

7. Safety Guidelines

Students should be aware that safety issues are of the utmost importance in the laboratory. Time should be spent during the first laboratory meeting to familiarize students with the placement of eye wash-stands, showers, fire extinguishers, fire exits, and hazardous waste disposal sites.

1. Prepare for each laboratory period by reading each exercise and becoming familiar with the principles and methods involved. By being familiar with the exercise, decrease the chances of an accident. Also, advance preparation allows us to use our time efficiently in the laboratory to complete the experiment.

2. No eating, drinking, or smoking is permitted in the laboratory.

3. Laboratory coats or aprons must be worn at all times in the laboratory. This is to ensure that culture material is not accidentally deposited on our clothes or skin, and as a safeguard to protect our clothes and ourself from chemical spills and stains.

4. Only those materials pertinent to laboratory work, such as laboratory manuals, laboratory notebooks, and other laboratory materials, should be brought to laboratory work space. All other items, such as coats, books, and bags, should be stored away from work area.

5. Begin each laboratory session by disinfecting work area. Saturate the area with a disinfectant, spread the disinfectant with a paper towel, and allow the area to dry. Repeat this procedure after have finishing the work to ensure that any material have deposited on the work surface is properly disinfected.

6. All culture material and chemicals should be properly labeled with name, class, date, and experiment. Labeling is critical to avoid improper use or disposal of material.

7. Be careful with Bunsen burners. To avoid injuries, burners should be turned off when not in use. When reaching for objects, be careful not to place hands into the flame.

8. All contaminated material must be disinfected before disposal or reuse. All material to be autoclaved should be placed in a proper receptacle for collection. Used pipets should be placed in disinfectant.

9. After the laboratory session, observe good hygiene by washing the hands before leaving the laboratory.

10. In the event of any accident or injury, report immediately to the laboratory instructor so that prompt and proper action can be taken.

8. Safe Handling of Microorganisms

Many of the procedures used in molecular biology research involve the use of live microorganisms. Whenever such organisms are used, it is essential that laboratory workers adhere rigidly to a microbiology laboratory code of practice and thereby significantly reduce the possibility of causing a laboratory-acquired infection. The safest way to approach work with live microorganisms is to make the following assumptions:

1. Every microorganism used in the laboratory is potentially hazardous.
2. Every culture fluid contains potentially pathogenic organisms.
3. Every culture fluid contains potentially toxic substances.

The basis of a laboratory code of practice is that no direct contact should be made with the experimental organisms or culture fluids e.g., contact with the skin, nose, eyes, or mouth. It must also be noted that a large proportion of laboratory-acquired infections result from the inhalation of infectious aerosols released during laboratory procedures. Below is a list of instructions that forms the basis of a laboratory code of practice microorganisms handling.

1. A laboratory coat that covers the trunk to the neck must be worn at all times.
2. There must be no eating, drinking or smoking in the laboratory.
3. There must be no licking of gummed labels.
4. Touching the face, eyes and so on should be avoided.
5. There must be no chewing or biting of pens or pencils.
6. Available bench space must be kept clear, clean, tidy, and free of unessential items such as books and handbags.
7. No materials should be removed from the laboratory without the permission of the laboratory supervisor or safety officer.
8. All manipulations, such as by pipet or loop, should be performed in a manner likely to prevent the production of an aerosol of the contaminated material.
9. Pipetting by mouth of any liquid is strictly forbidden. Pipet fillers, or automatic pipets, are used instead.
10. All manipulations should be performed aseptically, using plugged, sterile pipets, and the contaminated pipets should be immediately sterilized by total immersion in a suitable disinfectant.
11. Contaminated glassware and discarded petri dishes must be placed in lidded receptacles provided for their disposal.
12. All used microscope slides should be placed in receptacles containing disinfectant.

13. It must be recognized that certain procedures or equipment e.g., agitation of fluids in flasks, produce aerosols of contaminated materials. Lids should be kept on contaminated vessels, when possible.

14. All accidents, including minor cuts, abrasions, and spills of culture fluids and reagents, must be reported to the laboratory super-visor or safety officer.

15. Before leaving the bench, swab the working area with an appropriate disinfectant fluid.

16. Before departure from the laboratory, wash the hands with a germicidal soap and dry them with paper towels. Laboratory coats should be removed and stored for future use or laundered. Do not under any circumstances wander into an office or rest-room area wearing a potentially contaminated laboratory coat.

9. Preparation of Buffers and Solutions

When making up solutions, observe the following guidelines:

1. Use the highest grade of reagents, when possible.

2. Prepare all solutions with the highest quality distilled water available.

3. Autoclave solutions when possible. If the solution cannot be autoclaved and wish to store it, sterilize by filtration through a 0.2-2 nm filter.

4. Check the pH meter carefully, using freshly prepared solutions of standard pH, before adjusting the pH of buffers.

5. Always label the container with the name of the solution, the percentage or concentration, name/course and date. For highly basic solutions, such as 1M NaOH, be sure to use plastic containers as glass is corroded by bases.

6. Store solutions cold when possible.

Time can be saved by making up concentrated stock solutions e.g., 1M Tris that can be used to make up a range of different solutions.

Percentage Solution

A percentage solution is one in which the exact concentration of the solute is known in 100 mL of a liquid or solution. The concentration may be expressed or determined by weight or volume; it may be written out in grams and milliliters and expressed as follows:

Percentage (w/v) = weight (in grams) in 100 mL volume of solution.

Percentage (v/v) = volume (in milliliters) in 100 ml total volume of solution

Examples by Weight

For a 1% (w/v) aqueous solution of sodium chloride, weigh out 1 g of sodium chloride (NaCl) and add to 100 mL of distilled water, or 10 mg of NaCl per milliliter.

For a 5% (w/v) aqueous solution of sodium chloride, weigh out 5 g of sodium chloride and add to 100 mL of distilled water.

For 1000 mL of a 5% (w/v) aqueous solution of sodium chloride, use 10 times the above amounts, that is, 50 g of sodium chloride in 1000 mL of distilled water.

Example by Volume

The percentage of the solution is stated on the label, and a percentage solution should be determined from this value. For example, the percentage on a bottle of commercial strength hydrochloric acid varies from 36 to 40%. If we want a 1% solution of HCl, it is erroneous to take 1 mL of 36-40% HCl and add it to 99 mL of distilled water. An acceptable and correct formula for determining the amount of 36% (v/v) HCl needed to make up 100 mL of a 1% (v/v) aqueous solution of HCl is as follows:

$$36 \times X = 1 \times 100$$

$$36X = 100$$

$$X = 100/36$$

X = 2.78 mL of 36% (v/v) HCL in 97.22 mL of distilled water

Dilutions for Solutions (Percentage by Volume)

The most accurate formula for making dilutions of solutions is the following:

Percentage (%) of solution X Unknown volume (mL) = Percentage (%) Needed X Volume (mL) Wanted

Example of Preferred Method

To make up 1000 mL of 70% (v/v) ethanol from 95% (v/v) ethanol, substitute the known amounts in the above formula:

$$95 \times X = 70 \times 1000$$

$$9SX = 70,000$$

$$X = \frac{70,000}{95}$$

X = 736.8 mL of 95% (v/v) ethanol in 263.2 mL of distilled water. Although the above method is preferred, we can use a generally accepted method of subtracting the percentage required from the percentage strength of the solution that is to be diluted. The difference will be the amount of water that is to be used.

Example of Subtraction Method

The percentage required is 70% (v/v) ethanol and the solution to be diluted is 95% (v/v) ethanol. As 95 –70 = 25, 70 parts of 95% (v/v) ethanol and 25 parts of distilled water are the amounts to be combined. To make up approximately 1 liter of 70% (v/v) ethanol, simply place 700 mL of 95% ethanol in a 1000 mL graduated cylinder and fill to the 950mL mark with distilled water.

Molar Solutions

A molar (mole, molecular) solution is one in which 1 liter (1000 mL) of the solution contains the number of grams of the solute equal to its molecular weight (sum of atomic weights).

Examples of Molar Solutions

To make up a 1M solution of NaCl (sodium chloride):

1. Obtain the atomic weights of the elements.

   Sodium (Na) = 22.997 Chlorine (Cl) = 35.459

2. Obtain the sum of the atomic weights from the formula for molecular weight.

   Molecular weight of NaCl = 22.997 + 35.459 = 58.456

3. Weigh 58.46 g of NaCl and make up to a total volume of 1000 mL with distilled water.

To make up 100 mL of a 1 M solution of NaCl:

1. Same as Step 1 above.

2. Same as Step 2 above.

3. 58.46 = 5.85

4. Weigh 5.85 g of NaCl and make up to a total volume of 100 mL with distilled water.

10. DNA Extraction from Agarose Gel

Introduction

There are many different methods of extracting DNA bands from an agarose gel. Important consideration is the yield/purity of the DNA after extraction. Agar various impurities which may inhibit downstream reactions if not efficiently removed from the DNA. We used to give the generic term hoonose to the unspecified carbohydrates that co purified along with the DNA and inhibited enzyme reactions.

Cutting out the DNA band

Most of the methods require cutting out the band. It must visualize the band, in an ethidium bromide stained gel, in a dark-room on a UV light-box. The UV is dangerous, wear gloves, long sleeves and face protection. Never look at UV with unprotected eyes. If possible, set the trans-illuminator to long-wavelength UV and minimize the amount of time the DNA is exposed. This is because the UV mutagenesis the DNA at a measurable rate. Use a scapel blade to cut around the band of interest. Switch off the transilluminator, switch on the white light and carefully remove the band from the gel and place it on the glass. It is good to trim off as much empty agarose as possible so go back to UV illumination briefly to do this. Place the excised band in a 1.5 mL microfuge tube.

Three representative methods

Spin-columns (Nucleic acid purification columns)

1. These are excellent for extracting DNA. Manufacterers include Qiagen, Sigma, Novagen. Everything need comes with the kit, including protocol, but to summarise;

2. Dissolve the gel-slice in 3 volumes of chaotropic agent at 50°C for 10 minutes Apply the solution to a spin-column and spin for 1 minute (DNA remains in the column).

3. Wash the column by passing 70% ethanol through (DNA remains in the column, salt and impurities are washed out) Elute the DNA in a small volume (30µL) of water or buffer, spin to collect.

Dialysis tubing (semi-permeable membrane, Visking tubing)

1. Freeze the gel slice at –20°C for 30 minutes.

   This is to make it easier to handle the gel slice

2. Cut a 5 cm length of dialysis tubing and rinse it inside and out with distilled water. Then rinse it with the same buffer used for the gel e.g., 0.5 x TBE and leave it submerged in a small beaker of this buffer. Seal one end with a dialysis clip.

   Dialysis tubing is purchased in rolls (dried), prepared by boiling and stored submerged in buffer at 4°C.

3. Insert the frozen gel-slice into the tubing and add 200–400µL of buffer e.g., 0.5 x TBE. Seal the other end of the tubing with a second dialysis clip.

   The buffer around the gel-slice must be the same as the buffer inside the gel.

4. immerse the sealed tubing in an electrophoresis tank so that the DNA band is parallel to the electrodes and apply 5V/cm electric field. The DNA will migrate out if the gel towards the positive electrode. It will be retained by the dialysis tubing. We can see this happening under long-wavelength UV. It takes about 10–15 minutes.

5. Remove the buffer from the tubing and place into a 1.5 mL microfuge tube.

6. Phenol/chloroform extract and ethanol precipitate the DNA. Re-dissolve the DNA pellet in an appropriate volume of water or TE buffer e.g., 10µL. The pellet is often so small that it is invisible.

Paper strip method

1. Using a scalpel blade, cut a slit immediately in front of the band to be extracted.

   Do not remove the band from the gel.

2. cut a piece of filter paper e.g., 3 MM paper to size to fit inside the slit. For example, 3mm x 10mm

3. Place the paper strip in the slit, return the gel to the electrophoresis tank (submerged in buffer) and switch on the current for 2–5 minutes.

   The DNA runs onward into the paper and is delayed in the smaller mesh size of the paper.

   Eventually the DNA will pass through so we have to keep checking it under long-wavelength UV so as not to leave it too long.

4. Remove the strip of paper (carrying at least some of the DNA) and place into a 0.5 mL microfuge tube, DNA side down.

5. Make a tiny hole in the bottom of the tube using a needle.

6. Place the 0.5 mL tube inside a 1.5 mL tube and spin for 30 seconds.

    We may have to remove the lid of the 1.5 mL tube. The buffer and DNA are retained in the larger tube. We can add 100μL of TE to the paper and re-spin to get a little more DNA out.

7. Phenol/chloroform extract and ethanol precipitate the DNA. Re-dissolve the DNA pellet in an appropriate volume of water or TE buffer e.g., 100μL. The pellet is often so small that it is invisible.

11. Preparation of Glycerol Stocks

Glycerol stocks can be prepared from an overnight culture grown from a single colony picked from the plates prepared above in the transformation step. These stocks allow us to keep transformed bacterial cultures at -70°C for prolonged periods of time negating the need to perform transformations every time fresh plasmid are required. The eppendorf of glycerol stock is removed briefly from the freezer and a sterile toothpick is used to scrape some slithers of cells onto a LB-antibiotic selective plate which is then incubated overnight as before. These plates allow us to grow up large culture volumes from which fresh plasmid are purified.

Materials / Solutions

1. Glycerol

2. Culture

Protocol

1. Equal volume of 100% autoclaved glycerol was added to the culture.

2. They were mixed by gentle pipetting.

3. The mixture was poured into pre labeled cryotubes to half of its volume.

4. It was immediately transferred to dry ice and allowed to settle for an hour or so.

5. Thereafter it was stored at - 80°C.

12. Using the Microscope

Setting up: Acquire a microscope from the cabinet first. Carrying a microscope is a two-handed job. Embrace the arm of the scope with one hand and as you remove the scope from the shelf place the other hand under the base. Notice how the electrical cord is wrapped around the neck of the microscope. The cord should be tightly wrapped. In addition, the nosepiece should be adjusted to place the 4× lens in the locked position and the stage should be lowered. Move the nosepiece if this is not the case. Raise the stage and unwrap the cord. Turn the rheostat to 1, the lowest power level, plug the microscope in and flip the toggle to on. We always begin with the rheostat turned low in increase the working life of the bulb. Spend a few moments familiarizing you with the mechanical controls of the microscope. Observe how the stage moves when you turn the focus knobs, and movement of the slide holder, and how the condenser is raised and lowered.

Examining Samples: We frequently examine eukaryotic cells using a wet mount. In a wet mount, the cells being examined are suspended in water or stain and covered with a cover slip. The cover slip keeps the sample in place and undisturbed while also protecting the lens from the sample.

Positioning and Focusing: Begin with the stage in the lowered position. Rotate the nosepiece of the microscope until the 4× objective is in the locked position. Place the slide into the holder and use the coarse focus to raise the stage to the highest position. Do not raise the stage using the coarse focus if the 40× or 100× objectives is in place. Adjust the rheostat to an intermediate position so that the light is neither glaringly bright nor dim. Look through the ocular lenses and lower the stage using the coarse focus until the sample comes into focus.

Adjusting Ocular Lenses: The intra-ocular distance is adjusted simply by pulling the eyepieces apart or pushing them together. When you have the intra-ocular distance set correctly, you should see a single image of your sample. The left ocular lens has a separate focus adjustment (diopter adjustment ring) so you can set the ideal focus for both eyes. Once you have the sample close to being in focus, close left eye and use the fine control to focus for right eye as well as possible. Then close your right eye and use the diopter adjustment ring to focus the image for left eye. Note the setting of the ring where you focus well so you can turn to that setting if the ring gets moved for other users.

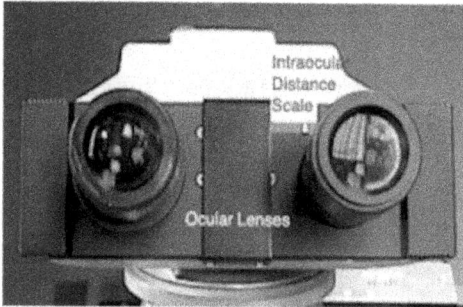

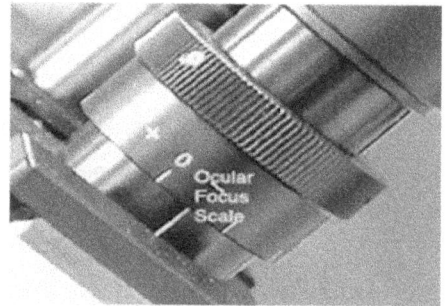

Putting Microscope Away

Turn the rheostat to 1 and then toggle the light off. Turn the nosepiece to the 4× objective and raise the stage to a high position. Wrap the electrical cord snugly around the arm and then lower the stage to help hold the cord in place. Using both hands to carry the scope, return it to the numbered slot in the microscope cabinet.

Using Oil Immersion Lens

To examine bacteria and other very small objects, we will need to use the oil immersion (100× lens). Special techniques must be used when using the 100× objective. With the 10-fold increase in magnification provided by the ocular lens, we are approaching the theoretical limit of light microscopy so must obtain the best possible resolution in order to get a clear image the sample. Because light travels more slowly through glass and most other media than it does through air, light leaving air and passing though glass is bent. You have probably observed this bending phenomenon when looking at objects in water whose position and appearance seem distorted. To prevent this distortion from occurring between the sample and the objective lens, we fill the space between with immersion oil which has the same optical properties as glass. Without immersion oil, objects seen under the 100× lens will appear fuzzy even at the best possible focus.

Before placing oil on the slide, focus on your sample as well as possible with the 40× objective. Make sure the light coming through the sample is optimal as well. If you are looking at bacteria, which may be very hard or impossible to see at 40×, you may find it useful to place a small grease pencil mark on the slide to focus on. Put the mark your sample from the distance so that it does not come into contact with the immersion oil as the oil will dissolve the mark and you will have nasty black junk floating around the sample. When you have set the light and focus as well as possible using the 40× objective, rotate the lenses half-way to the 100× position. Place a drop of immersion oil on your sample and then rotate the 100× into position. You should be able to see the immersion oil making direct contact with the lens. Look through the eyepiece and perfect the focus using the fine focus only. After you are though with this lens, remove the slide and rotate the objective to the side and clean off any remaining oil using lens paper. Do not use any other cleaner than lens paper. Also, be careful not to rotate the 40× lens around while the slide is still in place because oil on this lens will destroy your field of view. If the 40× becomes oily, or if the view though the 100× is not clear, try cleaning them thoroughly with lens paper. If that does not solve the problem, ask your instructor for help.

13. Diluting Solutions

We commonly use multiple dilutions of a single sample in procedures for estimating concentrations of serum proteins or counting cells is suspension. Frequently, these will be very high dilutions. By making a series of small dilutions rather than one large dilution, we minimize the use of excess reagents and decrease the chance of making measurement errors. Serial dilutions are a series of equal small dilutions used to obtain a large final dilution. For example, we might want to do 5 serial two-fold dilutions. We could do this by adding 1 mL of solute to 1 mL of solvent, mixing, transferring 1 mL of this mixture to another mL of solvent, mixing, transferring to 1 mL of solvent and so on. The dilution would be 1/2 in the first tube, 1/4 in the second, then 1/8, 1/16 and finally 1/32 in the final tube. Likewise, we could perform serial 5-fold dilutions by transferring 1 mL of solute into 4 mL of solvent. The dilutions for 5 of these steps would be 1/5, 1/25, 1/125, 1/625 and 1/3125.

Fractions: Calculating dilutions is nothing more than the multiplication and division of fractions. Keep in mind that when multiplying fractions you multiply the numerators together and then the denominators e.g., $2/3 \times 5/6 = 10/18 = 5/9$. When dividing fractions, invert the fraction you are dividing by and then multiply e.g., $2/3 \div 1/6 = 2/3 \times 6/1 = 12/3 = 4$.

Dilution Factors: We sometimes see dilutions described as x-fold dilutions, sometimes as fractions. A 4-fold dilution is the same thing as a 1/4 dilution. The dilution factor is the inverse of this fractional dilution. For example, if you performed a 1/2000 dilution, the dilution factor would be 2000. Thus, if you had 1 mL of a cell suspension, performed a 1/2000 dilution and then counted 45 cells in 1 mL of the dilute suspension, you would calculate the number of cells in the original suspension by taking 45× dilution factor (2000) for 90,000 cells/mL. In these types of problems, students divide by the dilution factor and try to tell there were 0.02 cells/mL, a result that is obviously absurd.

14. Streak Plating

One bacterial cell will create a colony as it multiplies. The streak process is intended to create a region where the bacteria are so dilute that when each bacterium touches the surface of the agar, it is far enough away from other cells so that an isolated colony can develop. In this manner, spreading an inoculum with multiple organisms will result in isolation of the different organisms. Mesophilic bacteria are generally streaked onto media solidified with 1.5% agar or agarose. Gelatin can be used if a high enough concentration of gelatin protein or a low enough incubation temperature is used. Thermophiles and hyperthermophiles can also be streaked onto growth media solidified with agar substitutes, such as Gelrite and guar gum. One-hundred-mm-diameter petri dishes are the most commonly used size of plate for streaking. The agar surface of the plate should be dry without visible moisture such as condensation drops. Traditionally, inoculated petri dishes are incubated with the agar side up to prevent condensed moisture from falling onto the agar surface, which would ruin the isolation by allowing bacteria to move across the moist surface creating areas of confluent growth instead. The inoculum for a streak plate could come from any type of source, for example clinical specimen, sedimented urine, environmental swab, broth, or solid culture. The two most common streak patterns are the three sector T streak and the four sector quadrant streak. In a streak plate, dilution is achieved by first spreading the specimen over the agar surface of one sector. If a cotton swab or disposable loop or needle was used to inoculate the first sector, it is now discarded into an appropriate container, while reusable loops, usually with nichrome or platinum wire (24 gauge), are flamed to incinerate any organisms on the loop. When cooled, the sterile loop is streaked through the initial sector and organisms are carried into the second sector where they are spread using a zig-zag movement. In a similar manner, the organisms present on the loop are incinerated after the second sector is streaked, and the third sector is streaked. For a four quadrant plate, the process is carried an extra step.

Materials

- Specimen to be streaked;
- Transfer loop (usually nichrome, a nickel-chromium alloy, or platinum; it may also be a single-use disposable plastic loop, which would be discarded between sectors rather than resterilized).
- Bunsen burner.

- Sterile Petri dish with appropriate bacterial media, such as trypticase soy agar.

- Labeling pen.

- Sterile cotton swabs (if necessary to remove condensation from the agar surface and from around the inner rim of the petri dish).

A. Label a Petri dish: Petri dishes are labeled on the bottom rather than on the lid. In order to preserve area to observe the plate after it has incubated, write close to the edge of the bottom of the plate. Labels usually include the organism name, type of agar, date, and the plater's name or initials. Using sterile cotton swabs, remove any visible water on the agar in the plate or around the inner rim of the petri plate. Observe the plate and mentally divide it into three sectors, a T. The area above the T will become the first sector streaked. The plate will then be turned clockwise with the agar side up. The second sector will then be at the top for streaking and then the plate is turned again so that the third sector can be streaked.

B. Sterilize the transfer loop before obtaining a specimen: In order to streak a specimen from a culture tube, metal transfer loops are first flamed so that the entire wire is red-hot. When flaming, the wire loop is held in the light blue area of a bunsen burner just above the tip of inner flame of the flame until it is red-hot. If a hot incinerator is available, the loop may be sterilized by holding it inside the incinerator for 5 to 7 seconds. Once sterile, the loop is allowed to cool by holding it still. Do not wave it around to cool it or blow on it. When manipulating bacteria, transfer loops are usually held like a pencil. If plastic disposable loops are being utilized, they are removed from the packaging to avoid contamination and after being used, are discarded into an appropriate container. A new loop is recommended for each sector of an isolation streak plate.

C. Open the culture and collect a sample of specimen using the sterile loop: Isolation can be obtained from any of a variety of specimens. This protocol describes the use of a mixed broth culture, where the culture contains several different bacterial species or strains. The specimen streaked on a plate could come in a variety of forms, such as solid samples, liquid samples, and cotton or foam swabs. Material containing possibly infectious agents should be handled appropriately in the lab, only by students with appropriate levels of skill and expertise. Remove the test tube cap. It is recommended that the cap be kept in right hand (hand holding the sterile loop). Curl the little finger of right hand around the cap to hold it or hold it between the little finger and third finger from the back. Modern test tube caps extend over the top of the test tube, keeping the rim of the test tube sterile while the rim of the cap has not been exposed to the bacteria. The cap can also be placed on the disinfected table, if the test tube is held at an angle so that air contamination does not fall down into the tube and the test tube cap is set with the sterile rim on the table.

Insert the loop into the culture tube and remove a loopful of broth.

Replace the cap of the test tube and put it back into the test tube rack.

D. Streak the plate: Inoculating the agar means that the lid will have to be opened. Minimize the amount of agar and the length of time the agar is exposed to the environment during the streak process.

1. Streak the first sector

Raise the petri dish lid to insert the loop. Touch the loop to the agar area on the opposite side of the dish, the first sector. Bacteria on the loop will be transferred to the agar. Spread the bacteria in the first sector of the petri dish by moving the loop in a back and forth manner across the dish, a zig-zag motion. Make the loop movements close together and cover the entire first region. The loop should glide over the surface of the agar; take care not to dig into the agar.

2. Between sectors

Remove the loop from the petri dish and obtain a sterile loop before continuing to the second sector. Either incinerate the material on the loop or obtain a sterile loop if using plastic disposable loops. The loop must be cool before streaking can continue. Metal loops can be touched to an uninoculated area of agar to test whether they are adequately cooled. If the loop is cool, there will be no sizzling or hissing and the agar will not be melted to form a brand. If a brand is formed, avoid that area when continuing with the streaking process.

3. Streak the second sector

Open the petri dish and insert the loop. Touch the cooled loop to the first sector once, invisibly drawing a few of the bacteria from the first sector into the second sector. The second sector is streaked less heavily than the first sector, again using a zig-zag motion.

4. Obtain a sterile loop for the third sector

5. Streak the third sector

Open the petri dish and insert the loop. Touch the cooled loop (if loop has been flamed) once into the second sector and draw bacteria from the second sector into the third sector. Streak the third sector with a zig-zag motion. This last sector has the widest gap between the rows of streaking, placing the bacteria a little further apart than in the previous two sectors. Watch closely to avoid touching the first sector as the streak is completed.

6. Final step

Flame the loop to incinerate any bacteria that are left on the loop. Allow the loop to cool before placing it near anything that is flammable. Invert the Petri dish so that the agar side is up and incubate the plates.

15. Laboratory Notes for Microbiological Experiments

A. Alternate streak patterns and different culture media: A variety of alternate streak patterns exist. Some are used for specific inocula, such as a urine specimen. The patterns also differ in the number of sectors as well as in the number of times the loop is sterilized. The four quadrant streak pattern would be recommended for use when large amounts of bacteria are expected in the inoculum. The extra sector will provide additional dilution and increase the probability of isolated colonies on the plate. Sometimes, cultures will be streaked on enrichment media or various selective and differential media. For instance, a culture which is expected to have a gram-negative pathogen will be streaked on a MacConkey agar plate, which inhibits the growth of gram-positive organisms.

B. Incinerating material on transfer loops flaming: Reusable microbiological loops and needles are sterilized by flaming. A Bunsen burner is traditionally used for this process. Most microbiology manuals show the microbiologist positioned with his/her hand above the burner, with the loop placed into the flame. To avoid possible contact with the flame, the microbiologist might consider placing his/her hand below the flame with the loop/needle above the hand in the flame. The flame of the Bunsen burner should be adjusted to blue, with the darker blue cone of cooler air visible in the center of the flame. The loop or needle should be placed into the hotter part of the flame and kept there until it glows red. There is a possible aerosolization hazard if the loop or needle contains liquid or a bacterial clump. These loops and needles should be placed into the heat slowly so that the moisture evaporates rather than sputters. If an incinerator such as a Bacti-Cinerator is used to sterilize the loop, the loop is to remain inside the incinerator for 5 to 7 seconds. When warmed up (which will take 5 minutes), the temperature inside the incinerator is 815°C. The incinerator will take 5 to 10 minutes to warm up to working temperature.

C. Several techniques decontaminate transfer loops between sectors of a streak plate, flame, dig into agar, flame once and rotate loop: A variety of methods exist for removing organisms from the loop between sectors. Beginning students are generally taught to sterilize the loop between each sector by incinerating and then cooling the loop. Clinical microbiologists practice a variety of methods. Some flame once after the initial sector and then rotate the loop so that the next sectors can be streaked with an unused side of the loop.

D. Isolated colony appearances: Isolated colonies can be described using the traditional colony descriptions. The appearance of an organism can vary. For instance, a colony of an organism growing in a crowded sector of the plate will not grow as large as the identical organism growing in isolation. The media composition, pH, and moistness, as well as the length of time and temperature can all affect the organism's appearance. Colonies selected for sub culturing should be colonies which are isolated, *i.e.,* there is no other colony visibly touching the colony. Agar with a surface layer of water is not suitable for obtaining isolated colonies. The water drops should be removed from the surface of the plate and from the rim of the plate by using sterile cotton swabs. Plates should be incubated agar side up, to avoid condensation that would drop onto the growing colonies on the agar surface.

E. Flaming tube mouths: Many protocols suggest flaming the tube mouth before and after removing organisms from a tube. Flaming was important when test tubes were capped with a cotton plug. Flaming would still be appropriate if a foam plug were being used.

F. Rehearsing Streak Procedure: Some instructors should practice streaking procedure to the students on a piece of paper. The process helps the student visualize the completed product and practice the fine muscle movements that are required in successful streaking for isolation. Students may also find that they can visualize the pattern better if they mark the back of the petri-dish. Before learning to streak, students should have had the opportunity to work with 1.5% agar media. Ideally they had the opportunity to practice using a loop on a plate to determine the best angle of approach and the amount of force required to glide the loop over the surface of the agar without gouging the surface.

G. Holding plate while Streaking: If possible, adequate lighting should be available to help the microbiologist follow the tracings of the loop on the agar. For most labs, this means that the Petri dish should be held in one's hand while being streaked in order to reflect the light properly. Additionally, the length of time the Petri dish lid is removed should be minimized in order to limit contamination. There are several ways to hold the petri dish. Beginning students might find that they obtain the best results when they leave the plate on the lab bench and lifting the lid to work. Other students may find that they can place the plate upside down on the workbench and lift the agar containing bottom, hold it to streak and then quickly replace it into the lid.

Segment 1

Biophysical Technology and Cell Biology

Experiment-1. Preparation of Buffers at Desired pH.

Objectives: To become familiar with operating a pH meter and to learn how to use the Henderson-Hasselbalch equation to make buffer solutions at a desired pH value.

Introduction: A buffer system is a mixture of a weak acid or a weak base and its salt (conjugate base or conjugate acid) that permits solutions to resist large changes in pH upon the addition of small amounts of hydrogen ions (H^+) or hydroxide ions (OH^-). It means a buffer helps maintain a near constant pH upon the addition of small amounts of H^+ or OH^- to a solution. In the definition of a buffer system, it should be noted that reference is made to weak acids and bases. Strong acids e.g., HCl and bases e.g., NaOH almost completely ionize in water:

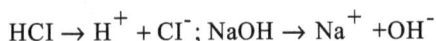

$$HCl \rightarrow H^+ + Cl^-; NaOH \rightarrow Na^+ + OH^-$$

Many acids and bases, however, do not undergo complete ionization in water. These compounds, then, are called weak acids and bases. Many organic acids are weak acids. Weak acids do not completely dissociate in water. The dissociation of an organic acid as follow as:

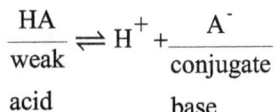

$$\underset{\text{weak}}{HA} \rightleftharpoons H^+ + \underset{\text{conjugate}}{A^-}$$

$$\underset{\text{acid}}{} \qquad \underset{\text{base}}{}$$

The unprotonated product of the acid dissociation reaction is referred to as a conjugate base. An acid is defined as a proton (H^+) donor, whereas the base is the H^+ acceptor. In a conjugate acid/base pair such as that indicated above, the weak acid always has one more H^+ than its conjugate base. Similarly, a weak base will have one less H^+ than its conjugate acid.

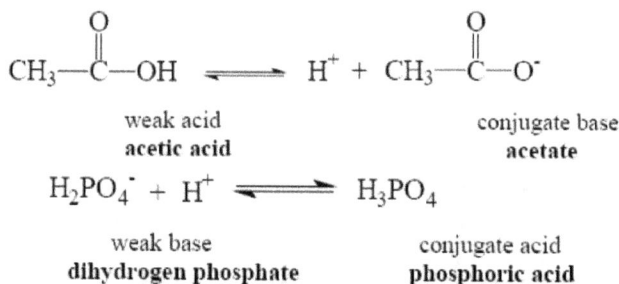

$$CH_3-\overset{\overset{\displaystyle O}{\|}}{C}-OH \;\rightleftharpoons\; H^+ + CH_3-\overset{\overset{\displaystyle O}{\|}}{C}-O^-$$

weak acid   conjugate base
acetic acid   acetate

$$H_2PO_4^- + H^+ \;\rightleftharpoons\; H_3PO_4$$

weak base   conjugate acid
dihydrogen phosphate   phosphoric acid

One can analyze the strength of a weak acid. This means that the amount of hydrogen ion released can be determined. To do this, one can use the following expression:

$$K_a \frac{[H^+][A^-]}{[HA]}$$

where K_a is defined as the acid dissociation constant.

More the value of K_a, the stronger the acid is. Because Ka values vary over a wide range, they are usually expressed using a logarithmic scale:

$$pK_a = -\log K_a$$

The hydrogen ion is one of the most important ions in biological systems. The concentration of this ion affects most cellular processes *e.g.*, the structure and function of most biological macromolecules and the rates of most biochemical reactions are strongly affected by $[H^+]$. The pH scale has been devised as a convenient method of expressing hydrogen ion concentration. The pH has been defined as the negative logarithm of the hydrogen ion concentration:

$$pH = -\log [H^+]$$

The Henderson-Hasselbalch equation provides a convenient way to think about buffers and pH:

$$pH = pK_a + \log \frac{[A^-]}{[HA]}$$

If one were examining the dissociation of acetic acid, Henderson-Hasselbalch relationship:

$$pH = pK_a + \log \frac{[CH_3COO^-]}{[CH_3COOH]}$$

The Henderson-Hasselbalch equation can be used to determine if an aqueous solution of a conjugate acid/base pair is functioning as a buffer. If the concentration of the weak acid is equal to that of its conjugate base, the ratio of these two components is one. When this is the case, the Henderson-Hasselbalch equation reduces to pH =

pKa because the log (1) is equal to zero. When the pH of the solution is equal to the pKa of the ionizing group, the solution is functioning at maximum buffering capacity. An aqueous solution of a conjugate acid/base pair functions as a good buffer when the ratio of the conjugate base to weak acid ranges from 1:9 to 9:1. Substituting these ratios into the Henderson-Hasselbalch equation, one finds that this aqueous solution functions as a good buffer when the pH of the solution is within approximately one pH unit of the ionizing group's pK_a.

$$pH = pK_a \pm 1$$

Because the log (1/9) is – 0.999 and the log of (9/1) is + 0.999.

Using the Henderson-Hasselbalch Equation

Example A: This is a two-component buffer system meaning that the weak acid and its conjugate base are added separately. How would you prepare 10 mL of a 0.01M phosphate buffer, pH 7.40, from stock solutions of 0.10 M KH_2PO_4 and 0.25 M K_2HPO_4? pK_a of KH_2PO_4 = 7.20. The following approach may be helpful in solving this type of buffer problem in which both the conjugate acid and base are added separately.

1. **Use the Henderson Hasselbalch equation to find the ratio of A⁻ to HA.**

   $$pH = pK_a + \log [A-] / [HA]$$

   $$7.40 = 7.20 + \log [A-] / [HA]$$

   $$0.20 = \log [A-] / [HA]$$

   $$1.584893192 = [A-] / [HA]*$$

   *Since [A-] / [HA] = 1.584893192, we can say that [A-] / [HA] = 1.584893192/ 1. In this case [A⁻] = 1.584893192; [HA] = 1.

2. **Calculate the decimal fraction (part/whole) of each buffer component.**

   A⁻ = 1.584893192 / (1.000 + 1.584893192)

   = 1.584893192 / 2.584893192= 0.61313682

   HA = 1.000 / 2.584893192= 0.38686318

3. **Find the molarity (M) of each component in the buffer by simply multiplying the molarity of the buffer by the decimal fraction of each component.**

   M_{A^-} = 0.01M x 0.61313682 = 0.006131368M

   M_{HA} = 0.01M x 0.38686318 = 0.003868632M

4. **Calculate the moles of each component in the buffer.**

   Moles = Molarity x Liters of buffer

   $Moles_{A^-}$ = 0.006131368 M x 0.01L = 6.131 x 10^{-5} moles

   $Moles_{HA}$ = 0.003868632 M x 0.01L = 3.869 x 10^{-5} moles

5. **Calculate the volume of each stock solution required to make the buffer**

   Liters of stock = moles of the buffer component / Molarity of the stock

   L_{A^-} = 6.131 x 10^{-5} moles / 0.25 M = 2.452 x 10-4 L = 245 μL

$L_{HA} = 3.869 \times 10^{-5}$ moles / 0.10 M = $3.869 \times 10\text{-}4$ L = 387µL

6. **To prepare this buffer, one would use appropriately-sized pipets to measure and transfer each component to a 10 mL volumetric flask and bring the solution to volume with dH$_2$O.**

Example B: This is a single component buffer system. This means that one component of the conjugate acid/base pair will be generated *in situ* (in solution). In the following example, the conjugate base will be generated by reaction between the weak acid (acetic acid) and strong base (sodium hydroxide). How would you prepare 10 mL of a 0.02 M acetate buffer, pH 4.30, from stock solutions of 0.05 M acetic acid (HAc) and 0.05 M NaOH? pKa acetic acid = 4.76.

1. **Use the Henderson Hasselbalch equation to find the ratio of A⁻ to HA.**

   pH = pK$_a$ + log [A⁻] / [HA]

   4.30 = 4.76 + log [A⁻] / [HA]

   -0.46 = log [A⁻] / [HA]

   0.34673685 = [A⁻] / [HA]

2. **Calculate the decimal fraction (part/whole) of each buffer component.**

   A⁻ = 0.34673685 / (1.00 + 0.34673685) = 0.34673685 / 1.34673685 = 0.257464441

   HA = 1.00 / 1.34673685 = 0.742535559

3. **Find the molarity (M) of each component in the buffer by simply multiplying the molarity of the buffer by the decimal fraction of each component.**

   M$_{A-}$ = 0.02M x 0. 257464441= 0.005149289 = 5.15×10^{-3} M

   M$_{HA}$ = 0.02M x 0. 742535559= 0.014850711 = 1.49×10^{-2} M

4. **Calculate the moles of each component in the buffer.**

   Moles = Molarity x Liters of buffer

   Moles$_A$- = 0.005149289 M x 0.01 L = 5.14929×10^{-5} moles

   Moles$_{HA}$ = 0.014850711M x 0.01 L = $1.485071.47 \times 10^{-4}$ moles

5. **Since this buffer is prepared by the reaction of a weak acid (HAc) with a strong base (NaOH), you must determine the total moles of the weak acid component needed because the conjugate base is made *in situ*.**

   Total moles = 5.15×10^{-5} moles NaOH + 1.49×10^{-4} moles HAc = 2.00×10^{-4} moles HAc. This sum indicates that, although in the buffer one only needs 1.49×10^{-4} moles HA, an additional 5.15×10^{-5} moles is needed to generate the conjugate base *in situ*.

6. **Calculate the volume of each stock solution required to make the buffer**

   Liters of stock = Moles of the buffer component / Molarity of the stock

   L$_{A-}$ = 5.14929×10^{-5} moles / 0.05 M = 1.03×10^{-3} L NaOH = 1.0 mL

   L$_{HA}$ = 2.00×10^{-4} moles / 0.05 M = 4.00×10^{-3} L CH$_3$COOH = 4.0 mL

7. **To prepare this buffer, one would use pipets to measure and transfer each component to a 10 mL volumetric flask and bring the solution to volume with dH$_2$O.**

Example C: What is the pH of a solution resulting from a mixture of 200 mL of 0.1 M NaOH and 100 mL of 0.3 M HAc? This problem is similar to Problem 3 in Experimental Procedures. It is a limiting reagent type problem.

1. **Calculate the initial moles of each reactant.**

   Moles = Molarity x Liters

   Moles$_{NaOH}$ = 0.1M x 0.2 L = 0.02 moles

   Moles$_{HAc}$ = 0.3M x 0.1 L = 0.03 moles

2. **Write the balanced equation for this reaction.**

   This is a neutralization reaction.

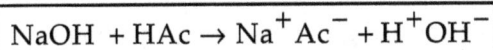

   $$NaOH + HAc \rightarrow Na^+Ac^- + H^+OH^-$$

3. **Determine the moles of each reactant remaining after the reaction.** This is a limiting reagent type problem. Since NaOH is present in the least amount and, according to the balanced equation the reactants react in a 1:1 ratio, the NaOH is completely consumed *i.e.*, zero moles of NaOH remain. Because the reactants react in a 1:1 ratio,

   Moles$_{HAc\ remaining}$ = Moles$_{HAc\ initial}$ − Moles$_{HAc\ reacted}$

   = 0.03 moles − 0.02 moles = 0.01 moles

4. **Determine the molarity of the buffer components *i.e.*, the conjugate acid-base pair.**

   M$_{HAc}$ = moles$_{HAc\ remaining}$ / Liters solution = 0.01 moles/0.3 L = 0.033 M

   The molarity of the conjugate base Ac- resulting from the dissolution of the product NaAc is:

   MAc- = moles formed / Liters solution = 0.02 moles / 0.3 L = 0.067 M

5. **Use the H-H equation to calculate the pH.**

   pH = pK$_a$ + log [A-] / [HA]

   = 4.76 + log (0.067/0.033)

   = 4.76 + log 2.02

   = 4.76 + 0.31

   = 5.07

Exercise: Determine the pH of a solution resulting from a mixture of 5 mL of 0.1 M KOH and 30 mL of 0.1 M HAc.

Procedure 1:

1. Prepare 10 mL of a 0.01 M phosphate buffer, pH 7.70, from stock solutions of 0.1 M K$_2$HPO$_4$ and 0.2 M KH$_2$PO$_4$. (pKa for the weak acid = 7.20).

A. Use the Henderson-Hasselbalch equation to calculate the volume of each stock solution needed.

$$pH = pK_a + \log [\text{conjugate base}] / [\text{weak acid}]$$

B. Cross check your calculations.

C. Make the solution and check the pH of a portion of your buffer solution using the pH meter.

2. Prepare 10 mL of 0.01 M acetate buffer, pH 3.80, from stock solutions of 0.1 M acetic acid and 0.02 M sodium hydroxide. $pK_{a\text{ acetic acid}} = 4.76$.

A.– C. Same as above.

D.Calculate the exact volume of the 0.01 M acetate buffer required to make 10 mL of a 0.0005 M acetate buffer.

Procedure 2:

1. Prepare this new buffer using the following equation to aid you in your calculations.

$$V1 = \frac{V_2 \times M_2}{M_1}$$

where V_1 = the volume of the concentrated solution (liters, L)

V_2 = the volume of the diluted solution (liters, L)

M_1 = the molar concentration of the concentrated solution (moles/L)

M_2 = the molar concentration of the diluted solution (moles/L)

2. Check the pH of this new buffer.

E. Calculate the exact volume of the 0.01 M acetate buffer required to make 10 mL of a 0.001 M acetate buffer.

(i) Prepare this new buffer.

(ii) Check its pH.

Experiment 2. Preparation of phosphate buffers.

Aim: Standardization buffers pH 4 and pH 7.

Phosphates

Phosphate salts are known by several names and the correct phosphate must be used to prepare buffer solutions. One phosphate cannot be substituted for another phosphate. Check formula of salt to be certain.

Table 1. Salts and their Formula

Formula	Name of salt	Other names
KH_2PO_4	Potassium dihydrogen phosphate	Potassium dihydrogen orthophosphate Monobasic potassium phosphate Monopotassium phosphate acid Potassium phosphate Potassium biphosphate
K_2HPO_4	Potassium hydrogen phosphate	Dipotassium hydrogen orthophosphate Dipotassium hydrogen phosphate Dibasic potassium phosphate Dipotassium phosphate
K_3PO_4	Potassium phosphate	Tribasic potassium Phosphate tripotassium phosphate

---

BOX 1
STANDARDIZATION BUFFERS

For pH=7.00: Add 29.1 mL of 0.1 molar NaOH to 50 mL 0.1 molar potassium dihydrogen phosphate.
Alternatively: Dissolve 1.20 g of sodium dihydrogen phosphate and 0.885 g of disdium hydrogen phosphate in 1 liter volume distilled water.
For pH= 4.00: Add 0.1 mL of 0.1 molar NaOH to 50 mL of 0.1 molar potassium hydrogen phthalate.
Alternatively: Dissolve 8.954 g of disodium hydrogen phosphste.12 H_2O and 3.4023 g of potassium dihydrogen phosphate in 1 liter volume distilled water.

Table 2. Range of common Buffer Systems

Buffering system	Useful buffering pH range (25°C)
Hydrochloric acid/ Potassium chloride	1.0 - 2.2
Glycine/ Hydrochloric acid	2.2 - 3.6
Potassium hydrogen phthalate/ Hydrochloric acid	2.2 - 4.0
Citric acid/ Sodium citrate	3.0 - 6.2
Sodium acetate/ Acetic acid	3.7 - 5.6
Potassium hydrogen phtaalate/ Sodium hydroxide	4.1 - 5.9
Disodium hydrogen phthalate / Sodium dihydrogen orthophosphate	5.8 - 8.0
Dipotassium hydrogen phthalate / Potassium dihydrogen orthophospate	5.8 - 8.0
Potassium dihydrogen orthophosphate / sodium hydroxide	5.8 - 8.00
Barbitone sodium / Hydrochloric acid	6.8 - 9.6
Tris (hydroxylmethyl) aminomethane / Hydrochloric acid	7.0 - 9.00
Sodium tetraborate/ Hydrochloric acid	8.1 - 9.2
Glycine/ Sodium hydroxide	8.6 - 10.6
Sodium carbonate/ Sodium hydrogen carbonate	9.2 - 10.8
Sodium tetraborate/ Sodium hydroxide	9.3 - 10.7
Sodium bicarbonate / Sodium hydroxide	9.60 - 11.0
Sodium hydrogen orthophosphate / Sodium hydroxide	11.0 - 11.9
Potassium chloride/ Sodium hydroxide	12.0 - 13.0

Table 3. Buffers 1.00 - 9.00

Buffer A pH 1.0 - 2.2		Buffer B pH 2.2 - 4.00		Buffer C pH 4.10 - 5.90		Buffer D pH 5.8 - 8.00		Buffer E pH 7.0 - 9.00	
50 mL 0.2 M KCl + mLs of 0.2 M HCl		100 mL 0.1 M potassium hydrogen phthalate + mLs of 0.1 M HCl.		100 mL 0.1 M potassium hydrogen phthalate + mLs of 0.1 M NaOH		100 mL 0.1 M KH_2PO_4 + mLs of 0.1 M NaOH.		100 mL 0.1 M tris (hydroxymethyl) aminomethane + mLs of 0.1 M HCl.	
pH	mLs of 0.2M HCl added	pH	mLs of 0.1M HCl added	pH	mLs of 0.1M NaOH added	pH	mLs of 0.1M NaOH added	pH	mLs of 0.1 M HCl added
1.00	134.0	2.20	99.0	4.10	2.6	5.80	7.2	7.00	93.2
1.10	105.6	2.30	91.6	4.20	6.0	5.90	9.2	7.10	91.4
1.20	85.0	2.40	84.4	4.30	9.4	6.00	11.2	7.20	89.4
1.30	67.2	2.50	77.6	4.40	13.2	6.10	13.6	7.30	86.8
1.40	53.2	2.60	70.8	4.50	17.4	6.20	16.2	7.40	84.0
1.50	41.4	2.70	64.2	4.60	22.2	6.30	19.4	7.50	80.6
1.60	32.4	2.80	57.8	4.70	27.2	6.40	23.2	7.60	77.0
1.70	26.0	2.90	51.4	4.80	33.0	6.50	27.8	7.70	73.2
1.80	20.4	3.00	44.6	4.90	38.8	6.60	32.8	7.80	69.0
1.90	16.2	3.10	37.6	5.00	45.2	6.70	38.6	7.90	64.0
2.00	13.0	3.20	31.4	5.10	51.0	6.80	44.8	8.00	58.4
2.10	10.2	3.30	25.8	5.20	57.6	6.90	51.8	8.l0	52.4
2.20	7.8	3.40	20.8	5.30	63.2	7.00	58.2	8.20	45.8
		3.50	16.4	5.40	68.2	7.10	64.2	8.30	39.8
		3.60	12.6	5.50	73.2	7.20	69.4	8.40	34.4
		3.70	9.0	5.60	77.6	7.30	74.0	8.50	29.4
		3.80	5.8	5.70	81.2	7.40	78.2	8.60	24.4
		3.90	2.8	5.80	84.6	7.50	82.2	8.70	20.6
		4.00	0.2	5.90	87.4	7.60	85.6	8.80	17.0
						7.70	88.4	8.90	14.0
						7.80	90.6	9.00	11.4
						7.90	92.2		
						8.00	93.4		

Table 4. Buffers 08 - 13

Buffer F pH 8.0 - 9.10		Buffer G pH 9.2 - 10.80		Buffer H pH 9.60 - 11.00		Buffer I pH 10.90 - 12.00		Buffer J pH 12.00 - 13.00	
100 mL 0.025 M $Na_2B_4O_7.10H_2O$ (borax) + mLs of 0.1 M HCl.		100 mL 0.025 M $Na_2B_4O_7.10H_2O$ (borax) + mLs of 0.1 M NaOH.		100 mL 0.05 M $NaHCO_3$ + mLs of 0.1 M NaOH.		100 mL 0.05 M Na_2HPO_4 + mLs of 0.1 M NaOH.		50 mL 0.2 M KCl + volume indicated (in mL) 0.2 M NaOH.	
pH	mLs of 0.1M HCl added	pH	mLs of 0.1M NaOH added	pH	mLs of 0.1M NaOH added	pH	mLs of 0.1M NaOH added	pH	mLs of 0.2M NaOH added
8.00	41.0	9.20	1.8	9.60	10.0	10.90	6.6	12.00	12.0
8.10	39.4	9.30	7.2	9.70	12.4	11.00	8.2	12.10	16.0
8.20	37.6	9.40	12.4	9.80	15.2	11.10	10.2	12.20	20.4
8.30	35.4	9.50	17.6	9.90	18.2	11.20	12.6	12.30	25.6
8.40	33.2	9.60	22.2	10.00	21.4	11.30	15.2	12.40	32.4
8.50	30.4	9.70	26.2	10.10	24.4	11.40	18.2	12.50	40.8
8.60	27.0	9.80	30.0	10.20	27.6	11.50	22.2	12.60	51.2
8.70	23.2	9.90	33.4	10.30	30.4	11.60	27.0	12.70	64.4
8.80	19.2	10.00	36.6	10.40	33.0	11.70	32.4	12.80	82.4
8.90	14.2	10.10	39.0	10.50	35.6	11.80	38.8	12.90	106.0
9.00	9.2	10.20	41.0	10.60	38.2	11.90	46.0	13.00	132.0
9.10	4.0	10.30	42.6	10.70	40.4	12.00	53.8		
		10.40	44.2	10.80	42.4				
		10.50	45.4	10.90	44.0				
		10.60	46.6	11.00	45.4				
		10.70	47.6						
		10.80	48.5						

Preparing a Buffer Solution

The preparation of buffers by mixing adjusters with a known volume of the primary salt solution and made up to 200 mL with distilled water.

Acetate buffer solutions pH 3 - 6

Make up the following solutions

(a) 0.1M acetic acid.

(b) 0.1M sodium acetate (tri-hydrate) (13.6g / l).

Mix in the following proportions to get the required pH.

pH	vol. of 0.1M acetic acid	vol. of 0.1M sodium acetate
3	982.3 mLs	17.7 mLs
4	847.0 mLs	153.0 mLs
5	357.0 mLs	643.0 mLs
6	52.2 mLs	947.8 mLs

Phosphate buffer solutions pH 7 - 11

Make up the following solutions

(a) 0.1M disodium hydrogen phosphate (14.2 g / l)

(b) 0.1M HCl

(c) 0.1M NaOH

Mix in the following proportions to get the required pH.

pH	vol. of phosphate	vol. of 0.1M HCl	vol. of 0.1M NaOH
7	756.0 mLs	244 mLs	
8	955.1 mLs	44.9 mLs	
9	955.0 mLs	45.0 mLs	
10	966.4 mLs		33.6
11	965.3 mLs		34.7

Addition of acid or base to a salt pH 3 - 11

The primary salt is a solid and is weighed out in grams. A measured amount of 0.1M HCl or NaOH is added, then made up to 1 liter to give the relevant buffer solution.

pH	Salt mixtureDilute each mixture to 1 liter solution with distilled water
3	10.21g potassium hydrogen phthalate and 223 mL of 0.10 M HCl
4	10.21g potassium hydrogen phthalate and 1 mL of 0.10M HCl
5	10.21g potassium hydrogen phthalate and 226 mL of 0.10 M NaOH
6	6.81g potassium dihydrogen phosphate and 56 mL of 0.10 M NaOH

7	6.81g potassium dihydrogen phosphate and 291mL of 0.10M NaOH
8	6.81g potassium dihydrogen phosphate and 467mL of 0.10M NaOH
9	4.77g sodium tetraborate and 46mL of 0.10M HCl
10	4.77g sodium tetraborate and 183mL of 0.10M NaOH
11	2.10g sodium bicarbonate and 227mL of 0.10M NaOH

Experiment 3. Qualitative tests of sugars

Introduction: A carbohydrate is an organic compound with the general formula $Cm(H_2O)n$, that is, consists only of carbon, hydrogen and oxygen, with the last two in the 2:1 atom ratio. Carbohydrates make up the bulk of organic substances on earth and perform numerous roles in living things. The carbohydrates (saccharides) are divided into four chemical groups: monosaccharides, disaccharides, oligosaccharides and polysaccharides. Polysaccharides serve for the storage of energy *e.g.*, starch in plants and glycogen in animals and as structural components *e.g.*, cellulose in plants and chitin in arthropods. Structural polysaccharides are frequently found in combination with proteins (glycoproteins or mucoproteins) or lipids (lipopolysaccharides). The 5-carbon monosaccharide ribose is an important component of coenzymes *e.g.*, ATP, FAD and NAD and the backbone of the genetic molecule known as RNA. The related deoxyribose is a component of DNA. Saccharides and their derivatives include many other important biomolecules that play key roles in the immune system, fertilization, preventing pathogenesis, blood clotting and development.

Tests on Carbohydrates

1. Molisch's Test

Molisch's Test is a sensitive chemical test for all carbohydrates and some compounds containing carbohydrates in a combined form, based on the dehydration of the carbohydrate by sulfuric acid to produce an aldehyde either furfural or a derivative, which then condenses with the phenolic structure resulting in a red or purple-coloured compound.

Procedure

- Apply the test for two different carbohydrate solutions of choice, preferably to one monosaccharide and one polysaccharide.

- Place 2 mL of a known carbohydrate solution in a test tube, add 1 drop of Molisch's reagent (10% α-naphthol in ethanol).

- Pour 1-2 mL of conc. H_2SO_4 down the side of the test tube, so that it forms a layer at the bottom of the tube.

- Observe the colour at the interface between two layers and compare your result with a control test.

A brown colour due to charring must be ignored and the test should be repeated with a more dilute sugar solution.

2. Solubility Tests

- Apply this test to all carbohydrates provided.
- Observe the solubility of the carbohydrates both in water and ethanol.

Do not depend on your solubility observations during identification of your unknown compound.

3. Carbohydrates as Reducing Sugars

A reducing sugar is any sugar that, in a solution, has an aldehyde or a ketone group. The enolization of sugars under alkaline conditions is an important consideration in reduction tests. The ability of a sugar to reduce alkaline test reagents depends on the availability of an aldehyde or keto group for reduction reactions. A number of sugars especially disaccharides or polysaccharides have glycosidic linkages which involve bonding a carbohydrate (sugar) molecule to another one and hence there is no reducing group on the sugar; like in the case of sucrose, glycogen, starch and dextrin. In the case of reducing sugars, the presence of alkali causes extensive enolization especially at high pH and temperature. This leads to a higher susceptibility to oxidation reactions than at neutral or acidic pH. These sugars, therefore, become potential agents capable of reducing Cu^{+2} to Cu^{+}, Ag^{+} to Ag and so fort. Most commonly used tests for detection of reducing sugars are Fehling's Test, Benedict's test and Barfoed's Test.

(a) Fehling's Test

Fehling's Solution (deep blue coloured) is used to determine the presence of reducing sugars and aldehydes. Perform this test with fructose, glucose, maltose and sucrose.

Procedure

- To 1 mL of Fehling's solution A (aqueous solution of $CuSO_4$) add 1 mL of Fehling solution B (solution of potassium tartrate).
- Add 2 mL of the sugar solution, mix well and boil.
- See red precipitate of cuprous oxide that forms at the end of the reaction.

(b) Barfoed's Test

Barfoed's reagent, cupric acetate in acetic acid, is slightly acidic and is balanced so that is can only be reduced by monosaccharides but not less powerful reducing sugars. Disaccharides may also react with this reagent, but the reaction is much slower when compared to monosaccharides. Perform this test with glucose, maltose and sucrose.

Procedure

- To 1-2 mL of Barfoed's reagent, add an equal volume of sugar solution.
- Boil for 5 min. in a water bath and allow standing.
- Observe a brick-red cuprous oxide precipitates if reduction has taken place.

(c) Seliwanoff's Test

Seliwanoff's Test distinguishes between aldose and ketose sugars. Ketoses are distinguished from aldoses via their ketone/aldehyde functionality. If the sugar contains a ketone group, it is a ketose and if it contains an aldehyde group, it is an aldose. This test is based on the fact that, when heated, ketoses are more rapidly dehydrated than aldoses. Perform this test with glucose, fructose, maltose and sucrose.

Procedure: Heat 1 mL of sugar solution with 3 mL Seliwanoff's reagent (0.5 g resorcinol per liter 10% HCl) in boiling water. In less than 30 seconds, a red coloir must appear for ketoses. Upon prolonged heating, glucose will also give an appreciable colour.

(d) Bial's Test

Bial's Test is to determine the presence of pentoses (5C sugars). The components of this reagent are resorcinol, HCl and ferric chloride. In this test, the pentose is dehydrated to form furfural and the solution turns bluish and a precipitate may form. Perform this test with ribose and glucose.

Procedure: To 5 mL of Bial's reagent, add 2-3 drops of sugar solution and boil. Upon boiling, note the green-blue colour formed.

4. Action of Alkali on Sugars

Procedure

- Heat 1 mL glucose solution with 1 mL 40% NaOH for 1 min.
- Cool and apply test for reducing sugars e.g., Fehling's Test.
- Apply a control test with glucose solution to observe the difference.

5. Inversion of Sucrose

Sucrose is a disaccharide, which means that it is a molecule that is derived from two simple sugars (monosaccharides). In the case of sucrose, these simple sugars are glucose and fructose. Inverted sugar is a mixture of glucose and fructose. It is obtained by splitting sucrose into these two components. The splitting of sucrose is a hydrolysis reaction which can be induced simply by heating an aqueous solution of sucrose. Acid also accelerates the conversion of sucrose to invert.

Procedure

- Add 5 mL of sucrose solution to two test tubes.
- Add 5 drops of conc. HCl to one test tube.
- Heat both tubes in boiling water bath for 10 min.
- Cool and neutralize with diluted NaOH (use litmus paper).
- Test both solutions for the presence of reducing sugar with Fehling's Test.

6. Iodine Test

Iodine test is an indicator for the presence of starch. Iodine solution (iodine dissolved in an aqueous solution of potassium iodide) reacts with starch producing a blue-black colour. Apply this test to all the polysaccharides provided.

Procedure

- To 2-3 mL of polysaccharide solution, add 1-2 drops of iodine solution.
- Observe the different colours obtained for each of the polysaccharide solutions.

7. Unknown Part

Take an unknown solid from your assistants and not forget to write unknown number in lab reports. Carry out the carbohydrate tests in a reasonable sequence to determine the unknown.

Experiment 4. Estimation of sugar by Anthrone method.

Introduction: Carbohydrates are the important components of storage and structural materials in the plants. They exist as free sugars and polysaccharides. The basic units of carbohydrates are the monosaccharides which cannot be split by hydrolysis into simpler sugars. The carbohydrate content can be measured by hydrolyzing the polysaccharides into simple sugars by acid hydrolysis and estimating the resultant monosaccharides.

Principle: Carbohydrates are first hydrolysed into simple sugars using dilute hydrochloric acid. In hot acidic medium glucose is dehydrated to hydroxymethyl furfural. This compound forms with anthrone a green coloured product with an absorption maximum at 630 nm.

Materials

(a) HCl-2.5 N

(b) *Anthrone Reagent:* Dissolve 200 mg anthrone in 100 mL of ice cold 95% H_2SO_4. Prepare fresh before use.

(c) *Standard Glucose:* Stock – Dissolve 100 mg in 100 mL water. Working standard – 10mL of stock diluted to 100mL with distilled water. Store refrigerated after adding a few drops of toluene.

Procedure

1. Weigh 100 mg of the sample into a boiling tube.
2. Hydrolyse by keeping it in boiling water bath for 3 hours with 5mL of 2.5 N-HCl and cool to room temperature.
3. Neutralise it with solid sodium carbonate until the effervescence ceases.
4. Make up the volume to 100 mL and centrifuge.
5. Collect the supernatant and take 0.5 and 1mL aliquots for analysis.
6. Prepare the standards by taking 0, 0.2, 0.4, 0.6, 0.8 and 1 mL of the working standard. '0' serves as blank.
7. Make up the volume to 1 mL in all the tubes including the sample tubes by adding distilled water.
8. Then add 4 mL of anthrone reagent.

9. Heat for eight minutes in a boiling water bath.

10. Cool rapidly and read the green to dark green colour at 630 nm.

11. Draw a standard graph by plotting concentration of the standard on the X-axis versus absorbance on the Y-axis.

12. From the graph calculate the amount of carbohydrate present in the sample tube.

Calculation

Amount of carbohydrate present in 100 mg of the sample

$$= \frac{\text{mg of Glucose}}{\text{Volume of Test sample}} \times 100$$

Volume of test sample

Precaution: Cool the contents of all the tubes on ice before adding ice-cold anthrone reagent.

Experiment 5. Qualitative tests of Amino Acids.

1. Solubility Tests: The solubility of amino acids and proteins is largely dependent on the solution pH. The structural changes in an amino acid or protein that take place at different pH values alter the relative solubility of the molecule. In acidic solutions, both amino and carboxylic groups are protonated. In basic solutions, both groups are deprotonated. Amino acids are essentially soluble in water. Their solubilities in water dilute alkali and dilute acid vary from one compound to the other depending on the structure of their side chains. Apply this test to glycine, tyrosine, glutamic acid and cysteine.

Procedure

- Note the solubility of amino acids in water and alcohol by placing a small amount in a test tube, adding a few mL of solvent and warming if necessary.

- Determine the amino acid solution is acidic or basic by using a litmus paper while testing the solubility in water.

- Repeat the solubility test using dilute HCl and dilute NaOH.

2. Ninhydrin Test: Ninhydrin (triketohydrindene hydrate) is a chemical used to detect ammoniaor primary and secondary amines. Amino acids also react with ninhydrin at pH = 4. The reduction product obtained from ninhydrin then reacts with NH_3 and excess ninhydrin to yield a blue coloured substance. This reaction provides an extremely sensitive test for amino acids. Avoid spilling ninhydrin solutions on skin, as the resulting stains are difficult to remove. (Ninhydrin is the most commonly used method to detect fingerprints, as the terminal amines or lysine residues in peptides and proteins sloughed off in fingerprints react with ninhydrin).

Procedure

- To 1 mL amino acid solution add 5 drops of 0.2% ninhydrine solution in acetone.

- Boil over a water bath for 2 min.
- Allow to cool and observe the blue colour formed.

3. Stability to Alkali: Amino acids, unlike amides and volatile amines, do not evolve NH_3 or alkaline vapor when boiled with alkali. This method can be used to differentiate amino acids from amines and amides. Apply this test to the provided amine or amide and also to glycine.

Procedure

- Pipette 1 mL 1% glycine and the amide or amine solution into separate test tubes.
- Add 1 mL dilute NaOH to each test tube and boil.
- Test the vapor from each boiling tube with wet litmus paper.

4. Specific Reactions for Individual Amino Acids

(a) Xanthoproteic Test: Some amino acids contain aromatic groups that are derivatives of benzene. These aromatic groups can undergo reactions that are characteristics of benzene and benzene derivatives. One such reaction is the nitration of a benzene ring with nitric acid. The amino acids that have activated benzene ring can readily undergo nitration. This nitration reaction, in the presence of activated benzene ring, forms yellow product. Apply this test to tyrosine, tryptophan, phenylalanine and glutamic acid.

Procedure

- To 2 mL amino acid solution in a boiling test tube, add equal volume of concentrated HNO_3.
- Heat over a flame for 2 min and observe the colour.
- Now cool thoroughly under the tap and cautiously run in sufficient 40% NaOH to make the solution strongly alkaline.
- Observe the colour of the nitro derivative of aromatic nucleus.

(b) Millon's Test: Millon's test is specific to phenol containing structures (tyrosine is the only common phenolic amino acid). Millon's reagent is concentrated HNO_3, in which mercury is dissolved. As a result of the reaction a red precipitate or a red solution is considered as positive test. A yellow precipitate of HgO is not a positive reaction but usually indicates that the solution is too alkaline. Apply this test to tyrosine, phenylalanine, glycine and α-naphtol.

Procedure

- To 2 mL amino acid solution in a test tube, add 1-2 drops of Millons reagent.
- Warm the tube in a boiling water bath for 10 min.

  A brick red colour is a positive reaction.

Note that this is a test for phenols and the ninhydrin test should also be positive if it is to be concluded that the substance is a phenolic amino acid.

(c) **Hopkin's Cole Test:** The indole group of tryptophan reacts with glyoxylic acid (glacial acetic acid, which has been exposed to light, always contains glyoxylic acid CHOCOOH as an impurity) in the presence of concentrated H_2SO_4 to give a purple colour. Apply this test to glycine, tryptophan and tyrosine.

Procedure

- To a few mL of glacial acetic acid containing glyoxylic acid, add 1-2 drops of the amino acid solution.
- Pour 1-2 mL H_2SO_4 down the side of the sloping test tube to form a layer underneath the acetic acid.
- The development of a purple colour at the interface proves a positive reaction.

(d) **Lead-Sulfide Test:** When cystine is boiled with 40% NaOH, some of sulfur in its structure is converted to sodium sulfide (Na_2S). The Na_2S can be detected by using sodium plumbate solution which causes the precipitation of PbS from an alkaline solution. In order to apply this test, first the sodium plumbate solution should be prepared. This test for cysteine and cystine.

Procedure

- Sodium Plumbate Solution Preparation:

    Add 5 mL dilute NaOH to 2 mL dilute lead acetate.

    A white precipitate of lead hydroxide forms.

    Boil until the precipitate dissolves with the formation of sodium plumbate.
- Boil 2 mL amino acid solution with a few drops of 40% NaOH for 2 min.
- Cool and add a few drops of the sodium plumbate solution.
- A brown colour or precipitate is a positive test for sulfides.

(e) **Ehrlich Test:** Aromatic amines and many organic compounds (indole and urea) give a coloured complex with this test. Apply this test to tryptophan, urea and glycine.

Procedure

- Put 0.5 mL of the amino acid solution to a test tube.
- Add 2 mL Ehrlich reagent and observe the colour changes.
- Repeat the test with urea solution.

(f) **Sakaguchi Test:** The Sakaguchi reagent is used to test for a certain amino acid and proteins. The amino acid that is detected in this test is arginine. Since arginine has a guanidine group in its side chain, it gives a red colour with α-naphthol in the presence of an oxidizing agent like bromine solution. Apply this test to arginine.

Procedure

- 1 mL NaOH and 3 mL arginine solution is mixed and 2 drops of α-naphthol is added.

- Mix thoroughly and add 4-5 drops of bromine solution under the hood.
- Observe the colour change.

(g) Nitroprusside Test: The nitroprusside test is specific for cysteine, the only amino acid containing sulfhydryl group (-SH). This group reacts with nitroprusside in the presence of excess ammonia. Apply this test cysteine, cystine and methionin.

Procedure

- Put 2 mL amino acid solution into the test tube.
- Add 0.5 mL nitroprusside solution and shake thoroughly.
- Add 0.5 mL ammonium hydroxide.
- Observe the colour change.

Experiment 6. Qualitative tests for Proteins.

(a) Biuret Test: The Biuret Test positively identifies the presence of proteins (not less than two peptides). The reaction in this test involves the complex formation of the proteins with Cu^{2+} ions in a strongly alkaline solution. Apply this test to gelatin, casein and albumin.

Procedure

- To 2 mL protein solution, add 5-6 drops of dilute $CuSO_4$ (Fehling's solution A diluted 1/10 with water).
- Add 3 mL 40% NaOH solution.
- Observe the colour change.

  If the protein tested is insoluble in water, then apply the procedure given below:

- Measure 3 mL acetone and 1.5 mL water into a test tube.
- Add 1 drop of dilute NaOH and a little piece of protein to be tested.
- Boil continuously over a small flame for 2 min and cool.
- Add 0.5 mL 40% NaOH and 2 drops of a 1/10 diluted Fehling's solution A.
- Observe the colour change.

(b) Ninhydrin Test: This test is given by only amino acids and proteins which contain free $-NH_2$ groups in their structure. Apply this test for all the proteins provided.

(c) Test for Amino Acids: Perform the tests for individual amino acids on the provided proteins e.g., Xanthoproteic Test, Millon's Test, Hopkin's Cole Test and Lead Sulphite Test.

(d) Precipitation of Proteins: The precipitation of a protein occurs in a stepwise process. The addition of a precipitating agent and steady mixing stabilizes the protein solution. Mixing causes the precipitant and the target product to collide. Enough mixing time is required for molecules to diffuse across the fluid.

I. By Neutral Salts: The precipitation of a protein by neutral salt is commonly known as salting-out method. Addition of a neutral salt, such as ammonium sulfate, compresses the solvation layer and increases the protein-protein interaction. As the salt concentration of a solution is increased, more of the bulk water becomes associated with the ions. As a result, less water is available to take part in the solvation layer around the protein, which exposes hydrophobic parts on the protein surface. Therefore, proteins can aggregate and form precipitates from the solution. The amount of neutral salt required to cause protein precipitation varies with the nature of the protein and the pH of the solution. Apply this test to all the proteins provided.

Procedure

- Add solid ammonium sulfate to about 5 mL of protein solution in a test tube (the salt should be added in quantities of approximately 1 g at a time)

- Agitate the solution gently after each addition to dissolve the ammonium sulfate.

II. By salts of Heavy Metals: Heavy metal salts usually contain Hg^{2+}, Pb^{2+}, Ag^+, Tl^+, Cd^{2+} and other metals with high atomic weights. Since salts are ionic, they disrupt salt bridges in proteins. The reaction of a heavy metal salt with a protein usually leads to an insoluble metal protein salt. Apply this test to all the proteins provided.

Procedure

- Treat 3 mL of the protein solution with a few drops of mercuric nitrate.

- A white precipitate formation should be observed.

III. By Acid Reagents: The precipitation of a protein in the presence of acid reagents is probably due to the formation of insoluble salts between the acid anions and the positively charged protein particles. These precipitants are only effective in acid solutions. Apply this test to all the proteins provided.

Procedure

- Treat 3 mL of protein solution provided with a few drops of trichloroacetic acid solution.

- Note the protein precipitate formed.

IV. Unknown Part: Take an unknown solid from your assistants and please do not forget to write your unknown number in your lab reports.

- Carry out the amino acid and protein tests in a reasonable sequence to determine your unknown solid.

Experiment 7. Estimation of protein by Lowry's method

Principle: The principle behind the Lowry method of determining protein concentrations lies in the reactivity of the peptide nitrogen with the copper [II] ions under alkaline conditions and the subsequent reduction of the Folin-Ciocalteay phosphomolybdicphosphotungstic acid to heteropolymolybdenum blue by the copper-catalyzed oxidation of aromatic acids. The Lowry method is sensitive to pH changes and therefore the pH of assay solution should be maintained at 10 - 10.5. The Lowry method is sensitive to low concentrations of protein. Dunn in 1992 suggests concentrations ranging from 0.10 - 2 mg of protein per mL while Price in 1996 suggests concentrations of 0.005 - 0.10 mg of protein per mL. The major disadvantage of the Lowry method is the narrow pH range within which it is accurate. However, we will be using very small volumes of sample which will have little or no effect on pH of the reaction mixture. A variety of compounds will interfere with the Lowry procedure. These include some amino acid derivatives, certain buffers, drugs, lipids, sugars, salts, nucleic acids and sulphydryl reagents. Price notes that ammonium ions, zwitterionic buffers, non-ionic buffers and thiol compounds may also interfere with the Lowry reaction. These substances should be removed or diluted before running Lowry assays.

Reagents

A. 2% Na_2CO_3 in 0.1 N NaOH

B. 1% NaK Tartrate in H_2O

C. 0.5% $CuSO_4.5\,H_2O$ in H_2O

D. 48 mL of A, 1 mL of B, 1 mL C

E. Phenol Reagent - 1 part Folin-Phenol [2 N] : 1 part water

Note: Reagents A, B and C may be stored indefinitely.

BSA Standard-1 mg/mL: Bovine Serum Albumin: 5 mg in 5 mL of water [1µg/µl]. Freeze 1 mL aliquots.

Procedure

Note: Run triplicate determination for all samples.

1. Set up eleven sets of three 16 × 150 mm test tubes in rack.
2. Add BSA [0, 10, 20, 30, 40, 50, 60, 70, 80, 90, 100 µl] to these tubes.
3. Add 2 mL of solution D to each test tube.
4. Incubate for 10 minutes at room temperature.
5. Add 0.2 mL of dilute Folin-phenol solution to each tube.
6. Vortex each tube immediately.
7. Incubate at room temperature for 30 minutes.
8. Determine absorbance of each sample at 600 nm.
9. Plot absorbance *vs* mg protein to obtain standard curve.
10. Set up triplicate assays for all unknowns.

Observation:

BSA (mL)	Water (mL)	Sample conc. (mL)	Sample vol. (mL)	Alk. CuSO₄ (mL)	Lowry reagent (mL)	O.D.600 nm
0.25	4.75	0.05	0.2	2	0.2	
0.5	4.5	0.1	0.2	2	0.2	
1	4	0.2	0.2	2	0.2	
2	3	0.3	0.2	2	0.2	
3	2	0.4	0.2	2	0.2	
4	1	0.5	0.2	2	0.2	
5	0	1.0	0.2	2	0.2	

Experiment 8. Estimation of proteins by Bradford method.

Aim: To estimate the amount of protein in the given sample by Bradford Assay.

Principle: The protein in solution can be measured quantitatively by different methods. The methods described by Bradford uses a different concept-the protein's capacity to bind to a dye, quantitatively. The assay is based on the ability of proteins to bind to coomassie brilliant blue and form a complex whose extinction coefficient is much greater than that of free dye.

List of Reagents and Instruments

A. Equipment
(i) Test tubes
(ii) Graduated cylinder
(iii) Weight Balance
(iv) UV spectrophotometer

B. Reagents
(i) Dissolve 100 mg of Coomassie-Brilliant blue G250 in 50 mL of 95% Ethanol.
(ii) Add 100 mL of 85% phosphoric acid and make up to 600 mL with distilled water.
(iii) Filter the solution and add 100 mL of glycerol, then make upto 1000 mL.
(iv) The solution can be used after 24 hrs.
(v) BSA

Procedure
1. Prepare various concentration of standard protein solutions from the stock solution (say 0.2, 0.4, 0.6, 0.8 and 1.0 mL) into series of test tubes and make up the volume to 1 mL .
2. Pipette out 0.2 mL of the sample in two other test tubes and make up the volume to 1 mL.
3. A tube with 1 mL of water serves as blank
4. Add 5.0 mL of coomassie brilliant blue to each tube and mix by vortex or inversion.
5. Wait for 10-30 minutes and read each of the standards and each of the samples at 595 nm.
6. Plot the absorbance of the standards verses their concentration.
7. Plot graph of optical density versus concentration. From graph find amount of protein in unknown sample.

Obervations:

BSA (mL)	Conc of BSA (mg/mL)	Distilled Water (mL)	Bradford Reagent (mL)	Incubate for 10 minutes	O.D. at 595nm

Calculations

Result: The amount of protein present in the given sample was found to be ......

Experiment 9. Estimation of DNA by diphenylamine method.

Principle: When DNA is treated with diphenylamine under acidic conditions, a blue compound is formed with the sharp observation maximum at 595nm. This reaction is produced by 2 deoxypentose in general and is not specific for DNA. In acid solution the straight from the deoxypentose is converted to the highly reactive b-hydroxy lerulin aldehyde, which reacts with diphenylamine to produce a blue complex. In DNA, only deoxyribose of purine nucleotide reacts so that the value obtained represents one half of the total deoxyribose produced.

Aim: To estimate the concentration of DNA by diphenylamine reaction.

Principle: This is a general reaction given by deoxypentoses. The 2-deoxyribose of DNA, in the presence of acid, is converted to ù-hydroxilevulinic aldehyde, which reacts with diphenylamine to form a blue coloured complex, which can be read at 595 nm.

Requirements:

1. Standard DNA solution: Dissolve calf thymus DNA (200µg/mL) in 1N perchloric acid/buffered saline.

2. Diphenylamine solution: Dissolve 1g of diphenylamine in 100 mL of glacial acetic acid and 2.5 mL of concentrated H_2SO_4. This solution must be prepared fresh

3. Buffered Saline: 0.5 mol/litre NaCl; 0.015 mol/litre sodium citrate, pH 7.

Procedure:

1. Pipette out 0.0, 0.2, 0.4, 0.6, 0.8 and 1 mL of working standard in to the series of labelled test tubes.

2. Pipette out 1 mL of the given sample in another test tube.

3. Make up the volume to 1 mL in all the test tubes. A tube with 1 mL of distilled water serves as the blank.

4. Now add 2 mL of DPA reagent to all the test tubes including the test tubes labeled 'blank' and unknown.

5. Mix the contents of the tubes by vortexing / shaking the tubes and incubate on a boiling water bath for 10 min.

6. Then cool the contents and record the absorbance at 595 nm against blank.

7. Then plot the standard curve by taking concentration of DNA along X-axis and absorbance at 595 nm along Y-axis.

8. Then from this standard curve calculate the concentration of DNA in the given sample.

Observations and Calculations

Volume of Standard (200 µg/ml) DNA (ml)	Volume of distilled Water (ml)	Concent ration of DNA (µg)	Volume of DPA reagent (ml)	Incubate in boiling water bath for 10 Min & Cool	A_{595}
0.0	1.0	00	2		0.00
0.2	0.8	40	2		
0.4	0.6	80	2		
0.6	0.4	120	2		
0.8	0.2	140	2		
1.0	0.0	200	2		
1.0 unknown	0.0	?	2		

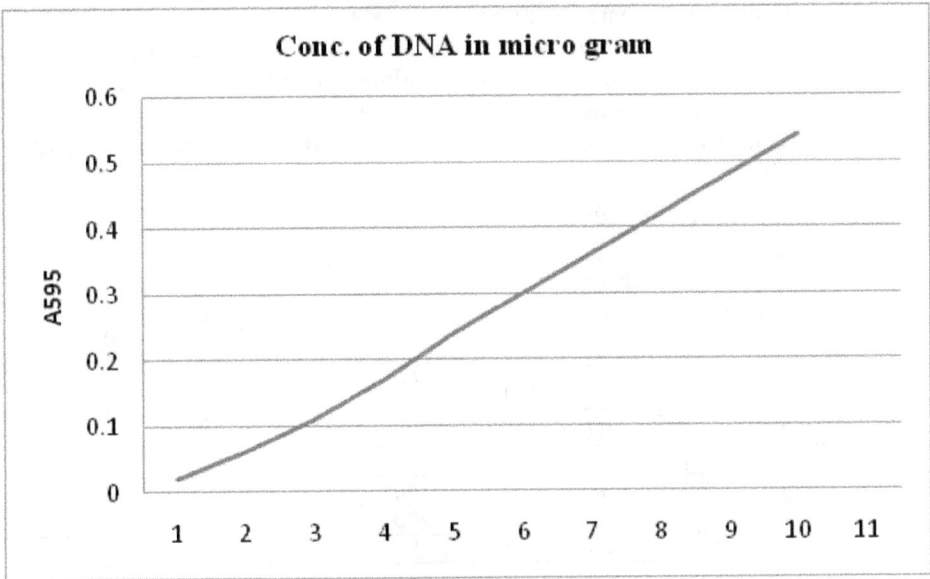

Standard curve for DNA estimation by DPA method

µ **Result:** The given unknown sample contains ——————————µg DNA/ mL.

Experiment 10. Estimation of RNA by Orcinol method.

Aim: To estimate the concentration of RNA by orcinol reaction.

Principle: This is a general reaction for pentoses and depends on the formation of furfural when the pentose is heated with concentrated hydrochloric acid. Orcinol reacts with the furfural in the presence of ferric chloride as a catalyst to give a green colour, which can be measured at 665 nm.

Requirements

1. Standard RNA solution- 200µg/mL in 1 N perchloric acid/buffered saline.

2. Orcinol Reagent- Dissolve 0.1g of ferric chloride in 100 mL of concentrated HCl and add 3.5 mL of 6% w/v orcinol in alcohol.

3. Buffered Saline- 0.5 mol/litre NaCl; 0.015 mol/litre sodium citrate, pH 7.

Procedure

1. Pipette out 0.0, 0.2, 0.4, 0.6, 0.8 and 1 mL of working standard in to the series of labeled test tubes.
2. Pipette out 1 mL of the given sample in another test tube.
3. Make up the volume to 1 mL in all the test tubes. A tube with 1 mL of distilled water serves as the blank.
4. Now add 2 mL of orcinol reagent to all the test tubes including the test tubes labeled blank and unknown.
5. Mix the contents of the tubes by vortexing / shaking the tubes and heat on a boiling water bath for 20 min.
6. Then cool the contents and record the absorbance at 665 nm against blank.
7. Then plot the standard curve by taking concentration of RNA along X-axis and absorbance at 665 nm along Y-axis.
8. Then from this standard curve calculate the concentration of RNA in the given sample.

Observations and Calculations

Volume of Standard (200 µg/ml) DNA (ml)	Volume of distilled Water (ml)	Concentration of DNA (µg)	Volume of DPA reagent (ml)	Incubate in water bath for 10 min & Cool	A_{665}
0.0	1.0	00	2		0.00
0.2	0.8	40	2		
0.4	0.6	80	2		
0.6	0.4	120	2		
0.8	0.2	140	2		
1.0	0.0	200	2		
1.0 unknown	0.0	?	2		

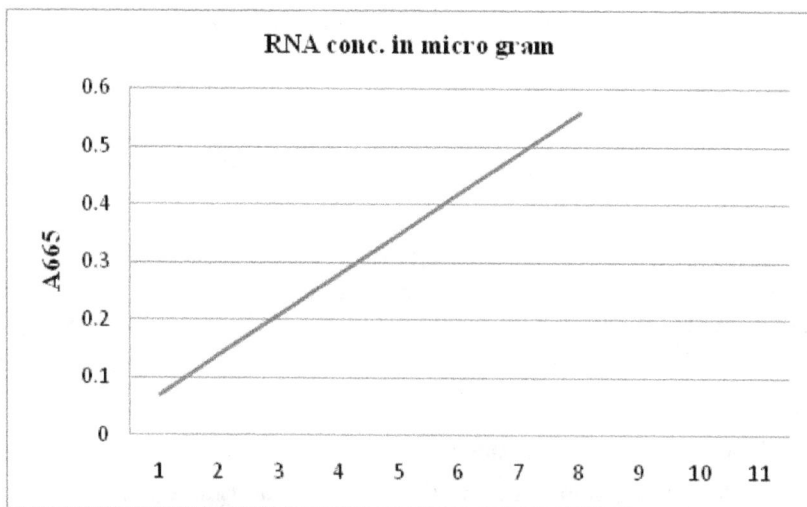

RNA conc. in micro gram

Standard curve for RNA estimation by Orcinol method

Result: The given unknown sample contains ———————————µg RNA/mL.

Experiment 11. Group analysis and Gravimetry.

Qualitative analysis is used to separate and detect cations and anions in a sample substance. In an educational setting, it is generally true that the concentrations of the ions to be identified are all approximately 0.01 M in an aqueous solution. The semimicro level of qualitative analysis employs methods used to detect 1-2 mg of an ion in 5 mL of solution.

First, ions are removed in groups from the initial aqueous solution. After each group has been separated, then testing is conducted for the individual ions in each group. Here is a common grouping of cations:

Group I: Ag^+, Hg_2^{2+}, Pb^{2+}

Precipitated in 1 M HCl

Group II: Bi^{3+}, Cd^{2+}, Cu^{2+}, Hg^{2+}, (Pb^{2+}), Sb^{3+} and Sb^{5+}, Sn^{2+} and Sn^{4+}

Precipitated in 0.1 M H_2S solution at pH 0.5

Group III: Al^{3+}, (Cd^{2+}), Co^{2+}, Cr^{3+}, Fe^{2+} and Fe^{3+}, Mn^{2+}, Ni^{2+}, Zn^{2+}

Precipitated in 0.1 M H_2S solution at pH 9

Group IV: Ba^{2+}, Ca^{2+}, K^+, Mg^{2+}, Na^+, NH_4^+

Ba^{2+}, Ca^{2+} and Mg^{2+} are precipitated in 0.2 M $(NH_4)_2CO_3$ solution at pH 10; the other ions are soluble. Many reagents are used in qualitative analysis, but only a few are involved in nearly every group procedure. The four most commonly used reagents are 6M HCl, 6M HNO_3, 6M NaOH, 6M NH_3. Understanding the uses of the reagents is helpful when planning an analysis.

Table 5. Common Qualitative Analysis Reagents

Reagent	Effects
6M HCl	Increases [H$^+$] Increases [Cl$^-$] Decreases [OH$^-$] Dissolves insoluble carbonates, chromates, hydroxides, some sulfates Destroys hydroxo and NH_3 complexes Precipitates insoluble chlorides
6M HNO_3	Increases [H$^+$] Decreases [OH$^-$] Dissolves insoluble carbonates, chromates and hydroxides Dissolves insoluble sulfides by oxidizing sulfide ion Destroys hydroxo and ammonia complexes Good oxidizing agent when hot
6 M NaOH	Increases [OH$^-$] Decreases [H$^+$] Forms hydroxo complexes Precipitates insoluble hydroxides
6M NH_3	Increases [NH_3] Increases [OH$^-$] Decreases [H$^+$] Precipitates insoluble hydroxides Forms NH_3 complexes Forms a basic buffer with NH_4^{+s}

1. Flame Test Introduction

The flame test is used to visually determine the identity of an unknown metal or metalloid ion based on the characteristic colour the salt turns the flame of a bunsen burner. The heat of the flame excites the metals ions, causing them to emit visible light. The characteristic emission spectra can be used to differentiate between some elements.

Classic Wire Loop Method: Take a clean wire loop. Platinum or nickel-chromium loops are most common. They may be cleaned by dipping in hydrochloric or nitric acid, followed by rinsing with distilled or deionized water. Test the cleanliness of the loop by inserting it into a gas flame. If a burst of colour is produced, the loop is not sufficiently clean. The loop must be cleaned between tests.

The clean loop is dipped in either a powder or solution of an ionic (metal) salt. The loop with sample is placed in the clear or blue part of the flame and the resulting colour is observed.

Wooden Splint or Cotton Swab Method: Wooden splints or cotton swabs offer an inexpensive alternative to wire loops. To use wooden splints, soak them overnight in distilled water. Pour out the water and rinse the splints with clean water, being careful to avoid contaminating the water with sodium (as from sweat on your hands). Take a damp splint or cotton swab that has been moistened in water, dip it in the sample to be tested and wave the splint or swab through the flame. Do not hold the sample in the flame as this would cause the splint or swab to ignite. Use a new splint or swab for each test.

Interpretation of Result: The sample is identified by comparing the observed flame colour against known values from a table or chart.

Red

Carmine to Magenta: Lithium compounds. Masked by barium or sodium.
Scarlet or Crimson: Strontium compounds. Masked by barium.
Red: Rubidium (unfiltered flame).
Yellow-Red: Calcium compounds. Masked by barium.

Yellow

Gold: Iron
Intense Yellow: Sodium compounds, even in trace amounts. A yellow flame is not indicative of sodium unless it persists and is not intensified by addition of 1% NaCl to the dry compound.

White

Bright White: Magnesium
White-Green: Zinc

Green

Emerald: Copper compounds, other than halides. Thallium.
Bright Green: Boron

Blue-Green: Phosphates, when moistened with H_2SO_4 or B_2O_3.

Faint Green: Antimony and NH_4 compounds.

Yellow-Green: Barium, manganese(II), molybdenum.

Blue

Azure: Lead, selenium, bismuth, cesium, copper(I), $CuCl_2$ and other copper compounds moistened with hydrochloric acid, indium, lead.

Light Blue: Arsenic and come of its compounds.

Greenish Blue: $CuBr_2$, antimony.

Purple

Violet: Potassium compounds other than borates, phosphates and silicates masked by sodium or lithium.

Lilac to Purple-Red: Potassium, rubidium and/or cesium in the presence of sodium when viewed through a blue glass.

Limitations of Flame Test

❖ The test cannot detect low concentrations of most ions.

❖ The brightness of the signal varies from one sample to another. For example, the yellow emission from sodium is much brighter than the red emission from the same amount of lithium.

❖ Impurities or contaminants affect the test results. Sodium, in particular, is present in most compounds and will colour the flame. Sometimes a blue glass is used to filter out the yellow of sodium.

❖ The test cannot differentiate between all elements. Several metals produce the same flame colour. Some compounds do not change the colour of the flame at all.

Table 6. Flame Test Colours

Symbol	Element	Colour
As	Arsenic	Blue
B	Boron	Bright green
Ba	Barium	Pale/Yellowish Green
Ca	Calcium	Orange to red
Cs	Cesium	Blue
Cu(I	Copper(I)	Blue
Cu(II)	Copper(II) non-halide	Green
Cu(II)	Copper(II) halide	Blue-green
Fe	Iron	Gold
In	Indium	Blue
K	Potassium	Lilac to red
Li	Lithium	Magenta to carmine

Contd.....

Table 6 Contd...

Symbol	Element	Colour
Mg	Magnesium	Bright white
Mn(II)	Manganese(II)	Yellowish green
Mo	Molybdenum	Yellowish green
Na	Sodium	Intense yellow
P	Phosphorus	Pale bluish green
Pb	Lead	Blue
Rb	Rubidium	Red to purple-red
Sb	Antimony	Pale green
Se	Selenium	Azure blue
Sr	Strontium	Crimson
Te	Tellurium	Pale green
Tl	Thallium	Pure green
Zn	Zinc	Bluish green to whitish green

2. Qualitative Analysis-Bead Tests

The bead test, sometimes called the borax bead or blister test, is an analytical method used to test for the presence of certain metals. The premise of the test is that oxides of these metals produce characteristic colours when exposed to a burner flame. The test is sometimes used to identify the metals in minerals. In this case, a mineral-coated bead is heated in a flame and cooled to observe its characteristic colour.

Procedure: First make a clear bead by fusing a small quantity of borax (sodium tetraborate: $Na_2B_4O_7 \bullet 10H_2O$) or microcosmic salt ($NaNH_4HPO_4$) onto a loop of platinum wire in a Bunsen burner flame. Sodium carbonate (Na_2CO_3) is used sometimes for the bead test, too. After the bead has been formed, coat it with a dry sample of the material to be tested and reintroduce the bead into the burner flame. The inner cone of the flame is the reducing flame; the outer portion is the oxidizing flame. Observe the colour and match it to the corresponding bead type and flame portion. The bead test is not a definitive method for identifying an unknown metal, but may be used to quickly eliminate or to narrow possibilities.

Colours indicators: The following abbreviations are used in the tables:

❖ *h*: hot

❖ *c*: cold

❖ *hc*: hot or cold

❖ *ns*: not saturated

❖ *s*: saturated

❖ *sprs*: supersaturated

Table 7. Borax beads

Colour	Oxidizing	Reducing
Colourless	*hc*: Al, Si, Sn, Bi, Cd, Mo, Pb, Sb, Ti, V, W*ns*: Ag, Al, Ba, Ca, Mg, Sr	Al, Si, Sn, alk. earths, earths*h*: Cu *hc*: Ce, Mn
Gray/Opaque	*sprs*: Al, Si, Sn	Ag, Bi, Cd, Ni, Pb, Sb, Zn *s*: Al, Si, Sn *sprs*: Cu
Blue	*c*: Cu *hc*: Co	*hc*: Co
Green	*c*: Cr, Cu *h*: Cu, Fe+Co	Cr*hc*: U*sprs*: Fe*c*: Mo, V
Red	*c*: Ni *h*: Ce, Fe	*c*: Cu
Yellow/Brown	*h*, *ns*: Fe, U, V*h*, *sprs*: Bi, Pb, Sb	W*h*: Mo, Ti, V
Violet	*h*: Ni+Co*hc*: Mn	*c*: Ti

Table 8. Microcosmic salt beads

Colour	Oxidizing	Reducing
Colourless	Si (undissolved)Al, Ba, Ca, Mg, Sn, Sr*ns*: Bi, Cd, Mo, Pb, Sb, Ti, Zn	Si (undissolved)Ce, Mn, Sn, Al, Ba, Ca, MgSr (*sprs*, not clear)
Gray/Opaque	*s*: Al, Ba, Ca, Mg, Sn, Sr	Ag, Bi, Cd, Ni, Pb, Sb, Zn
Blue	*c*: Cu *hc*: Co	*c*: W *hc*: Co
Green	U*c*: Cr *h*: Cu, Mo, Fe+(Co or Cu)	*c*: Cr *h*: Mo, U
Red	*h*, *s*: Ce, Cr, Fe, Ni	*c*: Cu*h*: Ni, Ti+Fe
Yellow/Brown	*c*: Ni*h*, *s*: Co, Fe, U	*c*: Ni*h*: Fe, Ti
Violet	*hc*: Mn	*c*: Ti

3. Identify an Unknown Chemical Mixture

Aim: To practice using the scientific method. To learn how to record observations and apply the information to perform more complex tasks.

Materials

Each group will need:

(a) plastic cups

(b) magnifying glass

(c) 4 unknown powders in 4 plastic baggies:

(i) sugar

(ii) salt

(iii) baking soda

(iv) corn starch

For the entire class; water, vinegar, heat source, iodine solution will be required.

Activitiy: Unknown powders are similar in appearance; each substance has characteristic properties that make it distinguishable from the other powders. Explain how the students can use their senses to examine the powders and record properties.

Have them use sight (magnifying glass), touch and smell to examine each powder. Observations should be written down. Introduce heat, water, vinegar and iodine. Explain the concepts of chemical reactions and chemical change. A chemical reaction takes place when new products are made from the reactants. Signs of a reaction could include bubbling, temperature change, colour change, smoke or change in odor. You may wish to demonstrate how to mix chemicals, apply heat or add indicator. If desired, use containers with labeled volume measurements to introduce students to the importance of recording quantities used in a scientific investigation. Students can put a specified amount of powder from the baggie into a cup e.g., 2 scoops, then add vinegar or water or indicator. Cups and hands are to be washed between experiments. Make a chart with the following:

(a) What was the appearance of each powder?

(b) What happened when water was added to each powder?

(c) What happened when vinegar was added to each powder?

(d) Did all powders produce the same response?

(e) What happened when iodine solution was added to each powder?

(f) Why do you think this happened?

(g) If you predicted the identity of the powders, were your predictions correct? If not, how were they different?

(h) What are true identities of the mystery powders A-D?

(i) How did you determine the correct answer?

Now, give the students a mystery powder made up using at least two of the four pure substances. They are to test this mixture using the procedures they used on the pure substances. In addition, they may wish to design new experiments.

Assessment: Students may be evaluated on their ability to correctly identify the final unknown mixture. Points may be awarded for teamwork, staying on task, submission of data or a lab report and ability to follow directions and follow safety rules.

Experiment 12. Assay of salivary Amylase activity.

When cells need to undertake a chemical reaction they cannot use the same tools as the organic chemist. They cannot use the extremely rare or reactive chemicals that are commonplace in organic synthesis and the range of temperatures and pH's available have to be within a more narrow range than what can be made to occur in a glass reaction flask. What we find in nature is a highly refined and complex system to get and efficiently extract raw materials needed to survive. This fantastically engineered system does its work at low temperature and high efficiency. The chemical reactions are carried out by micromachines (protein catalysts) called enzymes. Enzymes are all made up with the same 20 building blocks called amino acids. Human cells have some 30,000 different enzymes in them. Enzymes are of fundamental importance in almost all of the chemical reactions which take place in living organisms. When digestion occurs, enzymes released into the mouth, stomach and intestines catalyze or accelerate reactions which result in the breakdown of large food molecules into small building block molecules the body can more readily use. The following four digestive enzymes are:

- **Salivary amylase:** Breaks down starch into maltose.
- **Gastric pepsin:** Breaks down protein into amino acids.
- **Pancreatic chymotrypsin:** Breaks down protein into amino acids.
- **Pancreatic lipase:** Breaks down fats into fatty acids.

Salivary amylase is a typical human enzyme, it is made up of about 500 amino acid building blocks with a total molecule weight (MW) of about 60,000 (about 170 times more than its product, maltose, (MW 360.31).Approximately one litre of saliva is secreted into the human mouth each day by three pairs of salivary glands. Saliva contains many enzymes, including salivary amylase, the enzyme we will be assaying today. The substrate for amylase is starch, a polysaccharide. The product of the amylase reaction is maltose, a disaccharide made from two glucose molecules. Amylase is an enzyme that hydrolysis alpha-bonds of large alpha-linked polysaccharides such as starch and glycogen, yielding maltose and dextrin. It is the major form of amylase found in humans and other mammals. Amylase is found in saliva called ptyalin. The enzyme randomLy affects α-1-4 bonds, belonging to the amylose structure of starch and maltose units form. Amylase does not affect the α-1-6 bonds that belong to the amylopectin structure of starch. As a result of hydrolysis carried out with α-amylase, besides the maltose and glucose units, a large branched dextrin structure is formed in the media.

The optimum conditions for α- amylase:

Optimum pH: 5.6-6.9

- Human body temperature: 37 ^{0}C
- Presence of certain anions and activators:
- Chloride and bromide- most effective
- Iodide- less effective
- Sulphate and phosphate- least effective

Preparation of saliva solution: Obtain an unsalted cracker from your instructor, place it on your tongue and without chewing, and allow it to dissolve in your saliva. Note the time when you perceive a faint sweet taste.

Saliva: Have one partner chew on a clean rubber band and drool into a test tube until you have 5 mL of saliva. Note the sex and age of the spitter.

Diluted Saliva: Transfer 3 mL of the saliva to a fresh beaker and add 7 mL of tap water to the saliva and mix well with a pipet until homogeneous.

Diluted Saliva ready for reaction: Take 3 mL of the diluted solution and put it either in a test tube or in a small graduated cylinder.

Procedure

1. Add 1 mL of 1% starch solution and 1 mL phosphate buffer solution (pH=6.8) into 4 test tubes.

- Place each test tube into water baths at 0°C, 25°C, 37°C and 95°C, respectively.
- Wait for a few minutes and add 1 mL diluted (1/10) saliva into each test tube.
- Place 1 drop of iodine solution on 4 watch glasses and take 1 drop from each test tube to observe if there is any starch left (Starch gives blue colour with iodine solution).
- Record the time for the hydrolysis of 1 mL starch in each test tube.

2. Take 7 test tubes and prepare the following solutions.

Observation

Material	1	2	3	4	5	6	7
1% Starch solution	0.2	0.5	1	2	3	4	5
Distilled water	4.8	4.5	4	3	2	1	0
Phosphate buffer	1	1	1	1	1	1	1
Saliva (1/20) diluted	1	1	1	1	1	1	1

3. Shake each test tube thoroughly. Check each mixture for colour with iodine per minute.

4. Record colour changes.

Experiment 13: Isolation of Casein and Lactose from Milk.

Introduction: Milk is the most nutritionally complete food found in nature. All kinds of milk, human or animal, contain vitamins (thiamine, riboflavin, pantothenic acid and vitamins A, B_{12}, D), minerals such as calcium, potassium, sodium, phosphorus and trace metals, protein mostly casein, carbohydrates (principally lactose) and lipids (fats). Whole milk is an oil-in-water emulsion, containing its 3.9% fat dispersed as microsized globules. The fat emulsion is stabilized by complex phospholipids and proteins that are adsorbed on the surfaces of the globules. The fat in milk is so finely dispersed; it is digested more easily than fat from any other source. The globules are lighter than water, thus colesce on standing and eventually rise to the surface of the milk as cream. Vitamins A and D are fat-soluble substances and are thus concentrated in the cream. The fats in milk are primarily triglycerides, which are esters of saturated and unsaturated carboxylic acids with glycerol, a tri-alcohol. There are three kinds of proteins in milk *i.e.* casein, lactalbumins and lactoglobulins. All three are globular proteins, which tend to fold back on themselves into compact, nearly spheroidal units and are more easily solubilizied in water as collodial suspensions than fibrous proteins are. They are complete proteins, so called because they contain all the amino acids essential for building blood and tissue and they can sustain life and provide normal growth even if they are the only proteins, but they can contain greater amounts of amino acids than the proteins in egg and meat.

Casein, the main protein in milk, is a phosphoprotein. The phosphate groups are attached to the hydroxyl groups of some of the amino acid side chains. Casein exists in milk as the calcium salt, calcium caseinate. It is actually a mixture of at least three similar proteins which differ primarily in molecular weight and the amount of phosphorus groups they contain (α, β and k caseins), they form a micelle or a solublized unit. Neither α nor β casein is soluble in milk and neither is soluble either singly or in combination. If k casein is added to either one or to a combination of the two, the result is a casein complex that is soluble owing to the formation of the micelle. A structure proposed for casein micelle is shown below:

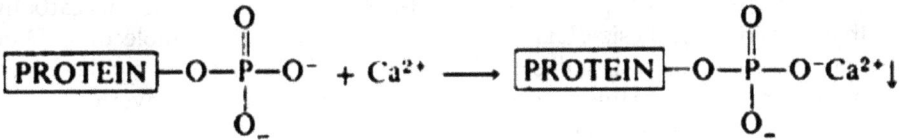

$$\boxed{\text{PROTEIN}}-\text{O}-\overset{\overset{\displaystyle O}{\|}}{\underset{\underset{\displaystyle O_-}{|}}{P}}-\text{O}^- + \text{Ca}^{2+} \longrightarrow \boxed{\text{PROTEIN}}-\text{O}-\overset{\overset{\displaystyle O}{\|}}{\underset{\underset{\displaystyle O_-}{|}}{P}}-\text{O}^-\text{Ca}^{2+}\downarrow$$

Casein

Calcium caseinate has an isoelectric point of pH 4.6. Therefore, it is insoluble in solutions of pH less than 4.6. The pH of milk is about 6.6; therefore, casein has negative charge at this pH and is solubilized as a salt. If acid is added to milk, the negative charges on the outer surface of the casein micelles are neutralized by protonation of the phosphate groups and the neutral protein precipitates, with the calcium ions remaining in solution:

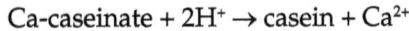

$$\text{Ca-caseinate} + 2\text{H}^+ \rightarrow \text{casein} + \text{Ca}^{2+}$$

A natural example of this process occurs when milk get sour. The souring of milk is an intricate process started by the action of microorganisms on the principal carbohydrate in milk, lactose. The microorganisms hydrolyse the lactose into glucose and galactose. Once galactose has been formed, *lactobacilli*, a strain of bacteria present in milk, convert it to the sour-tasting lactic acid. Since the production of the lactic acid also lowers the pH of the milk, the milk clots when it sours due to the precipitation of casein.

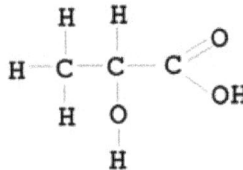

$$\text{H}-\overset{\overset{\displaystyle H}{|}}{\underset{\underset{\displaystyle H}{|}}{C}}-\overset{\overset{\displaystyle H}{|}}{\underset{\underset{\underset{\displaystyle H}{|}}{O}}{C}}-\text{C}\overset{\displaystyle O}{\underset{\displaystyle OH}{}}$$

Lactic acid

When the fats and proteins have been removed from milk, the carbohydrates remain in the whey, as they are soluble in aqueous solution. The main carbohydrate in milk is lactose.

α-Lactose:
D·Galactose + D·Glucose

Lactose

Lactose (4-O-(β-D-galactopyranosyl)-D-glucopyranose) is the only carbohydrate that mammals synthesize. It is a dissacharide consisting of one molecule of D-glucose and one molecule of D-galactose joined in 1, 4 fashion and is synthesized in the mammary glands. In this process, one molecule of glucose is converted to galactose and joined to another of glucose.

Melting Point: A melting point can be used to identify a substance and to get an indication of its purity. The melting point or freezing point of a solid is the temperature at which the solid exists in equilibrium with its liquid state under an external pressure of one atmosphere. More precisely, it is the temperature at which the vapour pressure of the solid phase becomes equal to the vapour pressure of the liquid phase. It is extremely difficult to establish the exact temperature at which this equilibrium is established; therefore, the temperature range over which liquid and solid are found to coexist is called the melting point. For example, a solid may be reported to have a 'melting point' of 100-101°C; this means that, on heating slowly, the first droplet of liquid was observed at 100°C and the last crystal of solid disappeared at 101°C. To determine the melting point of a crystalline substance, a small amount of the finely powdered crystals is introduced into a thin walled capillary tube; the latter is placed on an electrically heated hot-stage and heated. Two temperatures are recorded, the temperature at which the substance begins to liquefy and that at which it becomes completely liquefied. The observed melting point range is the interval between these two temperatures.

Melting point bath   Long necked Flask   Thiele Apparatus   Electrically sealed melting point block

Melting point determination apparatus

Equipment

Beaker 100 mL	Thrompt
Beaker 25 mL	Hot plate
Erlenmeyer Flask 50 mL	Thermometer
Graduated cylinder 10 mL	Dropper
Graduated cylinder 25 mL	Rubber tubing
Filtering Flask	Paper towels
Buchner Funnel	Glass rod

Chemicals

Acetic Acid, CH_3COOH

Ethyl ether, $C_4H_{10}O$

Ethanol, C_2H_5OH

Milk

Procedure

1. Measure 50 mL milk by a graduated cylinder and put it in a 100 mL beaker.
2. Heat the solution on a hot plate to bring the temperature to 55°C, control the temperature with thermometer.
3. Prepare 20 mL, 10 % acetic acid solution in a 25 mL beaker.
4. Add dropwise the 10% acetic acid solution while stirring. Do not add the acid too rapidly.
5. Keep the beaker on the hot plate, until the liquid becomes transparent and the casein no longer precipitates.

Isolation of Casein

1. Collect the casein with suction filtration and place the casein in a 100 mL beaker.
2. Prepare 20 mL 1:1 ethyl ether - ethanol solution in a 25 mL beaker and then add this mixture to the casein precipitate. Stir the solution for a few minutes.
3. Weigh the fitler paper and collect the casein by suction filtration.
4. Place the casein between several layers of paper towels to dry.
5. Keep the casein and allow it to dry for three days to determine its melting point and calculate the yield of our experiment.

Melting Point Determination

1. Fill a melting point tube with the sample (a thin-walled capillary tube) sealed at one end.
2. Attach the capillary tube to a thermometer.

3. Place the capillary in the melting point stage with oil bath.

4. Turn on the power and allow the hot-stage temperature to rise fairly rapidly to within 15-20°C below the expected melting point of the compound.

5. During the determination of the actual melting point range, heat the melting point hot-stage slowly at a uniform rate, about 2 degrees per minute.

6. Note the temperature at which the substance begins to liquefy and that at which it becomes completely liquefied.

Expected Results and Calculations

Melting point of casein: 280 °C

Melting point of casein: 342.3 °C

Percentage yield:

$$\text{Percentage of Product} = \frac{\text{Amount of product recovered}}{\text{Weight of Milk}} \times 100\%$$

Segment 2

Biochemistry, Bioenergetics and Physiology

Experiment 1: Expressing Concentration of Solutions.

Concentration of solutions should be accurately expressed for the appropriate use in the desired procedures. The units may generally be expressed in physical units, chemical units and proper name.

Physical Units: Weight of solute per unit volume of solution (weight per volume or w /v).

Example: 40 g% w / v glucose solution means, 40 g of glucose is dissolved in 100 mL of a given solvent to give a 40 % solution.

2. Weight of solute per weight of solvent (weight per weight or w / w).

Example: 30 g% w / w hydrochloric acid means, each 100 g of hydrochloric acid solution contains 30 g% of hydrochloric acid and the rest 70 g is the solvent (dw).

3. Volume of solute per volume of solvent (volume per volume or v / v).

Example: 90% v / v ethanol means 90 mL of absolute ethanol is mixed with 10 mL of distilled water.

Chemical units: Most common acids and some basic solutions like ammonium hydroxide are usually found with their concentrations expressed in specific gravity and percentage by weight of the specific solution. These two information (specific gravity and percentage by weight) should be changed to the commonly known expressions of concentration, like morality and normality. A molar solution is a solution that contains one mole of the solute in one liter of solution *e.g.*, molar weight of sulfuric acid (H_2SO_4) is 98. Therefore, one mole of H_2SO_4 contains 98 gm of H_2SO_4 per liter of solution. A normal solution is a solution that contains one gram equivalent weight of the solute in one liter of solution. The equivalent weight of H_2SO_4 is 98 divided for 2 (valancy of H_2SO_4), which is 49. Therefore, one normal solution of H_2SO_4 contains 49 gram of H_2SO_4 per liter of solution. To convert the given concentration to the form of molarity, the following steps should be applied.

1. Calculate the density of that solution from the specific gravity.
2. Find the amount of substance per liter of solution (multiply density with percentage by weight).
3. Calculate the molar concentration using the following formula:

$$\text{Molarity} = \frac{\text{Number of moles of solute}}{\text{Volume of solution in liter}}$$

or

$$\frac{\text{Amount of substance (Weight)}}{\text{Molar weight x Volume of solution in liter}}$$

Molarity (M) is amount of substance per unit mass of solvents and it is commonly expressed as mole/kg. If the information about a solution in a given bottle is in the form of percentage (weight by volume or w / v %), the concentration can be changed to molar solution using the following formula:

$$\text{Molarity (Mol/liter)} = \frac{\text{Gm \%} \left(\dfrac{W}{V} \times 10 \right)}{\text{Molar mass}}$$

Example: Convert 4% (w /v) NaOH into mol/liter of solution?

$$M = \frac{4\% \times 10}{40 \text{ (Molar mass of NaOH)}}$$

M = 1M solution

$$\text{Normality} = \frac{\text{Number of grams equivalent of solute}}{\text{Volume of solution in liter}}$$

$$= \frac{\text{Amount of Substance}}{\text{Equivalent weight x Volume of solution in liter}}$$

$$\text{Equivalent weight} = \frac{\text{Molecular weight}}{\text{Valency}}$$

Proper name: There are few instances where a solution is described by proper name as far as its concentration is concerned.

Example: Benedict's solution, copper sulfates hydrated, sodium citrate, sodium carbonate and distilled water.

Experiment 2: Determination of Urine Urea Nitrogen.

Principle: Urea is the major end product of protein and amino acid catabolism and is generated in the liver through the urea cycle. From the liver, urea enters the blood to be distributed to all intracellular and extracellular fluids, since urea is freely diffusible across most cell membranes. Most of the urea is ultimately excreted by the kidneys, but minimal amounts are also excreted in sweat and degraded by bacteria in the intestines. The urease specifically hydrolyzes urea to form ammonia and carbon dioxide. The ammonia is utilized by enzyme of glutamate dehydrogenase (GLDH) to reductively aminate α-ketoglutamate (α-KG) with simultaneous oxidation of reduced nicotinamide-adenine dinucleotide (NADH).

Clinical Significance: The urine urea nitrogen test to estimate of glomerular filtration rate. The excretion of urea is influenced by tubular re-absorption as well as filtration, the latter being influenced by urinary flow. In addition, urea production is affected by ingestion, catabolism and/or loss of proteins into the gastrointestinal tract. Because of the variability in metabolism and renal handling, elevations of circulating urea concentrations do not always correlate well with renal parenchymal function. Accordingly, a rise in urea can be attributed to pre-renal cause excess urea production, diminished renal blood flow or both, to post-renal causes obstruction along the genitourinary tract or to kidney perturbations (parenchymal kidney damage). If excessive production is the only factor elevating urea, the blood urea nitrogen rarely exceeds 40 mg/dL. Values beyond this usually indicate renal damage, urinary tract obstruction and diminished renal blood flow.

Specimen: 2 mL aliquot of a 24-hour urine collection. Proper 24 hour urine collection procedure should be followed and collection container should be refrigerated at 2-6°C during collection. It should be well-mixed and measured in a graduated cylinder. The total volume should be recorded.

Procedure

This method is based on the decomposing of urea $(NH_2)_2CO$ into N_2, H_2O and Na_2CO_3 by sodium hypobromite. The resulting N_2 is measured into Kowarski apparatus. The N_2 volume is transformed into N_2 grams (Avogadro's law) and the N_2 grams into urea grams.

1. Add tricloracetic acid to urine to precipitate the proteins (2.5 mL +2.5 mL).
2. Fill the apparatus with Kowarski solution over the superior tap and close it.
3. Add 3 mL of urine, open the tap and let only 2, 5 mL flow.
4. Add 7 mL of sodium hypobromite and let only 6 mL flow.
5. After each operation clean the reservoir of the apparatus.
6. There will be a gas buildup at the top of the apparatus that will read as N_2 volume (cm³) after 10-15 minutes.

Calculation: N_2 resulted from the reaction with V, in the reaction there were 1.25 mL of urine involved and 1.25 mL of tricloracetic acid.

V mL N_2................................1, 25 mL urine

X mL..1000 mL urine   X= V x 800

28g N_2..22400 mL N_2

Y mg..V x 800   Y= V

As there are 2 N_2 in urea, in 1000 mL of urine there are 2 x V grams of urea.

Normal value: 15-35 g/L

Experiment 3: Calculating Acid Number of Fats.

Light, heat, humidity and bacterial processes cause fats to hydrolyze leading to a bad odour due to the formation of fatty acids. Unsaturated fatty acids are oxidized by oxygen in air to form peroxides. The amount of free acid is a criterion for evaluating the quality and freshness of fats. There are antioxidants in several natural fats that prevent the oxidation of acids. Naphthols and phenols are of this class. The most prominent antioxidant is Vitamin E. It is used as an additive in food products to prevent oxidation. The stability and freshness of fat depends on the amount of antioxidant it contains.

Aim: To calculate the acid number and compare with the known oil types.

Procedure:

(i)   Weigh 5 g fat in an Erlenmeyer flask.

(ii) Dissolve the fat in the fat dissolver solution.

(iii) Add 1 mL of phenolphthalein as an indicator.

(iv) Titrate the solution with 0.1 M NaOH.

(v)   Record the end point.

(vi) Calculate the acid number by using the end point.

Results:

Experiment 4: Calculation of Saponification Number and Average Molecular Weight of Triacylglycerols.

The simplest lipids constructed from fatty acids are the triacylglycerols, also referred to as triglycerides, fats or neutral fats. Triacylglycerols are composed of three fatty acids each in ester linkage with a single glycerol. Triacylglycerols are major components of the natural lipid in biological tissue. Depending on the nature of the constituent fatty acids, they may be either oils or low melting point solids. Plant triacylglycerols generally tend to be oils, reflecting a relatively high content of saturated fatty acids, whereas animal triacylglycerols are usually solid. Information about the structure of triacylglycerols can be obtained by two parameters:

(a) Saponification Number

(b) Iodine Number

The saponification number gives an indication of the average molecular weight of the triacylglycerols, while the iodine number gives a relative measure of the degree of unsaturation. Analysis of acylglycerols can be achieved by hydrolysis followed by isolation and characterization of products. Hydrolysis of acylglycerols is most easily accomplished in hot alkali (saponification) but as lipids.

Aim: To calculate the saponification number of the oil sample and the average molecular weight of triacylglycerols.

Procedure:

(i) Get a round bottom flask (RBF). Clean RBF, rinse it with distilled water, then with acetone and allow drying in the oven.

(ii) After RBF cool down, weight it and record the weight value.

(iii) Measure 2 mL of oil with a graduated cylinder.

(iv) Place the oil into to RBF, weigh RBF once again and record the difference as the weight of oil sample.

(v) Set up a reflux apparatus (RBF+ condenser). Do not forget to add boiling chips.

(vi) Add 20 mL of 0.5M ethanolic NaOH into the RBF.

(vii) Refluxes for 30 min. Do not forget to flow water through the condenser.

(viii) After reflux, transfer the solution into an erlenmeyer flask and add 1-2 drops of phenolphthalein as an indicator.

(ix) Titrate the solution with 0.5M HCl.

(x) Record the end-point.

Results:

Experiment 5: Salting in, Salting Out and Dialysis of Proteins.

Salting in: The effects of salts such as sodium chloride on increasing the solubility of proteins is known as salting in. When low concentrations of salt are added to a protein solution, the solubility increases. Salt molecules stabilize protein molecules by decreasing the electrostatic energy between the protein molecules which increase the solubility of proteins.

Salting out: When the ionic strength of a protein solution is increased by adding salt, the solubility decreases and protein precipitates. The salt molecules compete with the protein molecules in binding with water. Some salts, such as high concentrations of ammonium sulfate, have general effects on solvent structure that lead to decreased protein solubility and salting out. In this case, the protein molecules tend to associate with each other because protein-protein interactions become energetically more favorable than protein-solvent interaction. Proteins have characteristic salting out points and these are used in protein separations in crude extracts. The most effective region of salting out is at the isoelectric point of the protein because all proteins exhibit minimum solubility in solutions of constant ionic strength at their isoelectric points. The salt commonly used is ammonium sulphate because:

(a) Its large solubility in water.

(b) Its relative freedom from temperature effects.

(c) It has no harmful effects on most of the proteins.

Dialysis: Separation of dissolved small molecules from macromolecules by virtue of their molecular dimensions through a semi permeable dialysis bag is called dialysis. One application of dialysis is desalting a solution. The salt molecules move from the more concentrated solution from inside the dialysis bag to the less concentrated solution e.g., distilled water. Factors affecting the rate of dialysis:

(a) The ratio of the higher to the lower concentration of that molecule on the two sides of the membrane to maximize the rate of movement it's necessary to stir the buffer.

(b) The pore size of the membrane.

(c) The size and charge of the dialyzable molecule.

In this experiment, myoglobin is isolated from skeletal muscle by salting out technique which discards up to 75% of the crude proteins in the protein purification process. We usually measure the total concentration of proteins rather than its type by using a general protein detection method as Biuret Test in addition of a specefic prorein test after each step of protein purification as salting out to follow the purification steps of the target protein, here we take one purification step (Part 1) with only the Biuret Test (Part 2).

Part 1: Salting Out Technique

Materials and Apparatus: Skeletal muscle, Waring Blender, Solid ammonium sulphate, Magnatic stirrer, Spectrophotometer and pH meter.

Procedure:

(i) Cut skeletal muscle (100 g) into small pieces.

(ii) Homogenize it for 10 seconds in 100 mL distilled water at room temperature in a blender.

(iii) Divide the homogenate in 5 equal parts.

(iv) Allow the homogenate to stand for 20 min. and then Centrifuge at 2000 rpm 4°C for 10 min.

(v) Discard the residue (palette) and adjust pH of supernatant to pH 7.0 by adding ammonium hydroxide solution (2M). We used sodium hydroxide (0.1M) much diluted strong base in replace of ammonium hydroxid solution.

vi) Measure the volume of the sample (supernatant 4 mL).

(vii) Calculate the required grams of ammonium sulfate salt needed to saturate the solution to 35 % of salt. By using the attached table called as Nomograme, then-

X_1 g ————< it is found in 1000 mL of protein solution, so:

in ? g >———— in 4 mL (supernatant volume)

? = N_1 g of salt.

(viii) Add (N) g of salt to the protein solution very slowly and mix during the addition, for best results the addition should be very slowly with constant stirring. To get a 0-35% saturation of the solution.

(ix) Centrifuge the tube sample at 3500 rpm for 10 minutes.

(x) Discard the pellet and measure the volume of the supernatant, record the volume (3.5mL)

(xi) Calculate again the required amount of salt to be added to saturate the protein solution to 55 % of salt.

X_2 g ————> in 1000 mL of protein solution.

? ————> 3.5 mL.

? = N_2 g of salt.

(xii) Add a (N_2) g of salt to the supernatant (solution) slowly while mixing.

(xiii) Centrifuge the sample at 3500 rpm for 10 minutes also.

(xiv) Discard the supernatant and dissolve the pellet which contains the desired protein (Myoglobin) 10 mL of distilled water.

Desalting:

(i) Remove the ammonium sulphate used in the salting out procedure by dialysis using dialysis tubing (bag).

(ii) Place the protein solution in the dialysis bag made by tying knots in the end of cellulose dialysis tubing.

(iii) Put the sealed bag in a large volume of cold water which is being moderately remove and the protein solution is equilibrated with water at least 6-8 hours are required for complete dialysis or overnight.

(iv) After that, transport the remaining protein solution into new centrifuge tube and store it at 4-8°C temperature until use.

(v) Find out the amount of protein in the dialyzed sample using Biuret Method.

Part 2: Biuret Assay of Protein Biuret Test.

Objective: This test used to detect and determine the protein concentration. So, it can be used for both qualitative and a quantitative analysis of protein.

Principle: This test or reaction is given by peptides containing at least tow peptide bonds, *i.e.,* it is not given by dipeptides and most of the free amino acids in general except histidine, serine and therionine which give a reaction. The principle underlying the test can be demonstrated with the chemical compound biuret which, just as proteins, is able to complex copper (II) ions to give a violet coloured complex. The biuret assay does not in fact use biuret, but is also named as it detects the peptide bond between the urea molecules or between the amino acids. So, the biuret reaction takes its name from the fact that biuret itself, obtained by heating urea gives a similar coloured complex with cupric ions.

$$2NH_2 - CO - NH_2 \;\;\xrightarrow{\text{heating}}\; NH_3 \;+\; NH_2 - CO - NH - CO - NH_2$$

    (Urea)   **(Biuret)**

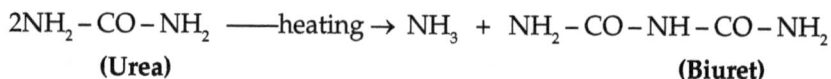

Not all Biuret Test actually require the same reagent. Rather, the term biuret test' is a generic term for testing of proteins by using copper (II) sulphate solution in an alkaline environment.

Biuret Reagent *(Alkaline Copper Sulphate)*: It is made of potassium hydroxide (KOH) or sodium hydroxide (NaOH) and copper sulphate ($CuSO_4$), together with potassium sodium tartarate. The blue reagent turns violet in the presence of proteins and changes to pink when combined with short chain polypeptides. The potassium hydroxide does not participate in the reaction at all, but is merely there to provide an alkaline medium so that the reaction can take place. This reagent is commonly used in a biuret protein assay, a colourimetric assay. The biuret reagent reacts with peptides and proteins to give a violet coloured Cu^{+2} peptide complex. This coloured complex can be measured quantitatively by spectrophotometer in the visible region. The colour obtained is directly proportional to the number of peptide bond present in the protein. In this experiment the amount of isolated protein from skeletal muscle is determined by the Biuret assay and from the standard curve of Bovine Serum Albumin (BSA).

Materials and Method:

(1) Standard Protein (5 g/L of Bovine serum albumin).

(2) Myoglobin Protein Sample 1 isolated from skeletal muscle by salting out technique.

(3) New Protein sample 2 (BSA).

(4) Label 11 test tubes and add to each tube the solutions as the following table:

Tube	1	2	3	4	5	6	7	8	9	10	11 (Blank)
Standard	0.1	0.2	0.4	0.6	0.8	1					
Distilled Water	0.9	0.8	0.6	0.4	0.2	0					1
Sample 1							1				
Sample 1'								1			
Sample 2									1		
Sample 2'										1	
Biuret Reagent	4	4	4	4	4	4	4	4	4	4	4

(5) Mix well all the test tubes.

(6) Allow to stand for 20 min.

(7) Read the absorbance at 540 nm against the blank.

(8) Record the results in the observation table.

(9) Plot a standard curve (graph) using concentration of bovine serum albumin against the absorbance at 540 nm.

(10) Determine the concentration of protein present in sample 1, 1' and 2, 2'.

(11) Record the concentration in the observation table.

(12) Calculate the average of the two concentration of sample 1 (1 & 1') and sample 2 (2 & 2').

Calculation:

1. **Calculation of Standard Protein serial concentrations:** By using the dilution law (Dilution Equation) as following:

$$C_1 \times V_1 = C_2 \times V_2$$

When C_1 and V_1 = main standard concentration and its required volume to be diluted until one (1) mL. of volume (V_2) with distilled water to give C_2 concentration (unknown concentration). So, to calculate the concentration of diluted standard protein in tube no. one, which prepared by take 0.1 mL of main standard protein (stock Std. protein) with 0.9 mL of distilled water:

$$C_1 = 5 \, g/L, \, V_1 = 0.1, \, C_2 =?, \, V_2 = 1 \, mL$$

$$C_1 \times V_1 = C_2 \times V_2$$

$$5 \times 0.1 = C_2 \times 1$$

$$C_2 = 5 \times 0.1 / 1 \longrightarrow C_2 = 0.5 \, g/ L.$$

2. **Concentration of samples (1 & 2):** From the standard curve, protein concentration in sample 1.............g/L and in sample 2...g/L. The average value is......

Observations

Tube No.	Absorbance (nm)	Protein conc. (g/L)	Average (g/L)
Blank (11)		0.0	
1		0.5	
2		1.0	
3		2.0	
4		3.0	
5		4.0	
6		5.0	
7 (sample 1)		? (From std. curve)	* (C of tube 7 + 8)/ 2
8 (sample 1')		?	
9 (sample 2)		?	* (C. of tube 9 +10)/ 2
10 (sample 2')		?	

Results:

Experiment 6: Determination of Serum Albumin by Bromocresol Green Method.

Serum albumin measurements are used in the diagnosis of numerous diseases. Elevated serum albumin levels are usually the result of dehydration. Decreased serum albumin levels are found in a number of conditions including kidney disease, liver disease, infections, severe burns and cancer. In 1965, Rodkey, introduced a convenient, direct method for determining albumin concentrations in serum utilizing a neutral buffered solution of bromocresol green (BCG) as the dye binding indicator. In 1971, Doumas et al. increased the sensitivity of the reaction by adding a nonionic surfactant to the reagent to prevent turbidity and improve linearity. This Albumin method is a modification of the Doumas and Rodkey procedures utilizing a different buffering system. At pH 4.2, bromocresol green reacts with albumin to form an intense green complex. The absorbance of the albumin-BCG complex is measured bichromatically (600/800nm) and is proportional to the albumin concentration in the sample.

pH 4.2

Albumin + Bromocresol---------------------->Green Complex

Reagents and materials:

(i)   A stock standard solution of albumin (100g/L)

(ii) A diluent solution (D)

(iii) Bromocresol green (BCG) dye.

(iv) Control sample /Pateint 1 /Patient 2.

Procedure:

1.   Take six small plastic tubes (set A) and six large plastic tubes (set B), each set labeled 1-6.

2.   Take set A (1-6) and prepare albumin standards according to table below with six concentration points ranging from 0-100g/L.

Set (A) tubes 1-6	1A	2A	3A	4A	5A	6A
Std concentration g/l	0				80	100
µL of stock albumin	0				800	1000
µL of normal saline	1000				200	0
Total volume (mL)	1.0	1.0	1.0	1.0	1.0	1.0

3.   Cover each tube with parafilm and mix by gentle inversion 4 to 5 times.

4.   Transfer 25µL of albumin standards from set (A) to set (B), labeled 1-6 also.

5.   Take three more tubes and label them as Control, Patient 1 and patient 2.

6.   Now add 25µL of Control, patient sample 1 and patient sample 2 to appropriate tubes.

7.   To all the nine tubes add 5 mL of BCG dye solution.

8.   Cover each tube with parafilm and mix by gentle inversion.

9.   Set the spectrophotometer at 628 nm and set the absorbance at zero using distilled water.

10. Record the absorbance of each of the standard in observation table provided below.

11. Record the absorbance of Control and Patient samples 1 and 2 in table below.

12. Draw standard curve using graph paper provided.

Standard curve:

1. Write the title of the experiment on top and date of the experiment.

2. Write the concentrations of albumin standards on x-axis.

3. Write the absorbance of albumin standards on y-axis.

4. Clearly label x and y-axis.

5. Produce a linear curve, which may form a plateau at the last two points.

Observations:

Albumin std (g/L)	Absorbance
0	-
20	-
40	-
60	-
80	-
100	-

Samples	Absorbance	Conc. g/L	Condition
Control	-	-	-
Patient 1	-	-	-
Patient 2	-	-	-

Results:

Experiment 7: Determination of Total Cholesterol.

Measurement of cholesterol is used primarily in diagnosis and treatment of disorders involving excess cholesterol in the blood and lipid and lipoprotein metabolism disorders. Total serum cholesterol analysis has proven useful in the diagnosis of hyper lipoproteinemia, atherosclerosis, hepatic and thyroid diseases. Total and HDL cholesterols, in conjunction with a triglyceride determination, provide valuable information for the prediction of coronary heart disease.

Principle: The cholesterol esters are hydrolyzed to free cholesterol by cholesterol esterase (CE). The free cholesterol is then oxidized by cholesterol oxidase (CO) to cholesten-3-one with the simultaneous production of hydrogen peroxide. The hydrogen peroxide produced couples with 4-aminoantipyrine and phenol, in the presence of peroxidase, to yield a chromogen with maximum absorbance at 505 nm. The intensity of the colour produced is directly proportional to the concentration of total cholesterol in the sample.

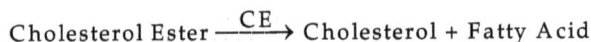

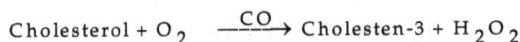

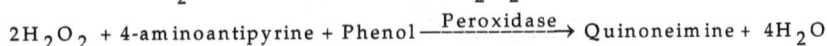

$$\text{Cholesterol Ester} \xrightarrow{\text{CE}} \text{Cholesterol} + \text{Fatty Acid}$$

$$\text{Cholesterol} + O_2 \xrightarrow{\text{CO}} \text{Cholesten-3} + H_2O_2$$

$$2H_2O_2 + \text{4-aminoantipyrine} + \text{Phenol} \xrightarrow{\text{Peroxidase}} \text{Quinoneimine} + 4H_2O$$

Reagents

Cholesterol Colour Reagent: A solution containing phosphate buffer (pH 6.7 at 25°C) containing 1.6 mmol/L 4-aminoantipyrine, > 5560 U/L peroxidase (botanical), > 400 U/L cholesterol esterase (mammalian), > 400 U/L cholesterol oxidase (microbial), a preservative and a stabilizer.

Cholesterol Phenol Reagent: A solution containing 40 mmol/L phenol, a surfactant and a stabilizer.

Cholesterol Calibrator: 1 x 15 mL solution containing 193 mg/dL (5 mmol/L) cholesterol, a surfactant and a preservative.

Reagent Preparation and Storage: Prepare the required volume of working reagent by mixing equal volumes of colour reagent and phenol reagent. Mix gently and thoroughly. The reagents included are stable until the expiry date stated on the labels at 2-8°C. The prepared working reagent is stable for 4 weeks at 2-8°C or for 5 days at 18-26°C. The reagent solutions should be clear. Turbidity would indicate deterioration.

Specimen: Fresh, clear, unhemolysed serum. The specimen should be drawn in the morning following a 12 hour fast.

Sample Storage: Samples should be stored at 2-8°C for 1 week or minus 20°C for 4 weeks.

Materials

- Genzyme Diagnostics' total serum cholesterol reagents and calibrator.
- Automated analyzer capable of accurately measuring absorbance at appropriate wavelengths as per instrument application.
- Alternative calibration material.

Procedure

The test for total cholesterol using this reagent will be performed on an automated analyzer using an endpoint test mode, with a sample to reagent ratio of 1:100 and a wavelength reading of (primary/secondary) 505/600 nm. Calibration material should be used to calibrate the procedure. The frequency of calibration, if necessary, using an automated system is dependent on the system and the parameters used. The results should fall within the acceptable range as established by the laboratory. The analyzer automatically calculates the total serum cholesterol concentration of each sample. A sample with a total serum cholesterol concentration exceeding the linearity limit should be diluted with 0.9% saline and re-assayed incorporating the dilution factor in the calculation of the value.

Reference Intervals: Values for selecting adults at moderate and high risk of coronary artery disease who require treatment given below:

Age (Years)	Moderate Risk	High Risk
20-29	>200 mg/dL (5.17 mmol/L)	>222 mg/dL (5.74 mmol/L)
30-39	>220 mg/dL (5.69 mmol/L)	>240 mg/dL (6.21 mmol/L)
40 and over	>240 mg/dL (6.21 mmol/L)	>260 mg/dL (6.72 mmol/L)

Results: Total serum cholesterol concentration is reported as ... mg/dL or ....(mmol/L).

Experiment 8: Determination of Serum Glutamate oxaloacetate transaminase (SGOT).

Serum Glutamate oxaloacetate transaminase is an enzyme that is normally present in liver and heart cells. Glutamate-oxaloacetate transaminase (GOT), also known as Aspartate amino transferase (AST) is a transaminase (EC 2.6.1.1) similar to the more liver specific alanine transaminase (ALT). SGOT is released into blood when the liver or heart is damaged. The blood SGOT levels are thus elevated with liver damage from viral hepatitis or with an insult to heart from a heart attack. Some medications can also raise SGOT levels. Although commonly included clinically as part of a diagnostic liver function test, GOT has a broader clinical utility since it may also be elevated in diseases affecting other organs, such as the heart or muscles in myocardial infarction, also in acute pancreatitis, acute hemolytic anemia, severe burns, acute renal disease, musculoskeletal diseases and trauma. It catalyzes the reaction:

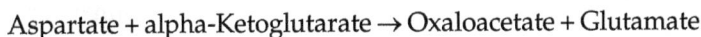

Aspartate + alpha-Ketoglutarate → Oxaloacetate + Glutamate

Diagnostically, it is almost always measured in units/liter (U/L).

Principle: Reitman and Frankel' described a calorimetric procedure for assaying GOT activities. End products of the transaminations react with di-nitrophenylhydrazine to form a hydrazone complex. This product yields a coloured complex when alkaline diluents are added. The colour intensity at 505 nm can be related to enzyme activity by reference to a standard curve.

Reagents:

GOT substrate: 200 mM aspartic acid and 1.8 mM ketoglutaric acid buffered at pH 7.5. Preservative added. Store at 2-8°C. Stable until expiration date if sealed tightly. The substrate should be a clear colourless solution. Turbidity would indicate deterioration.

Calibration Solution: 1.5 mM pyruvate buffered at pH 7.5. Preservative added. Store at 2-8°C. Stable until expiration date if sealed tightly. The calibration solution is a clear and colourless solution. Turbidity would indicate deterioration.

Colour Reagent: 1.0 mM 2, 4-dinitrophenylthydrazine in dilute acid. Avoid contact with eyes, skin and clothing. In case of contact, wash with large amount of water. Store at 2-8°C. Stable until expiration date if sealed tightly. The colour reagent is a clear yellow solution. Turbidity or a brown colour would indicate deterioration.

Instruments: Use a spectrophotometer or colourimeter calibrated at 490-520 nm.

Specimen Collection

(a) Use unhemolyzed serum separated from the blood clot as soon as possible.

(b) Plasma may be used.

(c) Grossly hemolyzed or lipemic samples should not be used.

Sample Storage: Serum transaminases appear stable for one week at 2-8°C. No special additives or preservatives are needed. Serum from patients receiving erythromycin may show elevated results.

Materials: 0.1 mL and 0.5 mL micropipettors, 5.0 mL pipettor, incubator capable of maintaining $37 \pm 0.5°C$.

Reaction Conditions:

    (a) Wavelength 490-520 nm

    (b) Incubation Temperature 37°C

    (c) Incubation Time: 60 min

    (d) Sample Volume 0.1 mL

    (e) Substrate Volume 0.5 mL

    (f) Colour Reagent Volume 0.5 mL

    (g) Alkaline Diluent Volume 5.0 mL

    (h) Total Volume 6.1 mL

Preparation of Alkaline Diluent: Dissolve 16 grams of sodium hydroxide in 1.0 L D-H_2O. Allow to cool before use.

Procedure

Preparation of Calibration Curve: All reagents should be at room temperature.

1. Calibration curves must be prepared. Use the specific substrate and set up the following tubes:

2. Arrange tubes and add materials as given in table below:

Tube	D-H_2O (mL)	Substrate (mL)	Cal.Ref.(mL)	GOT(U/mL)
1	0.2	1.0	0.0	0
2	0.2	0.9	0.1	22
3	0.2	0.8	0.2	55
4	0.2	0.7	0.3	95
5	0.2	0.6	0.4	150
6	0.2	0.5	0.5	215

3. Add 1 mL colour Reagent to each tube. Mix well and let stand for 5 minutes at room temperature.

4. Add 10 mL alkaline diluent to each tube. Mix well and let stand for 5 minutes at room temperature.

5. Zero instruments with D-H_2O at 505 nm (490-520 nm acceptable).

6. Read and record absorbance.

7. Plot enzyme activity versus absorbance. A non-linear curve is obtained with decreasing slope as enzyme activity increases.

8. Linearity extends to 215 U/mL for GOT. If enzyme activity exceeds these levels, dilute the specimen × 10 with isotonic saline and repeat the assay. Multiply the result × 10 to correct for dilution.

Performance

1. Dispense 0.5 mL substrate (GOT) into tubes labeled with Reagent, Blank, Cal. Soln., Control, Sample, etc.

2. Pre-warm at 37°C for 3 minutes.

3. At timed intervals, add 0.1 mL sample into appropriately labeled tube and mix well. Use D-H_2O as specimen into appropriately labeled tube and mix well. Use D-H_2O as specimen for Reagent Blank.

4. Incubate at 37°C for 60 minutes.

5. At timed intercals, add 0.5 colour reagent to each tube and mix well.

6. Allow to stand at room temperature for 20 minutes.

7. Add 5.0 mL Alkaline Diluent to each tube and mix well. Let stand for 5 minutes at room temperature.

8. Zero instruments with Reagent Blank at 505 nm (490-520 nm acceptable).

9. Read and record absorbance for *cal. soln., control, sample 1*, etc.

10. Determine enzyme activity from calibration curve.

Results:

Stability of Final Reaction Product: The test samples should be read within 30 minutes.

Calculation of Results: Determine enzyme activities using the calibration curves generated with GOT calibration solution.

Limitations: Detergent free glassware should be used.

Expected values: 8-40 U/mL

Normal: 5-40 U/mL

Experiment 9: Determination of Serum Glutamic Pyruvate Transaminase (SGPT).

Introduction: The term SGPT stands for Serum Glutamic Pyruvate Transaminase. This is an enzyme that is found in the cells of the liver. It is also commonly known as Alanine Transaminase, abbreviated as ALT. In a normally healthy individual, the level of SGPT is measurable in the blood. When there is acute liver damage, the level of SGPT tends to rise dramatically. It should be noted that the level of SPGT may be elevated in an individual who has recently performed physical exercise. An elevation in the level of ALT is not a confirmation of a diagnosis of liver damage. It is used in conjunction with other types of liver test to confirm whether the patient has indeed suffered from liver damage. The next stage of the liver test for SGPT is to understand the underlying cause of the liver damage. The liver could be damaged by an infectious disease such as mononucleosis or hepatitis. This damage is generally temporary and heals after the patient has recovered from the condition. The level of SGPT is also elevated in an individual who is suffering from bile related problems. Often the bile ducts leading out of the liver get blocked or infected. This could cause the level of ALT in a liver test to be elevated.

There are many different medications that are likely to cause an elevation in the level of SGPT in the blood. This elevation tends to be temporary and gets reversed as the patient's body absorbs the medication or passes it out of the system in the urine. When a drug overdose has occurred, the patient may suffer from liver damage which, apart from causing an elevation in the level of ALT also causes other typical symptoms of liver damage. The liver test for SGPT is diagnostically relevant and can be used with other tests such as the ALT or SGOT test. These tests can confirm whether the elevation in the level of SGPT is related to liver damage or related to bile duct problems. The liver test for SGPT is almost never conducted in isolation. The test forms a part of the standard liver panel test which is a test that is conducted over several different components that are supposed to be present in the liver with particular concentrations.

Principle: Reitman and Frankel' described a calorimetric procedure for assaying GPT activities. End products of the transaminations react with di-nitro phenylhydrazine to form a hydrazone complex. This product yields a coloured complex when alkaline diluent is added. The colour intensity at 505 nm can be related to enzyme activity by reference to a standard curve.

GPT Substrate: 200 mM alanine and 8 mM ketoglutaric acid buffered at pH 7.5. Preservative added. Store at 2-8°C. The substrate should be a clear and colourless solution. Turbidity would indicate deterioration.

Calibration Solution: 1.5 mM pyruvate buffered at pH 7.5. Preservative added. Store at 2-8°C. The calibration solution is a clear and colourless solution. Turbidity would indicate deterioration.

Colour Reagent: 1.0 mM 2, 4-dinitrophenylthydrazine in dilute acid. Avoid contact with eyes, skin and clothing. In case of contact, wash with large amount of water. Store at 2-8°C. The colour reagent is a clear yellow solution. Turbidity or a brown colour would indicate deterioration.

Instruments: Use a spectrophotometer or colourimeter calibrated at 490-520 nm.

Specimen Collection

(i) Use un-hemolyzed serum separated from the blood clot as soon as possible.

(ii) Plasma may be used.

(iii) Grossly hemolyzed or lipemic samples should not be used.

(iv) Serum transaminases appear stable for one week at 2-8°C.

(v) No special additives or preservatives are needed.

Materials: 0.1 mL and 0.5 mL micropipettors, 5.0 mL pipettor, Incubator capable of maintaining 37 ± 0.5°C.

Reaction Conditions:

(a) Wavelength 490-520 nm

(b) Incubation Temperature 37°C

(c) Incubation Time 30 min

(d) Sample Volume 0.1 mL

(e) Substrate Volume 0.5 mL

(f) Colour Reagent Volume 0.5 mL

(g) Alkaline Diluent Volume 5.0 mL

(h) Total Volume 6.1 mL

Preparation of Alkaline Diluent: Dissolve 16 grams of sodium hydroxide in 1.0 L D-H_2O. Allow to cool before use.

Procedure

Preparation of Calibration Curve: All reagents should be at room temperature.

1. Calibration curves must be prepared for GPT. Use the specific substrate and set up the following tubes:

2. Arrange tubes and add materials as given in table below:

Tube	D-H_2O (mL)	Substrate (mL)	Cal.Ref. (mL)	GPT (U/mL)
1	0.2	1.0	0.0	0
2	0.2	0.9	0.1	25
3	0.2	0.8	0.2	50
4	0.2	0.7	0.3	83
5	0.2	0.6	0.4	126
6	0.2	0.5	0.5	-

3. Add 1.0 mL colour Reagent to each tube. Mix well and let stand for 5 minutes at room temperature.

4. Add 10.0 mL alkaline diluent to each tube. Mix well and let stand for 5 minutes at room temperature.

5. Zero instrument with D-H_2O at 505 nm (490-520 nm acceptable).

6. Read and record the absorbance.

7. Plot enzyme activity versus absorbance. A non-linear curve is obtained with decreasing slope as enzyme activity increases.

8. Linearity extends to 126 U/mL for GPT. If enzyme activity exceeds these levels, dilute the specimen X 10 with isotonic saline and repeat the assay. Multiply the result X 10 to correct for dilution.

Performance:

1. Dispense 0.5 mL substrate (GPT) into tubes labeled as Reagent, Blank, Cal. Soln., Control, Sample, etc.

2. Prewarm at 37°C for 3 minutes.

3. At timed intervals, add 0.1 mL sample into appropriately labeled tube and mix well. Use D-H_2O as specimen into appropriately labeled tube and mix well. Use D-H_2O as specimen for reagent blank.

4. Incubate at 37°C for 30 minutes for GPT.

5. At timed intercals, add 0.5 colour Reagent to each tube and mix well.

6. Allow to stand at room temperature for 20 minutes.

7. Add 5.0 mL Alkaline Diluent to each tube and mix well. Let stand for 5 minutes at room temperature.

8. Zero instruments with Reagent Blank at 505 nm (490-520 nm acceptable).

9. Read and record absorbance for *cal. soln., control, sample 1,* etc.

10. Determine enzyme activity from calibration curve.

Results:

Stability of Final Reaction Product: The test samples should be read within 30 minutes.

Quality Control: The reliability of test results should be monitored routinely using suitable quality control materials (normal and abnormal) analyzed in the same manner used for the unknowns. The calibration curve should be validated with each run. This is accomplished by using the calibration solution in the performance of test and obtaining the value from the curve. The calibration solution has a GPT value equal to 132 U/mL.

Expected values: 5-30 U/mL

Normal: 5-35 U/mL (Highest levels seen in liver disease).

Experiment 10: Determination of Serum Bilirubin

Introduction: Like so many other substances measured in clinical chemistry laboratories, bilirubin is a waste product. Bilirubin, the principle pigment in bile, is derived from the breakdown of haemoglobin. After several degradation steps, free bilirubin becomes bound by albumin and is transported through the blood to the liver. This bilirubin is not soluble in water and is referred to as insoluble, indirect or unconjugated. In liver, bilirubin is rendered soluble by conjugation with glucuronide. The water-soluble bilirubin, called direct or conjugated, is transported along with other bile constituents into the bile ducts, then to the intestines. In the intestines, bacterial enzyme action converts bilirubin to several related compounds, collectively referred to as urobilinogen. Early methods for bilirubin estimation were based on measurement of its oxidation product, biliverdin or on assessment of the icteric index. Introduction of diazo reaction for bilirubin by van den Bergh in 1918 led to its widespread adoption for quantitating the pigment in serum. Van den Bergh and Muller found that bilirubin in normal serum reacted with Ehrlich's diazo reagent (diazotized sulfanilic acid) when alcohol was added. Their observation that bile pigment reacted with the diazo reagent without the addition of alcohol led to the recognition that some change in bilirubin had been affected by the liver. Bilirubin that reacts with the diazo reagent without the addition of alcohol is called direct or conjugated while the form that reacts only in the presence of alcohol is called indirect or unconjugated. A low concentration of bilirubin is found in normal plasma, almost all of which is indirect. The sum of the direct and indirect forms or conjugated and unconjugated is termed total bilirubin. Routine analytical procedures exist for the determination of total bilirubin and for the measurement of direct bilirubin. The indirect fraction is obtained by subtracting the direct value from the total value. The determination of direct as well as total bilirubin is used in differentiating certain types of jaundice.

There are two tests for bilirubin direct-reacting (conjugated) and indirect-reacting (unconjugated). Differentiating between the two is important diagnostically, as elevated levels of indirect bilirubin are usually caused by liver cell dysfunction *e.g.*, hepatitis, while elevations of direct bilirubin typically result from obstruction either within the liver (intrahepatic) or a source outside the liver e.g., gallstones or a tumor blocking the bile ducts. Bilirubin measurements are especially valuable in newborns, as extremely elevated levels of unconjugated bilirubin can accumulate in the brain, causing irreparable damage.

Clinical Significance: Any increase in formation or retention of bilirubin by the body may result in jaundice, a condition characterized by an increase in the bilirubin level in the serum and the presence of a yellowish pigmentation in the skin. Jaundice may be classified as prehepatic, hepatic or post-hepatic. In prehepatic jaundice, excess bilirubin production (haemolysis) is responsible. Hepatic jaundice occurs when either the removal of bilirubin from the blood or conjugation of bilirubin by the liver is defective. This can have organic or genetic causes. Post-hepatic jaundice refers to anatomic obstruction of the extrahepatic biliary tree. The most common causes of jaundice are liver disease and blockage of the common bile duct. It is necessary to distinguish between the causes of jaundice early in the disease prior to the onset of complications, as the course of treatment is dependent on the cause of the jaundice. Haemolytic jaundice is caused by overproduction of bilirubin due to excessive haemolysis and the inability of the liver to adequately remove this pigment from the blood. This condition is usually associated with elevated values of serum indirect bilirubin. Cirrhosis of the liver and infectious or toxic hepatitis are caused by some type of intrahepatic obstruction, where production of bilirubin is not increased, but accumulates and is discharged back into the blood. In these conditions, the indirect form of bilirubin predominates in the early phase, but as liver damage progresses the direct form also becomes elevated. Obstructive jaundice, caused by a post-hepatic blockage of the larger bile passages, particularly the common bile duct, results in a reflux of bilirubin into the blood. This condition, when uncomplicated, is associated with elevated serum bilirubin only of the direct type. Measurement of total bilirubin and determination of the direct and indirect fractions is important in routine screening for and the differential diagnosis of jaundice Specimens for bilirubin determination should be protected from light, since bilirubin is lightsensitive and will break down under exposure.

Methods of Determination

1. **Van den Bergh, Malloy and Evelyn Reaction:** In an aqueous solution, Ehrlich's diazo reagent reacts with the direct bilirubin in the serum to form a pink to reddish-purple coloured compound (azobilirubin). It is read at one minute. In a 50% methyl alcohol solution, Ehrlich's diazo reagent reacts with the total bilirubin in the serum to form a pink to reddish-purple coloured compound. (Read at 30 minutes.)

2. **Methods of Jendrassik and Grof:** Serum or plasma is added to a solution of sodium acetate and caffeine-sodium benzoate. The sodium acetate buffers the pH of the diazo reaction, while the caffeine-sodium benzoate accelerates the coupling of bilirubin with diazotized sulfanilic acid. The azobilirubin colour develops within 10 minutes. An accelerating agent facilitates the coupling of albumin-bound bilirubin with the diazo reagent.

3. Some other Methods

(a) Conjugated Bilirubin: Conjugated bilirubin reacts with DSA under acid conditions to form a red chromophore. The absorbance due to the chromophore is directly proportional to the conjugated bilirubin in the sample and is measured using a two-filter (540-600 nm) end point technique.

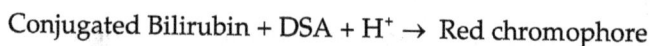

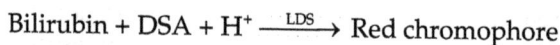

$$\text{Conjugated Bilirubin} + \text{DSA} + \text{H}^+ \rightarrow \text{Red chromophore}$$

(Non-absorbing at 540 nm)   (Absorbs at 540 nm)

(b) Total Bilirubin: Total bilirubin reacts with DSA under acid conditions to form a red chromophore. Lithium dodecyl sulfate (LDS) is employed to solubilize the unconjugated bilirubin. The absorbance due to the chromophore is directly proportional to the bilirubin in the sample and is measured using a two-filter (540-600 nm) end point technique.

$$\text{Bilirubin} + \text{DSA} + \text{H}^+ \xrightarrow{\text{LDS}} \text{Red chromophore}$$

(Non-absorbing at 540 nm)   (Absorbs at 540nm)

(c) Neonatal Bilirubin (up to 21 days): The absorbance of the sample, measured using a two-filter (452-540 nm) differential technique is directly proportional to the bilirubin concentration. Absorbance at 452 nm is due to the bilirubin concentration and, if present, haemoglobin. At 540 nm, bilirubin does not absorb, while hemoglobin exhibits the same absorbance as it does at 452 nm. The use of 540 nm as the blanking wavelength thus eliminates any hemoglobin contribution from the total absorbance at 452 nm. Bilirubin in newborn babies can be read in this direct spectrophotometric procedure in part due to the fact that the normal range is much higher than for adults. In addition, carotene and other dietary pigments prevent adult and specimens from older children from being suitable.

Principle of Reactions

Bilirubin is coupled with diazotized sulfanilic acid to form azobilirubin. The colour of this derivative is pH dependent, occurring as pink in acid or neutral medium and blue under alkaline conditions.

Direct (conjugated) bilirubin couples with diazotized sulfanilic acid (p-diazobenzenesulfonic acid), forming a blue colour at alkaline pH.

Direct Bilirubin (conjugated) + Diazotized Sulfanilic acid $\xrightarrow{\text{alkaline pH}}$ Blue colour Azobilirubin

Indirect (unconjugated) bilirubin is diazotized only in the presence of an accelerating agent, caffeine-benzoate-acetate mixture. Thus, the blue azobilirubin produced in mixtures containing accelerating agent originates from both the Direct and Indirect fractions and reflects the Total bilirubin concentration.

Total Bilirubin + Caffeine - benzoaten Acetate mixture + Diazotized Sulfanilic acid → Azobilirubin

Reagents

(a) Caffeine reagent (caffeine, sodium benzoate, sodium acetate)

(b) *Alkaline tartrate:* Avoid contact with skin and clothing.

(c) HCl (0.05 N)

(d) *Diazo Reagent (sulfanilic acid, sodium nitrite):* Reconstitute one vial Diazo with 6.0 mL HCl. Stable five days at 2-6°C.

(e) *Cysteine Reagent:* Prepare by adding 10.5 mL distilled water. Cap, shake. Stable three months (room temperature) in the dark.

(f) *Bilirubin reference:* Assayed dry preparation containing bilirubin in a protein base for use as a control or for calibration purposes. The actual bilirubin concentration appears on the vial label.

(g) Standard controls and unknowns.

Specimen Collection and Storage: Fresh serum is recommended, but heparinized plasma is also acceptable. Specimens must be protected from both artificial light and sunlight during processing and storage as bilirubin will undergo auto-oxidation to biliverdin. The use of a serum blank eliminates interference from hemolysis and lipemia.

Preparation of Calibration Curve

1. Reconstitute bilirubin reference with 3.0 mL water. Let stand for several minutes and swirl or invert to mix.

2. Number the three test tubes and pipette solutions as indicated in the table below:

Tube	Bilirubin Ref.	Water	Dilution factorm (F)	Bilirubin (mg/dL) – (F) x Listed Value of bilirubin Ref.	Absorbance
1	0.05 mL	0.15	0.25		
2	0.10 mL	0.10	0.50		
3	020 mL	-	1.00		

3. To each tube add in the sequence shown (mix after each addition)

(a) 1.0 mL caffeine reagent.

(b) 0.5 mL diazo reagent.

(c) 0.1 mL cysteine solution.

(d) 1.5 mL alkaline tartrate.

4. Transfer solutions to cuvettes and record absorbance of all tubes using water as a reference at 600 nm. Read within 30 minutes.

5. Calculate the bilirubin concentrations for each tube by multiplying the listed value for the bilirubin reference by the appropriate dilution factor and record.

6. Plot a calibration curve of the absorbance vs. concentration.

Procedure:

1. For screening purposes, the serum blank may be omitted, since the contribution by serum to the final absorbance in this procedure is generally minor.

2. A serum blank should be included primarily when assaying highly turbid sera or control or grossly haemolyzed specimens.

3. Results are not significantly affected by haemoglobin concentrations up to 280 mg/dL.

4. When the serum blank is omitted, the total and direct bilirubin tubes are read versus water as a reference.

5. Set up blank tube only on specimens that are hemolyzed or lipemic.

6. To appropriately labeled test tubes, add the following:

S.No.	Solution	Blank tube	Total tube	Direct tube
1.	Serum	0.2	0.2	0.2
2.	HCl	0.5	-	1.0
3.	Caffeine Reagent	1.0	1.0	-
4.	Diazo Reagent (Mix well)	-	0.5	0.5
5.	Cysteine Solution (Mix well)	0.1	0.1	0.1
6.	Alkaline Tartrate (Mix well)	1.5	1.5	1.5

7. Transfer to cuvettes and read absorbance of all tubes, including blank using Distilled water as a reference at 600 nm.

Results: Use the prepared calibration curve to determine the concentration of unknown samples. Determine total and direct bilirubin levels from the curve. The indirect bilirubin is the difference between the total and the direct. Record all results on worksheet.

Normal values	Total	Direct
Adults	0.2-1.2 mg/dL	0.3 mg/dL
Infants	1.0-12.0 mg/dL	—

Experiment 11: Blood Group Analysis.

Introduction: Since 1901, more than 20 distinct blood group systems have been identified and characterized. Yet, ABO system, the first described, remains the most clinically significant in blood transfusion and organ transplantation medicine. The

ABO antigens are the only cellular antigens which consistently produce a potent, naturally occurring antithetical antibody which circulates in the plasma of healthy individuals. ABO antigens are expressed on most blood cells organs and tissues and in most body fluids. The ABO antigens are primarily glycolipids which are found on the surface of human red blood cells as well as in association with other body tissues. These are two distinct parts to ABO grouping. The Direct or Forward grouping requires known anti-A and anti-B typing antiserums for testing unknown cells. The Indirect, Reverse or Back grouping requires a pool of known A and known group B cells. Both Forward and Reverse grouping is routinely carried out. The forward typing antigen-antibody reaction results in visible agglutination of the red blood cells determining the blood groups A and B and AB. No agglutination with anti-A, anti-B, determines the amorphous, group O. In the reverse typing reagent red blood cells agglutinate when antibodies in patient serum react with their corresponding antigenic determinants on the red blood cell. Anti-A and B antibodies in patient serum agglutinates red blood cells possessing A and/or B blood group antigens, while group O red blood cells will not react with the patient serum. The approximate frequency of each antigen on the erythrocytes of a Caucasian population is A-41%, B-9%, AB-4%, O-46%.

Principle: Compatibility between the blood groups of donor and recipient determines the success of a Blood transfusion. The ABO and Rh blood groups are looked at while conducting the test. In a diagnostic lab, Monoclonal antibodies are available for A, B and Rh antigen. Monoclonal antibody against Antigen A (also called Anti-A), comes in a small bottles with droppers; the monoclonal suspension being blue in colour. Anti-B comes in yellow colour. Anti-D (monoclonal antibody against Rh) is colourless. All the colour codes are universal standards. When the monoclonal antibodies are added one by one to wells that contain the test sample (blood from patient), if the RBCs in that particular sample carry the corresponding Antigen, clumps can be observed in the corresponding wells. A drop of blood is left without adding any of the antibodies; it is used as a control in the experiment. The monoclonal antibody bottles should be stored in a refrigerator. It is recommended to tilt the bottle a couple of times before use in order to re-suspend the antibodies that have settled at the bottom of the bottle. The two types of antigen present in blood cells are given below.

S.No.	Blood Group	Antigen	Antibody	Genotype
1.	A	a	b	I^aI^a/I^a
2.	B	b	a	I^bI^b/I^b
3.	AB	ab	-	I^aI^b
4.	O	-	ab	I^oI^o

Specimen Requirements: 10 mL red top serum tube without serum separator. Transport at room temperature. Do not use serum tubes with serum separator gel. This may interfere with results, causing false agglutination. All serum tubes received for ABO-RH typing with a serum separator will be rejected.

Procedure:

1. Bring reagents and samples to room temperature before use.

2. Wipe your finger with alcohol and prick with needle carefully. Prepare 33-45% suspension of test red blood cells in isotonic saline.

3. Place one drop of the Anti-A, Anti-B and Anti-D reagent at glass slide or ceramic tile at three different places.

4. Add one drop of prepared 33-45% suspension of test blood red blood cells to each drop of reagent on test slide.

5. Mix the red blood cells and reagents thoroughly over an approx. 20 mm circular area, using a separate, clean applicator stick for each reagent cell test.

6. Observe for 3-5 minutes.

7. Compare the results from image given below.

8. Record the results in observation table for each student group.

Observation: Agglutination reaction in the following table:

S.No.	Name	Anti-A	Anti-B	Anti-D	Blood Group
1.					
2.					
3.					
4.					
5.					
6.					
7.					
8.					
9.					
10.					

Experiment 12: Ouchterlony Double Diffusion Test

Aim: To determine the titer of Ag or Ab and to determine between the given Ag and Ab by ouchterlony double diffusion method.

Principle: In double diffusion method, the Ag and Ab diffuse radically through the agarose gel. If they are serologically related, they form precipitation line in the agarose gel. This serological method was designed by ouchterlony. Depending upon the pattern of (specific lines) precipitation lines formed, the identical nature of Ag *i.e.,* sharing similar type of epitopes is determined.

Requirements: Glass Plates, Pipettes, Glass Slides, Hot plate, micropipettes and tips.

Chemicals: Agarose, K_2HPO_4, Sodiumazide, NaCl, KH_2PO_4, acetic acid and ethanol.

Materials: Commercially available antibody and antigen solutions.

Reagents: 1% phosphate buffered saline buffer (1% PBS) is prepared by dissolving 315g of KH_2PO_4, 1.09 g of K_2HPO_4, 8.5 g of NaCl in 600 mL of distilled water and pH is adjusted to 7.2 with 0.1 N HCl. The total volume is made to 1000 mL using distilled water.

1.2% Agarose gel is prepared by dissolving 120 mg of agarose in 10 mL of 1% PBS buffer.

Procedure: The glass plates are washed and air dried. The test agarose solution which is at a temperature of 50-60°C is coated on cleaned glass plate. The agarose coated plates are now punched with agar punch to make 3 different wells on the gel plate. In one well 10 μL of antiserum containing Abs is added and in another 2 wells, 10 micro litre of each two different Ag solutions are added. After loading the wells with Ag and antiserum solutions, the agarose plate is now put under slightly moist conditions, incubated for 24 hrs at 35°C. After the incubation period, the slides are observed for the formation of precipitin lines.

Observation: The incubated agarose plates showed formation of different types of precipitin lines. The precipitin line formed in the first plate was U shaped or arc shaped. The precipitin line formed in the second plate was X-shaped or spur shaped. The precipitin line formed in the third plate was X or cross shaped.

Result: The arc shaped precipitin line formed confirms that the two antigens lobed are identical and they had specificity towards the antibodes loaded. The spur shaped precipitin line formed indicates that one of Ag is specific to Ab provided but the second type of Ag has few antigenic determinants common with that of first Ag type solution. The cross shaped precipitin line formed indicates that the two kinds of antigens loaded are unidentical to each other.

Experiment 13: Determination of Haemoglobin Content by Haemoglobinometer.

Principle: The basic principle for the estimation of haemoglobin is that haemoglobin is converted into acid hematin which is brown in colour. This colour is compared with the standard.

Material: 0.1 N HCl, Distilled water, Spirit or Dettol, Blood sample and Cotton.

Required tools: Pipette (with rubber pipe), Test tube, Haemoglobinometer, Dropper, Brush, Lancet, Glass rod. These things normally come along with the Haemoglobinometer kit.

Procedure:

1. Take 20 mL of 0.1 N HCl in a test tube, a special test tube with Hb level markings on it.

2. With the help of Dettol, disinfect the place where blood taking procedure will be carried out. Clean and disinfect the finger from which the blood sample will be taken. Also disinfect the tools those are going to use for the procedure.

3. With the help of lancet, remove blood through the finger (finger no. 4 from thumb) and take it on a glass slide.

4. Take 0.02 mL blood in a pipette from the glass slide.

5. Put that blood in the test tube in which 20 mL of 0.1N HCl.

6. Shake the test tube well so that blood and 0.1 N HCl will mix with each other properly.

7. Keep the test tube in haemoglobinometer for 5 minutes.

8. Check the colour of the solution in the test tube. It should match with the colours shown on both sides of the haemoglobinometer. To match the colour of solution present in the test tube, add drops of distilled water with help of dropper.

9. Now compare the colour. If it matches with the colour on sides, then take the reading on the test tube. This is Hb level in the blood.

Observation: The reading where the colour of acid hematin matched with that of standard. **Normal Haemoglobin Concentration:**

- ❖ **Men:** 14 to 18 g/dL.
- ❖ **Women:** 12 to 14 mg/dL.

Precautions:

- ❖ Use separate lancet for each person.
- ❖ Don't prick near nail, prick on tip of finger.
- ❖ Clean the pipette immediately after taking blood.
- ❖ Always take reading of haemoglobinometer in sunlight or in the bright light.
- ❖ Make sure that blood doesn't come in mouth while sucking from the pipette.

Segment 3

Biological Techniques and Biotechnology

Experiment 1: Culture of Bacteria on Solid and Liquid Medium.

Introduction

Bacteria will grow on practically any source of organic food which provides carbon compounds to be respired for energy and nitrogen compounds to be incorporated into proteins for growth. These substances are normally provided dissolved in water. However, in nature, bacteria can break down solid and insoluble substances by releasing enzymes into the substrate in which they are growing. These substances are thus broken down or digested to simpler substances and the process is called extracellular digestion because it takes place outside the bacterial cells. The two normal media used in bacteriology are a clear soup like liquid nutrient broth, usually in tubes and nutrient agar, which is set into a jelly by the addition of a seaweed extract called agar and when melted poured into glass or plastic Petri dishes also known as plates. Sometimes, substances are mixed into media, in o rder to suppress growth of other types of bacteria. There are many such selective media. A standard carbon source is glucose and nitrogen is often provided by peptones (partially digested proteins) or inorganic salts. Minerals and vitamins may also be provided, according to the growth requirements of the bacteria. Combinations of chemicals (buffers) may be used to keep the pH stable. Measured amounts of the concentrates are added to water and dissolved to reconstitute the media. These media must then be sterilized by heating in an autoclave like a pressure cooker at 121°C (pressure 1 bar or 15 lb/sq.in) for 15 minutes, which kills all living organisms, including spores. All apparatus used from this point onwards must be sterilized by heat (glassware 160°C for 2hrs) or exposure to radiation. Aseptic techniques must be used to reduce the likelihood of bacterial contamination. This usually involves disinfection of working areas, minimizing possible access by bacteria from the air to exposed media and use of flames to kill bacteria which might enter vessels as they are opened. Bacteria may be introduced to the media (inoculated) by various means. Usually the bacteria e.g., from a drop in a heat sterilized loop are spread on the surface of agar. A similar technique is used with broth cultures.

Composition of Culture media: Bacteria infecting humans (pathogens) are chemo-organoheterotrophs. When culturing bacteria, it is very important to provide similar environmental and nutritional conditions that exist in its natural habitat. Hence, an artificial culture medium must provide all the nutritional components that a bacterium gets in its natural habitat. Most often, a culture medium contains water, a source of carbon and energy, source of nitrogen, trace elements and some growth factors. Besides these, the pH of the medium must be set accordingly. Some of the ingredients of culture media include water, agar, peptone, casein hydrolysate, meat extract, yeast extract and malt extract.

Classification: Bacterial culture media can be classified in at least three ways; Based on consistency, based on nutritional component and based on its functional use.

Classification based on consistency

Culture media are liquid, semi-solid or solid and biphasic.

A. Liquid media: These are available for use in test-tubes, bottles or flasks. Liquid media are sometimes referred as broths *e.g.*, nutrient broth. In liquid medium, bacteria grow uniformLy producing general turbidity. Certain aerobic bacteria and those containing fimbriae (Vibrio and Bacillus) are known to grow as a thin film called 'surface pellicle' on the surface of undisturbed broth. Bacillus anthracis is known to produce stalactite growth on ghee containing broth. Sometimes the initial turbidity may be followed by clearing due to autolysis, which is seen in penumococci. Long chains of Streptococci when grown in liquid media tend to entangle and settle to the bottom forming granular deposits. Liquid media tend to be used when a large number of bacteria have to be grown. These are suitable to grow bacteria when the numbers in the inoculum is suspected to be low. Inoculating in the liquid medium also helps to dilute any inhibitors of bacterial growth. This is the practical approach in blood cultures. Culturing in liquid medium can be used to obtain viable count (dilution methods). Properties of bacteria are not visible in liquid media and presence of more than one type of bacteria cannot be detected.

B. Solid media: Any liquid medium can be rendered by the addition of certain solidifying agents. Agar agar (simply called agar) is the most commonly used solidifying agent. It is an unbranched polysaccharide obtained from the cell membranes of some species of red algae such as the genera Gelidium. Agar is composed of two long-chain polysaccharides (70% agarose and 30% agarapectin). It melts at 95°C (sol) and solidifies at 42°C (gel), doesn't contribute any nutritive property, it is not hydrolyzed by most bacteria and is usually free from growth promoting or growth retarding substances. However, it may be a source of calcium and organic ions. Most commonly, it is used at concentration of 1-3% to make a solid agar medium. New

Zealand agar has more gelling capacity than the Japanese agar. Agar is available as fibres (shreds) or as powders.

C. Semi-solid agar: Reducing the amount of agar to 0.2-0.5% renders a medium semi-solid. Such media are fairly soft and are useful in demonstrating bacterial motility and separating motile from non-motile strains (U-tube and Cragie's tube). Certain transport media such as Stuart's and Amies media are semi-solid in consistency. Hugh and Leifson's oxidation fermentation test medium as well as mannitol motility medium is also semi-solid.

D. Biphasic media: Sometimes, a culture system comprises of both liquid and solid medium in the same bottle. This is known as biphasic medium (Castaneda system for blood culture). The inoculum is added to the liquid medium and when subcultures are to be made, the bottle is simply tilted to allow the liquid to flow over the solid medium. This obviates the need for frequent opening of the culture bottle to subculture. Besides agar, egg yolk and serum too can be used to solidify culture media. While serum and egg yolk are normally liquid, they can be rendered solid by coagulation using heat. Serum containing medium such as Loeffler's serum slope and egg containing media such as Lowenstein Jensen medium and Dorset egg medium are solidified as well as disinfected by a process of inspissations.

Classification Based on Nutritional Component

Media can be classified as simple, complex and synthetic (or defined). While most of the nutritional components are constant across various media, some bacteria need extra nutrients. Those bacteria that are able to grow with minimal requirements are said to non-fastidious and those that require extra nutrients are said to be fastidious. Simple media such as peptone water, nutrient agar can support most non-fastidious bacteria. Complex media such as blood agar have ingredients whose exact components are difficult to estimate. Synthetic or defined media such as Davis and Mingioli medium are specially prepared media for research purposes where the composition of every component is well known.

Classification Based on Functional use or Application

These include basal media, enriched media, selective/enrichment media, indicator/differential media, transport media and holding media.

A. Basal media are basically simple media that supports most non-fastidious bacteria. Peptone water, nutrient broth and nutrient agar considered basal medium.

B. Enriched media: Addition of extra nutrients in the form of blood, serum, egg yolk etc, to basal medium makes them enriched media. Enriched media are used to grow nutritionally exacting (fastidious) bacteria. Blood agar, chocolate agar, Loeffler's serum slope etc are few of the enriched media.

C. Selective and enrichment media are designed to inhibit unwanted commensal or contaminating bacteria and help to recover pathogen from a mixture of bacteria. While selective media are agar based, enrichment media are liquid in consistency. Both these media serve the same purpose. Any agar media can be made selective by addition of certain inhibitory agents that don't affect the pathogen. Various approaches

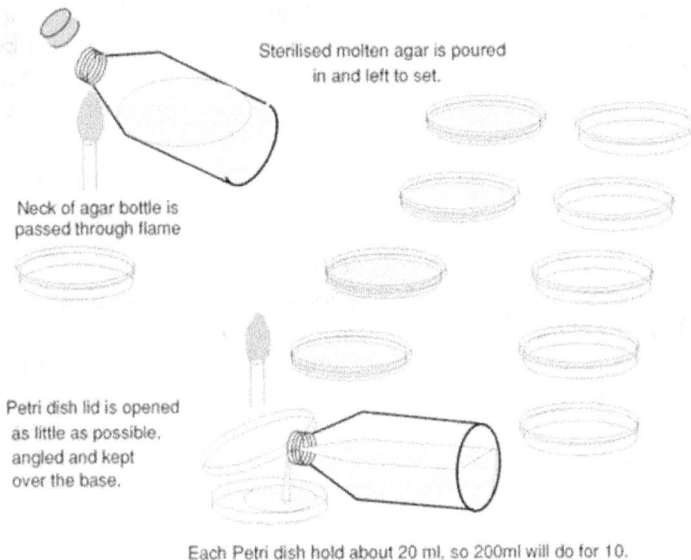

Sterilised molten agar is poured
in and left to set.

Neck of agar bottle is
passed through flame

Petri dish lid is opened
as little as possible,
angled and kept
over the base.

Each Petri dish hold about 20 ml, so 200ml will do for 10.

Pouring a Plate

to make a medium selective include addition of antibiotics, dyes, chemicals, alteration of pH or a combination of these.

D. Enrichment media: They are liquid media that also serves to inhibit commensals in the clinical specimen. Selenite F broth, tetrathionate broth and alkaline peptone water are used to recover pathogens from fecal specimens.

E. Differential media or indicator media: Certain media are designed in such a way that different bacteria can be recognized on the basis of their colony colour. Various approaches include incorporation of dyes, metabolic substrates etc, so that those bacteria that utilize them appear as differently coloured colonies. Such media are called differential media or indicator media. Exmples: MacConkey's agar, CLED agar, TCBS agar, XLD agar etc.

F. Transport media: Clinical specimens must be transported to the laboratory immediately after collection to prevent overgrowth of contaminating organisms or commensals. This can be achieved by using transport media. Such media prevent drying (desiccation) of specimen, maintain the pathogen to commensal ratio and inhibit overgrowth of unwanted bacteria. Some of these media (Stuart's and Amie's) are semi-solid in consistency. Addition of charcoal serves to neutralize inhibitory factors. Cary Blair medium and Venkatraman Ramakrishnan medium are used to transport feces from suspected cholera patients. Sach's buffered glycerol saline is used to transport feces from patients suspected to be suffering from bacillary dysentery.

G. Anaerobic media: Anaerobic bacteria need special media for growth because they need low oxygen content, reduced oxidation –reduction potential and extra nutrients. Media for anaerobes may have to be supplemented with nutrients like hemin and vitamin K. Boiling the medium serves to expel any dissolved oxygen. Addition of 1% glucose, 0.1% thioglycollate, 0.1% ascorbic acid, 0.05% cysteine or red hot iron filings can render a medium reduced. Robertson cooked meat that is commonly used to grow Clostridium spps medium contain a 2.5 cm column of bullock heart meat and 15 mL of nutrient broth. Before use the medium must be boiled in water bath to expel any dissolved oxygen and then sealed with sterile liquid paraffin. Methylene blue or resazurin is an oxidation-reduction potential indicator that is incorporated in the thioglycollate medium. Under reduced condition, methylene blue is colourless.

Preparation and Preservation

Care must be taken to adjust the pH of the medium before autoclaving. Various pH indicators that are in use include phenol red, neutral red, bromothymol blue, bromocresol purple etc. Dehydrated media are commercially available and must be reconstituted as per manufacturers' recommendation. Most culture media are sterilized by autoclaving. Certain media that contain heat labile components like glucose, antibiotics, urea, serum, blood are not autoclaved. These components are filtered and may be added separately after the medium is autoclaved. Certain highly selective media such as Wilson and Blair's medium and TCBS agar need not be sterilized. It is imperative that a representation from each lot be tested for performance and contamination before use. Once prepared, media may be held at 4-5°C in the refrigerator for 1-2 weeks. Certain liquid media in screw capped bottles or tubes or cotton plugged can be held at room temperature for weeks.

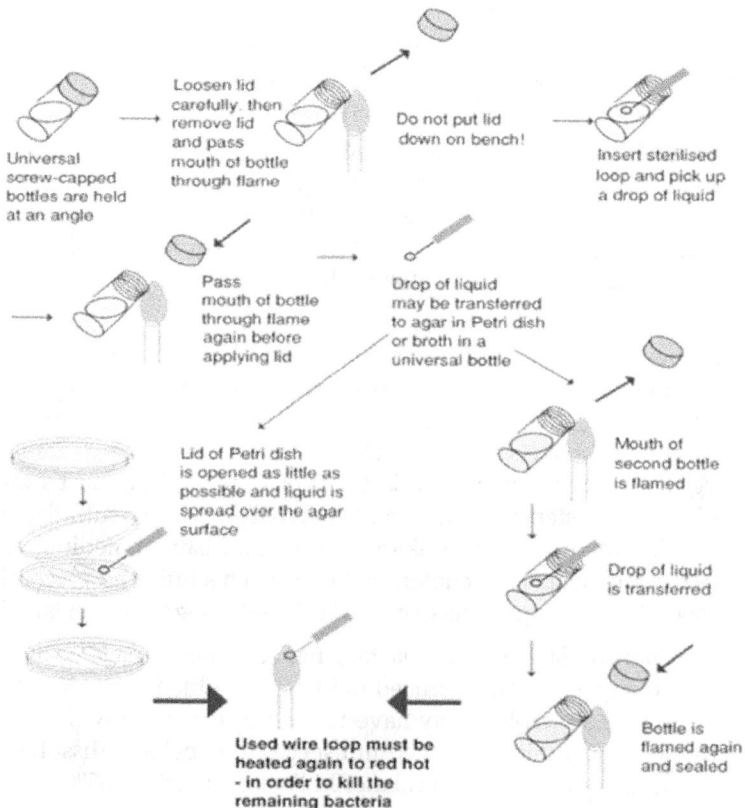

Experiment 2: Isolation of Bacteria.

Sampling and Inoculation

We frequently use sterile cotton-tipped swabs to collect bacteria from the environment. The swab is then used to transfer bacteria to an agar plate and a loop used to spread the bacteria over the remainder of the plate.

Swab: To remove the swab from the tube, grasp the tube in the left hand and the cap with the small and ring fingers of the right. Pull the cap off. By using these fingers, the thumb and remaining fingers are free to grab the swab and remove it from the tube. Return the cap to the tube. If the source to be sampled is dry, you will want to moisten the swab before collecting the sample. A moist swab will much more effectively pick up bacteria than a dry swab. Open a tube with sterile water and dip the swab into the water. Raise the swab above the level of the water and push it against the walls of the tube. Rotate the swab to force out excess water. You want the swab to be damp, but not dripping wet. To collect bacteria, rub the swab over the surface being sampled while rotate the swab handle between thumb and forefinger. You want to expose all surfaces of the swab to the surface, not just one spot. If you don't transfer the bacteria to an agar plate immediately, return the swab to its original tube for holding and transport.

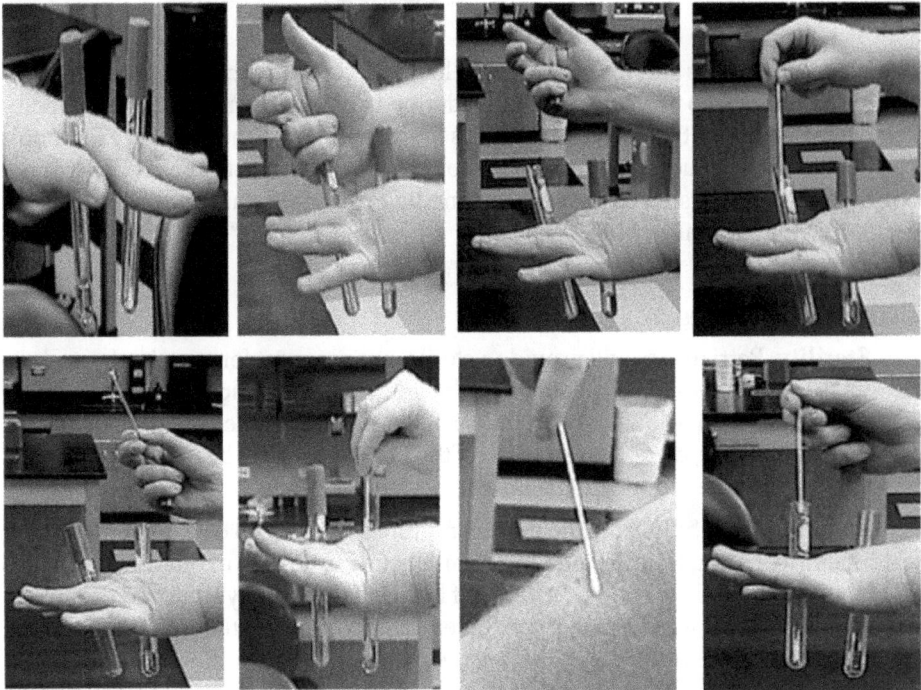

Loop: Loops are extremely useful tools for moving bacteria. Before acquiring bacteria, the loop is sterilized by holding it into a flame until the wire glows red from loop to holder. Once the loop has had few moments to cool, bacteria in suspension are picked up by dipping the instrument into the broth and picking up a single loop full of broth. Bacteria in colonies are picked up by touching the end of the loop to the colony. Do not need to pick up the whole colony. Each colony contains billions of bacteria so simply touching the colony will almost always give you plenty of bacteria to work with.

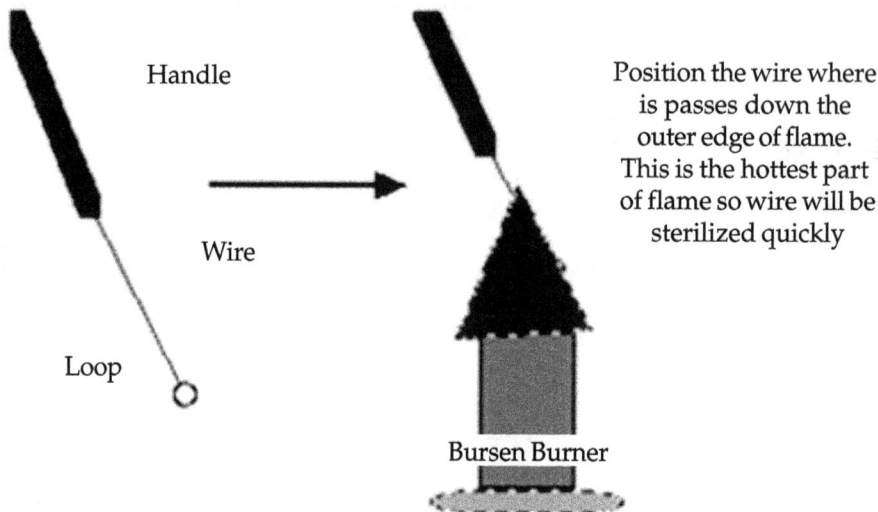

Handle

Wire

Loop

Position the wire where is passes down the outer edge of flame. This is the hottest part of flame so wire will be sterilized quickly

Bursen Burner

Needle: Needles are straight wires (no loop) used to pick up bacteria from closely packed colonies or to inoculate in a much defined area. We commonly used needles to inoculate semi-soft media. The needle is first sterilized as shown above for loops. The needle is then touched to the desired colony. Do not try to stir the needle around. The bacteria are transferred to the target media by a single stab, straight down and back up with minimal wobble.

Using Petri dishes

Sterility: Petri dishes will provide a sterile environment for growing bacteria as long as they are handled correctly. Keep the lid in place as much as possible. When streaking (described below) only lift the lid off enough to get the swab or loop under. As much as possible, do not take the lid off the plate to observe bacteria. Never carry the plate around the room with the lid off.

Labeling: Carefully label the plates and tubes. There will be a lot of plates and test tubes incubating together making clear labeling crucial to avoid chaos. Always label the bottom of the plate so that, even if lids get accidentally switched or broken, we will know what was in each plate. Likewise, do not label tubes on the cap. The label should include your name, the date the plate was struck and what was put into the plate.

Disposal: We may be using petridishes made of plastic or glass. Plastic dishes are disposable so when you have finished with them they are placed in the red disposal bin and are destroyed by autoclaving. Glass petridishes are reused. When you finish with a glass Petri dish, all writing and tape must be removed and the dish placed in the location. Failure to remove ID information from glass plates or other glassware will result in point deductions from your lab score.

Streaking for Isolation

There are several techniques for obtaining isolated bacterial colonies but this is the one your humble author has found most effective. Mentally or with a grease pencil or marker if helpful divide the plate into 3 equal sized sections as shown below.

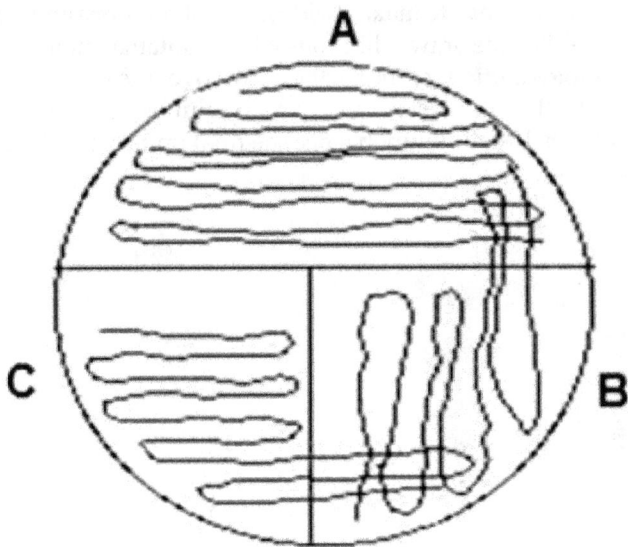

Start streaking with a loop or swab at the top of area A. Make as many streak lines as you can without overlapping. If you're using a swab, rotate it between thumb and forefinger as you streak to expose the entire swab surface to the plate. Inoculate bacteria into region B by moving a sterile loop once or twice through region A and then making more streak lines that neither overlap nor enter region A again. Sterilize the loop and inoculate region C using the same technique. If done carefully, this technique is guaranteed to produce isolated colonies in some area of the plate. If you have a mixture of bacteria on a plate, it becomes fairly simple to obtain a pure culture. Find a well isolated colony and touch the colony with a sterile loop. If the culture is not yet pure, repeat the isolation technique with another plate.

Quantifying Bacteria by Spread Plate

The number of bacteria in solution can be readily quantified by using the spread plate technique. In this technique, the sample is appropriately diluted and a small aliquot transferred to an agar plate. The bacteria are then distributed evenly over the surface by a special streaking technique. After colonies are grown, they are counted and the number of bacteria in the original sample calculated. The end point of our analysis is the number of colony forming units per mL (CFU/mL) since we are counting the number of colonies rather than the actual number of bacteria. We are assuming that the each viable bacterium in the suspension will form an individual colony, which is a valid assumption if we do all the techniques properly. CFU/mL is actually a more useful determination than counting all the bacteria under a microscope because in many bacterial populations some significant number will be dead cells and thus of no interest.

Diluting Bacteria: Bacteria commonly grow up to densities around 10^9 CFU/mL, although the maximum densities vary tremendously depending on the species of bacteria and the media they are growing in. Therefore, to get readily countable numbers of bacteria, we have to make a wide range of dilutions and assay all of them with the goal of having one or two dilutions with countable numbers. We do this by making serial 10-fold dilutions of the bacteria that cover the whole probably range of concentrations. We then transfer 0.1 mL of each dilution to an agar plate, which in effect makes another 10-fold dilution since the final units are CFU/mL and we are only streaking 0.1 mL.

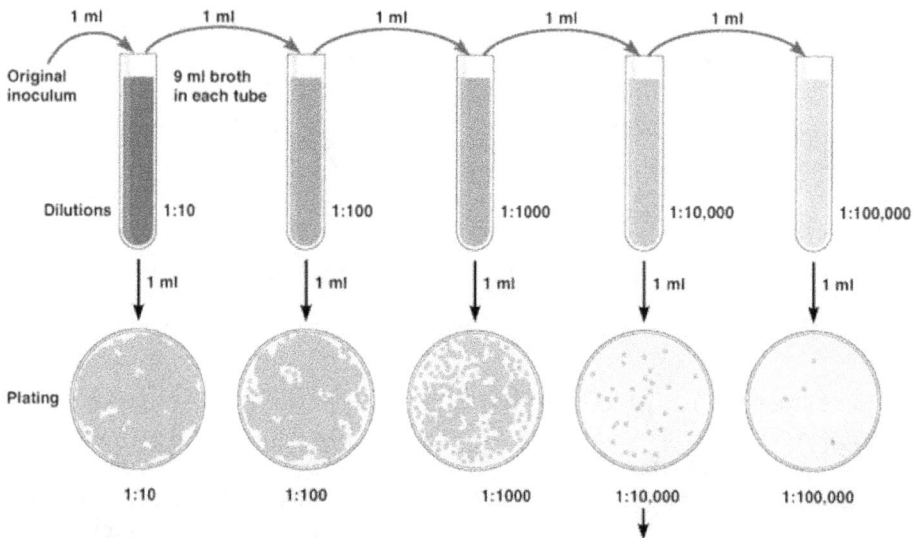

Calculation: Number of colonies on plate × reciprocal of dilution of sample = number of bacteria/ml

For example, if 32 colonies are on a plate of 1/10,000 dilution, then the count is 32 x 10,000 = 320,000/mL in sample.

Inoculating the Plate: Streaking in this technique is done using a bent glass rod. 0.1 mL of bacterial suspension is placed in the center of the plate using a sterile pipet. The glass rod is sterilized by first dipping it into a 70% alcohol solution and then passing it quickly through the Bunsen burner flame. The burning alcohol sterilizes the rod at a cooler temperature than holding the rod in the burner flame thus reducing the chance of you burning your fingers. When all the alcohol has burned off and the rod has air-cooled, streak the rod back and forth across the plate working up and down several times. Unlike streaking for isolation, you want to backtrack many times in order to distribute the bacteria as evenly as possible. Turn the plate 90 degrees and repeat the side to side, up and down streaking. Turn the plate 45 degrees and streak a third time. Do not sterilize the glass rod between plate turnings. Cover the plate and wait several minutes before turning it upside down for incubation. This will allow the broth to soak into the plate so the bacteria won't drip onto the plate lid.

Using Petri dishes 9-10 cm in diameter

↓

Add 15mL – 20 mL of medium at about 45°to each Petri dish and allow solidifying

↓

Spread a measured volume of not less than 0.1 mL of sample prepared as described earlier, over the surface of medium

↓

Invert the petridish and incubate at 30-35 °C for 48-72hrs.

↓

Examine the plate for growth. Count the number of colonies and express the average in terms of colony forming unit per mL (cfu/mL).

Flow Diagram of Spread Plate Method

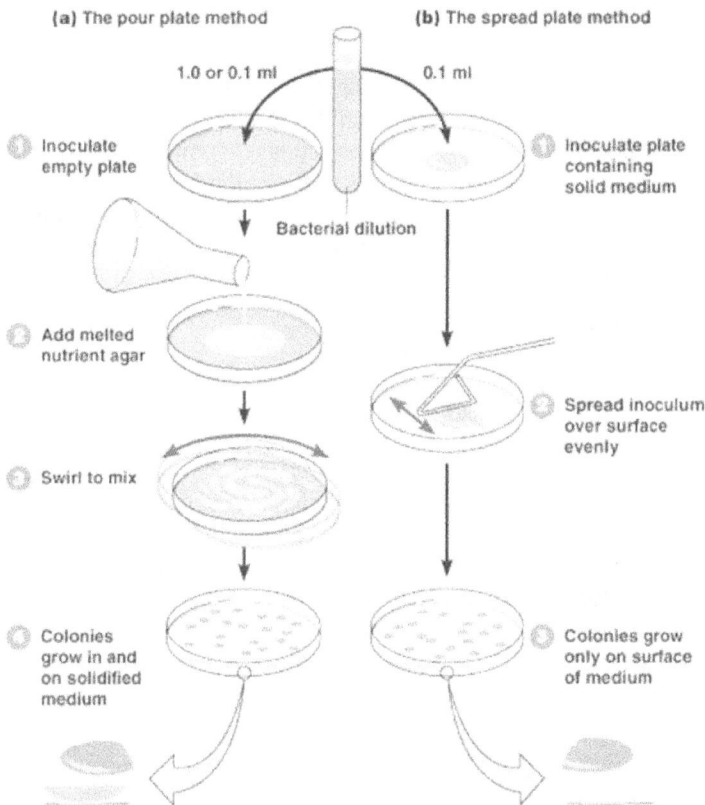

Pour Plate and Sperad plate methods

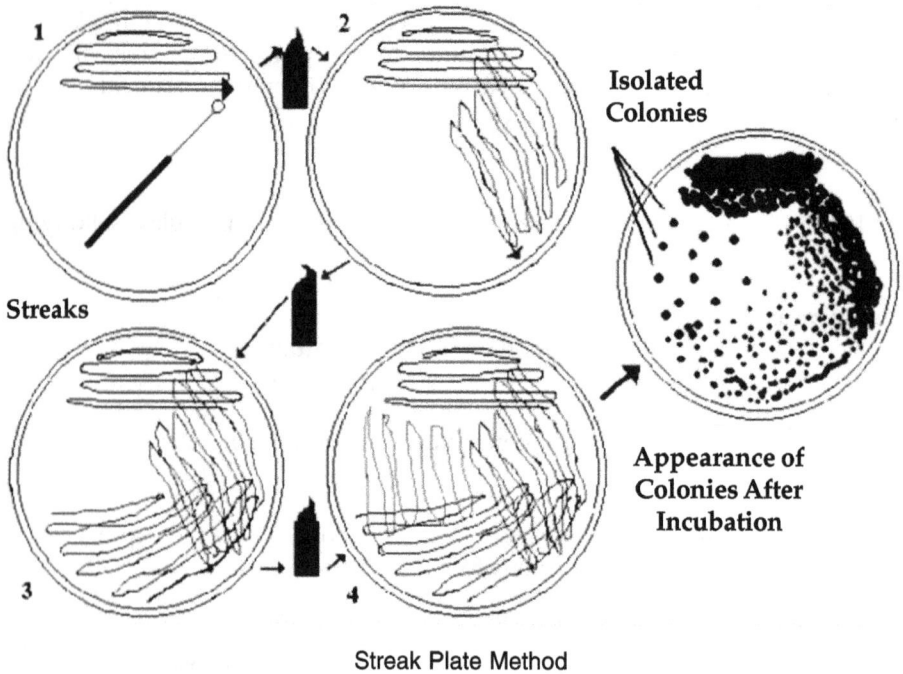

Streak Plate Method

Counting Bacteria: Colonies are most readily counted using a plate counter. The plate counter has a light source and a magnifying glass making colonies easier to see. If at all possible, you don't want to count plates with more than 300 or less than 30 colonies. In the former case, the colonies will be running together and in the latter there are too few to allow statistically accurate counts. Once you count the colonies, multiply by the appropriate dilution factor to determine the number of CFU/mL in the original sample.

Plate Assays for Exoenzymes

Bacteria degrade macromolecules by secreting exoenzymes, enzymes that have their action outside the cytoplasm. We can investigate a bacteria's ability to degrade specific macromolecules by mixing the macromolecule into the agar and checking for degradation following exposure to the bacteria. To ensure that we observe positive results, we inoculate these plates very heavily over a small area. Since we are not spreading bacteria over the whole plate, we can easily put two or three bacteria on a single plate. This allows us to put positive and negative controls on the plate with our unknown bacterium.

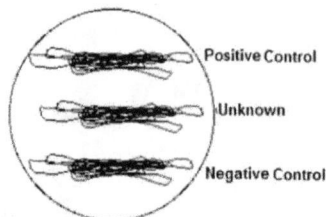

Using a sterile loop, streak the positive control, unknown and negative control onto a single plate. Put a lot of organisms in one place by moving the loop back and forth over the same area several times. Sterilize the loop between each organism. After 24 to 48 hours, exoenzymes will have had time to degrade the macromolecule in the area of the streak.

Starch plate: If we are looking for amylase activity breaking down starch in the media, we observe results by covering the plate with grams iodine. Iodine forms an insoluble purple complex with starch. If the starch has broken down, the area around the bacterial streak will remain clear after starch addition.

Inoculating Broth and Semi-solid Media

Many types of experiments are done in broth cultures. We must have pure cultures for doing work in broth in order to know which bacteria are responsible for the effects we observe. To inoculate a broth culture, hold a labeled broth tube in left hand and loop in right hand using the thumb and first two fingers. Flame sterilizes the loop. Remove the cap from the broth tube with the little finger of the right hand curling against your palm. Flame the opening of the broth tube. Touch the loop to the desired colony on the plate and then stir the loop around in the broth. Reflame the opening of the tube, return the cap and place the tube in a test tube rack. Flame sterilizes the loop.

Phenol red Broth: We can quickly differentiate between aerobic and facultative anaerobes based on whether they ferment sugars. The phenol red broth test is very useful for making this determination. Phenol red is a pH indicator which turns from red to yellow as the pH goes from alkaline to acidic. Any sugar (most often glucose since it is the most readily fermented sugar) can be added to provide a target for respiration. Fermentation of sugars other than glucose (lactose, sucrose, maltose, etc.) can be used to help differentiate between various fermentative bacteria. The phenol red broth also is a rich source of amino acids, needed for the growth of bacteria which do not ferment the sugars. Amino acid metabolism does not interfere with our results, however, because they are usually broken down in Kreb's cycle rather than glycolysis and so do not yield acidic waste products. In fact, amino acid utilization will usually make the media even brighter red due to the release of excess amine groups raising the pH of the media.

To inoculate phenol red broth, use the steps described in inoculating broth cultures. Colour changes should be apparent within 24 hours. If the media changes to a bright yellow colour, the test is positive for fermentation. If the colour is unchanged or red, the test is negative for fermentation and the bacteria are probably growing on amino acids, especially if the media becomes deep red. A pale orange colour indicates that there may be some slight fermentation going on, but not enough to call the test positive. Any bacteria that grow on TSA should also grow in a phenol red broth and therefore you probably did not get a good inoculation.

Inoculating on semi-solid media: We occasionally work with semi-solid media, which is much like any other agar media except that a smaller percentage of agar is present making the agar much softer. The agar is sufficiently soft that motile bacteria can swim through the media. We can use these properties to check for motility if we are careful in our inoculation technique. We use a needle (straight wire) rather than a loop, using one stab straight down through the media. Non-motile bacteria will only grow along the stab line but motile bacteria will swim through the soft agar making the whole tube turbid.

Experiment 3: Methods of Sterilization.

Sterilization is the destruction of all microbial forms including viruses and spores. It is a process that is intended to kill or remove all types of microorganisms, with an acceptably low probability of an organism surviving on any article. Various methods are currently being used for sterilization of orthodontic and endodontic instruments.

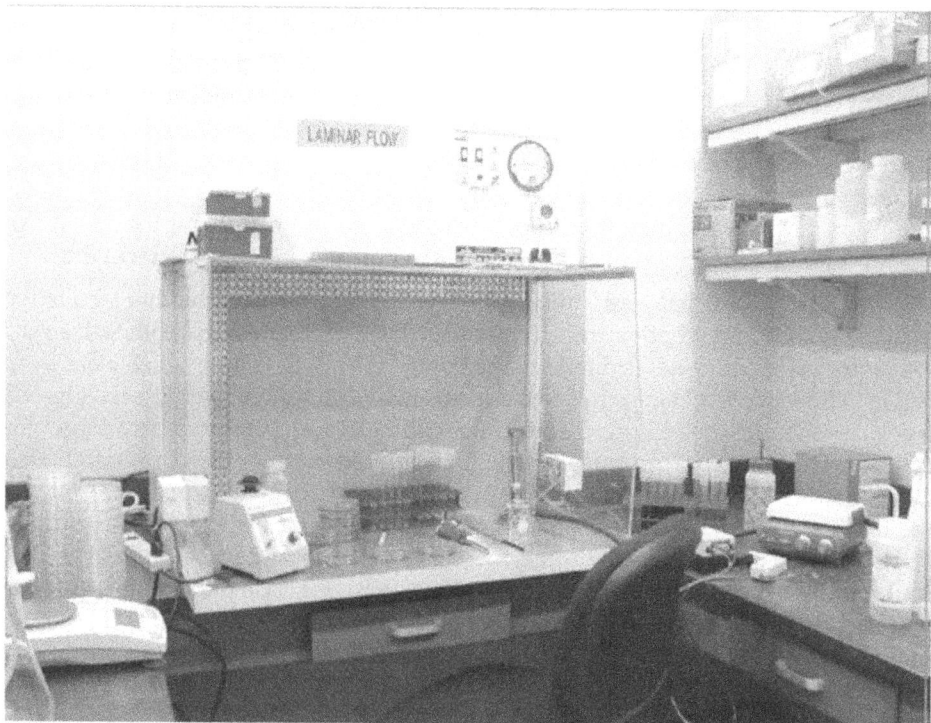

Microbiology Lab

Achieving sterilization is not only contingent on achieving these three essentials but it is also important that instruments and media are properly inspected, assembled, packaged and loaded into sterilizer in accordance with established procedures and techniques. This includes media, instruments, sterilants, sterilization systems and sterilizers. All methods of sterilization are intended to kill microorganisms. Therefore, one must be mindful that sterilants and sterilizing equipment can be hazardous. Sterilization can be achieved by high pressure steam (autoclave), dry heat (oven), chemical sterilants (glutaraldehydes or formaldehyde solutions) or physical agents (radiation). Because sterilization is a process, not a single event, all components must be carried out correctly for sterilization to occur. To be effective, sterilization requires time, contact, temperature and high pressure. The effectiveness of any method of sterilization is also dependent upon four other factors:

(a) **The type of microorganism present:** Some microorganisms are very difficult to kill. Others die easily.

(b) **The number of microorganisms present:** It is much easier to kill one organism than many.

(c) **The amount and type of organic material that protects the microorganisms:** Any chemical remaining on poorly cleaned instruments acts as a shield to microorganisms during the sterilization.

(d) **The number of cracks and crevices on an instrument that might harbor microorganisms:** Microorganisms collect in and are protected by scratches, cracks and crevices.

Sterilization Methods

Sterilization involves the use of a physical or chemical procedure to destroy all microbial life, including highly resistant bacteria spores. The major sterilizing agents commonly used in healthcare facilities are:

(a) Saturated steam and dry heat

(b) Ethylene oxide gas

(c) Hydrogen peroxide gas plasma

(d) Chemical Methods

(e) Other viz. UV, Ozone etc.

Saturated Steam and Dry Heat

High pressure, saturated steam uses an autoclave or dry heat using an oven, are the most common and readily available methods used for sterilization. High pressure steam sterilization is an effective method of sterilization but is the most difficult to do correctly. It is generally the method of choice for sterilizing instruments and other items used in healthcare facilities. Where electricity is a problem, instruments can be sterilized in a nonelectric steam sterilizer using kerosene or other fuel as a heat source. Dry heat sterilizers are good in humid climates but need a continuous supply of electricity, making them impractical in many remote areas. Furthermore, dry heat sterilization, which requires use of higher temperatures, can be used only with glass or metal objects, it will melt other substances. Saturated steam under pressure is the oldest and most widely used economical, effective and reliable method of sterilization available. The steam sterilizer consists of a pressurized chamber, increasing the pressure in chamber elevates and holds the temperature. The sterilizer chamber and all contents must be free of any air entrapment to ensure direct contact of the steam to all surfaces to be sterilized. Steam sterilizers are designed to eliminate all air from the chamber during the conditioning phase in the sterilization cycle. Steam is vaporized water and serves as the conduit to rapidly permeate packaging delivering high temperature moist heat to all contents and destroying microorganisms. Steam kills microorganisms by coagulating and denaturing the cell protein. Due to the very high temperatures and moisture associated with steam sterilization it may only be used with heat and moisture stable instruments and compatible materials.

The different types of steam sterilization processes include:

(a) Dynamic air removal process, also known as pre-vacuum, high vacuum or mechanical air removal. Dynamic air removal steam sterilizers utilize a mechanical vacuum pump to suck air from the sterilizer chamber during the condition phase of the sterilization cycle. Since the removal of air is mechanical the total cycle time is less than that of a gravity cycle.

(b) Gravity, downward air displacement process, relies on gravity to remove air from the sterilizer chamber. Since steam is lighter than air, as it enters the sterilizer chamber it rises to the top. As the chamber fills with steam, the steam forces the air down and out of the chamber drain.

(c) An abbreviated steam sterilization cycle, known as flash, can be accomplished in either a pre-vacuum or gravity displacement sterilizer. Flash sterilization is intended for emergency use when instrumentation is urgently needed and time does not allow for routine processing. Flash sterilized items are intended for immediate use.

Standard Conditions for Heat Sterilization

1. Steam sterilization (Gravity): Temperature should be 121°C (250°F); pressure should be 106 kPa (15 lbs/in^2); 20 minutes for unwrapped items; 30 minutes for wrapped items or at a higher temperature of 132°C (270°F), pressure should be 30 lbs/in^2; 15 minutes for wrapped items. Allow all items to dry before removing them from the sterilizer. Pressure settings (kPa or lbs/in^2) may vary slightly depending on the autoclave or sterilizer used.

2. Dry heat: 170°C (340°F) for 1 hour (total cycle time placing instruments in oven, heating to 170°C, timing for 1 hour and cooling is 2-2.5 hours) or 160°C (320°F) for 2 hours (total cycle time is 3-3.5 hours).

Sterile instruments and media should be used immediately unless they were wrapped in a double layer of muslin, paper or other appropriate material prior to sterilization or can be stored in a dry, sterile container with a tight fitting lid. The material used for wrapping instruments and other items must be porous enough to let steam through but tightly woven enough to protect against dust particles and microorganisms. Wrapped sterile packs should remain sterile until some event causes the package or container to become contaminated.

Sterilization by Steam: Steam is an effective sterilant for two reasons. First, saturated steam is an extremely effective carrier of thermal energy. It is many times more effective in conveying this type of energy to the item than is hot (dry) air. In a kitchen, potatoes can be cooked in a few minutes in a steam pressure cooker while cooking may take an hour or more in a hot air oven, even though the oven is operated at a much higher temperature. Steam, especially under pressure, carries thermal energy to the potatoes very quickly, while hot air does so very slowly. Second, steam is an effective sterilant because any resistant, protective outer layer of the microorganisms can be sends by the steam, allowing coagulation similar to cooking an egg white of the sensitive inner portions of the microorganism. However, certain types of contaminants especially greasy or oily materials can protect microorganisms against the effects of steam, thus hindering the process of sterilization. This reemphasizes the need for thorough cleaning of objects before sterilization. Steam sterilization requires four conditions: adequate contact, sufficiently high temperature, correct time and sufficient moisture. Although all are necessary for sterilization to take place, sterilization failures in clinics and hospitals are most caused by lack of steam contact or failure to attain adequate temperature. The essential conditions for steam sterilization are temperature, saturated steam, time and pressure. Recommended minimum sterilization times for wrapped instruments:

(a) **Prevacuum:** 270°F 4 min exposure; 30 min drying time

(b) **Gravity displacement:** 250°F 30 min exposure; 45 min drying time

(c) **Prevacuum:** 270°F 3 min exposure; no drying time

(d) **High-speed gravity:** 270°F 3 min exposure; no drying time

(e) **Prevacuum:** 270°F 4 min exposure; no drying time

(f) **High-speed gravity:** 270°F 10 min exposure; no drying time

Sterilization by Dry Heat: The dry heat is a practical way to sterilize needles and other instruments. A convection oven with an insulated stainless steel chamber and perforated shelving to allow the circulation of hot air is recommended, but Dry heat sterilization can be achieved with a simple oven as long as a thermometer is used to verify the temperature inside the oven. Dry heat sterilization is accomplished by thermal (heat) conduction. Initially, heat is absorbed by the exterior surface of an item and then passed to the next layer. Eventually, the entire object reaches the temperature needed for sterilization. Death of microorganisms occurs with dry heat by a process of slow destruction of protein. Dry heat sterilization takes longer than steam sterilization, because the moisture in the steam sterilization process significantly speeds up the penetration of heat and shortens the time needed to kill microorganisms. Dry heat sterilization should be used to sterilize anhydrous items that can withstand high temperatures. Dry heat sterilization may be used to sterilize instruments mainly not media. Dry heat sterilization is accomplished by conduction where heat is transferred from molecule to molecule or from the exterior surface of an item to its internal parts. The destruction of organisms occurs by oxidation, which is a slow burning up process of coagulating the cells protein. It is a long sterilization process due to the length of time it takes for objects to reach required temperatures; unlike steam sterilization there is no moisture present, which speeds up heat penetration. There are great variations in times and temperatures based on volume, density, packaging and sterilization apparatus. It is essential to follow the manufacturer's instructions for the items being sterilized and the sterilizer being utilized. Settings range from 30-minute exposure at 356° F to 6 hour exposure at 250°F.

Chemical Sterilization: An alternative to high pressure steam or dry heat sterilization is chemical sterilization. If objects need to be sterilized, but using high pressure steam or dry heat sterilization would damage them or equipment is not available, they can be chemically sterilized. Some high-level disinfectants will kill endospores after prolonged (10-24 hour) exposure. Common disinfectants that can be used for chemical sterilization include glutaraldehydes and formaldehyde. Sterilization takes place by soaking for at least 10 hours in 2-4% glutaraldehyde solution or at least 24 hours in 8% formaldehyde. Glutaraldehydes are only practical sterilants for some instruments which cannot be heated. Both glutaraldehydes and formaldehyde require special handling and leave a residue on treated instruments. Therefore, rinsing with sterile water is essential if the item must be kept sterile. Formaldehyde is less expensive than glutaraldehydes, it is also more irritating to the skin, eyes and respiratory tract and classified as a potential carcinogen. When using glutaraldehydes or formaldehyde, wear gloves to avoid skin contact, wear eyewear to protect from splashes, limit exposure time and use both chemicals only in well ventilated areas.

Liquid Chemical Sterilization: Liquid chemical sterilization is utilized for sterilization of heat sensitive instruments or media that can be immersed. This method employs the use of a germicidal solution and requires the complete immersion of items in the solution for a prescribed period of time to kill microorganisms. Peracetic acid is a liquid chemical sterilant used in conjunction with a self- contained automated processor designed for this method of sterilization. Glutaraldehyde is also a liquid chemical sterilant when used according to the manufacturer's directions for sterilization; however, it is usually used as a high level disinfectant. There are several disadvantages of using glutaraldehyde as a sterilant. A well ventilated work environment is required and personal protective equipment such as gloves, goggles, masks, aprons and gowns are necessary to protect the staff performing the process.

Conditions

(a) Items must be totally immersed in the chemical, allowing direct contact to all surfaces for a prescribed period of time to achieve sterilization.

(b) Peracetic acid comes in a single use, sealed container at a precise concentration.

(c) Peracetic acid requires 12 minutes of exposure and the temperature range is between 122°F to 131°F.

(d) Glutaraldehyde is activated once a container is opened, by adding pre-measured activating chemical, which comes with each bottle.

(e) Glutaraldehyde requires 10 hours of exposure.

Ultraviolet Light: Ultraviolet (UV) light has been used to help disinfect the air for very long time. For example, UV irradiation can interrupt transmission of airborne infections in enclosed indoor environments or laboratory. Because UV irradiation has very limited energy, UV light does not penetrate dust, mucous or water. Although in theory intense UV light can be both bactericidal and virucidal, in practice only limited disinfection of instruments can be achieved. This is because UV rays can kill only those microorganisms that are struck directly by UV light beams. For surfaces that cannot be reached by UV rays, any microorganisms present will not be killed.

Ozone: Ozone sterilization is the newest low temperature sterilization method recently introduced in the US and is suitable for many heat sensitive and moisture sensitive instruments. Ozone is a strong oxidizer and is generated within the sterilizer using grade oxygen, water and electricity. Ozone is inexpensive, non-toxic and environmentally friendly. Ozone sterilization is compatible with stainless steel instruments. Ozone sterilization is not cleared to glass or plastic ampoules, liquids or implants. Information regarding device compatibility should be obtained from manufacturer of device and sterilizer manufacturer. Packaging materials that can be used for ozone sterilization include anodized aluminum containers using non-cellulose disposable filters, polyethylene pouches and uncoated nonwoven wrap. The cycle time is approximately 4.5 hours, at a temperature of 85°F- 94°F.

Experiment 4: Sterilization of Nutrient Media.

Two methods viz. autoclaving and membrane filtration under positive pressure are commonly used to sterilize culture media. Culture media, distilled water and other stable mixtures can be autoclaved in glass containers that are sealed with cotton plugs, aluminium foil or plastic closures. However, solutions that contain heat labile components must be filter-sterilized. Generally, nutrient or plant tissue culture media are autoclaved at $1.05 \, kg/cm^2$ (15 psi) and 121°C. The time required for sterilization depends upon the volume of medium in the vessel. For small volumes of liquids (100 mL or less), the time required for autoclaving is 15-20 min, but for larger quantities (2-4 litre), 30-40 min is required. The pressure should not exceed 20 psi, as higher pressures may lead to the decomposition of carbohydrates and other thermo labile components of a medium. There is evidence that medium exposed to temperatures in excess of 121°C may not properly gel or may result in poor cell growth. Since many proteins, vitamins, amino acids, plant extracts, hormones and carbohydrates are thermolabile and may decompose during autoclaving, filter sterilization may be required. The porosity of the filter membrane should be no larger than 0.2 microns (μm). Empty glassware that is to hold media must be sterilized in an autoclave before filter sterilization. Nutrient media that contain thermo labile components can be prepared in several steps. A solution of the heat stable components is sterilized in the usual way by autoclaving and then cooled to 35°-50° C under sterile conditions; in a separate operation, solutions of the thermo labile components are filter sterilized. The sterilized solutions are combined under aseptic conditions to give the complete media.

Minimum Autoclaving Time

Volume of Medium per V essel (mL)	Minimum Autoclaving(min)	Volume of Medium per Vessel (mL)	Minimum Autoclaving (min)
25	20	500	35
50	25	1000	40
100	28	2000	48
250	31	4000	63

Bacteria live in soil, streams, food, in us and in virtually all habitable locations on earth. They can make us wine, yogurt and garden compost and without them we couldn't even digest our food. All nitrogen would eventually be lost to the atmosphere without them. Bacteria are increasingly used as research tools and in biotechnology, recombinant DNA technology, enzymes and designer drugs. Bacteria also can make breath stink, rot teeth, clog lungs, give Montezuma's revenge. Bacteria are ubiquitous and are of major importance to biological scientists, physicians, environmentalists, food preparers and brew masters. General and specialized media are required for bacterial growth and for characterization. The basic procedures can be applied to almost any type of assay or culture requirement for propagation of obligate aerobes or facultative anaerobes. Obligate anaerobes are poisoned by oxygen and specialized procedures are needed for their maintenance. Bacteria display a wide range of nutritional and physical requirements for growth including:

- ❖ Water
- ❖ Source of energy
- ❖ Sources of carbon, nitrogen, sulphur, phosphorus
- ❖ Minerals e.g., $Ca^{2+,}$ Mg^{2+}, Na^+
- ❖ Vitamins and growth factors

Microorganisms may be grown in liquid, solid or semisolid media. Liquid media are utilized for growth of large numbers of organisms or for physiological or biochemical studies and assays. Some species, such as *Streptococcus* or *Staphylococcus*, demonstrate typical morphologies only when grown in liquid media. Solid media are useful for observations of characteristic colonies, for isolation of pure cultures and for short term maintenance of cultures. Usually, the preparation of a solid medium for growth includes the addition of 1 to 2% agar to solution of appropriate nutrients. Agar is a complex carbohydrate extracted from marine algae that solidifies below temperatures of 45°C. It is not a nutritional component. Usually, bacteria are grown in complex media. Media contain nutrients in the form of extracts or enzymatic digests of meat, milk, plants or yeast. For fastidious organisms we must use delicious sounding concoctions such as tomato juice agar or chocolate agar or something less appetizing such as brain heart infusion broth or blood agar.

There is no single medium or set of physical conditions that permits the cultivation of all bacteria and many species are quite fastidious, requiring specific ranges of pH, osmotic strength, temperature and presence or absence of oxygen. The requirements for growth of bacteria under laboratory conditions are determined by trial and error. We can culture bacteria using a rich, complex medium, namely tryptic soy agar or broth, so that a wide variety of possible unknowns can be mixed into the same culture and grown on the same plates. Agar plates will be used for isolation and some assays and for short term maintenance of cultures. Agar slant tubes will be used for long term maintenance of isolates. Broths (liquid media) will be used to grow isolates for some assays or for the assays themselves. When fungal spores or bacteria-laden microscopic particles make contact with plates, broths and tubes colonies reproduce. We cannot recognize individual colonies when the plates are covered with fuzz. No untreated surface in the lab is sterile and nearly all dust and other particles have spores or active cells on their surfaces. All labware and media must be sterilized before use. Other methods including filtration, ethylene oxide, radiation or ultraviolet light, may be necessary if components are heat labile or materials are not heat resistant. An autoclave is designed to deliver steam into a pressure chamber, generating high heat and pressure at the same time. Heating media to above 121°C for 4 to 20 min. destroys nearly all living cells and spores. High pressure allows the temperature to exceed 100 degrees, which can't be accomplished with steam at one atmosphere. We use an autoclave that starts timing when the temperature reaches 121° and exhausts the steam slowly after the prescribed time above 121°. The autoclave is effectively a giant pressure cooker. To properly use an autoclave:

❖ Check the steam pressure and ensure that the instrument is set for slow exhaust if liquids are to be sterilized

❖ Ensure that door is closed properly and securely

❖ Check that the time and/or automatic cycle are set properly

❖ Ensure that the temperature is well below 100°C before attempting to open the door

❖ Crack the door to allow steam to vent, keeping face and hands well away from the opening

❖ Exposing tightly stopper bottles to variable pressures invites explosion and injury. When heating any liquids using any method, take care disturbing the flask or bottle. Material near the bottom may be superheated and boil over when moved. Stoppers, caps, cover, must be vented never make them fit tightly.

Experiment 5: Preparation of Agar plates.

Introduction: Traditional plates were reusable glass petridishes with lids. The plastic disposable petridishes are used now, typically 95 or 100 mm in diameter. When prepared for inoculation, a plate contains solid agar to provide a surface for growth, mixed with nutrient materials. We prepare agar media either by mixing 1 to 2% agar with individual components or by using a pre-mixed powder. Either way, the dry components must be heated to melt the agar and sterilized in a flask or bottle, then poured into the plates using aseptic technique, preferably in a sterile cabinet (laminar flow hood). Containers used for media must have vented tops and should be capable of holding at least 20% more than the intended volume of medium, to allow for expansion during sterilization. The 1L capped bottles to be very convenient for preparing large quantities. To facilitate cooling, handling and pouring, prepare them with 500 mL medium. Beware of vessels with narrow necks, surface area of the liquid should be large enough to prevent superheating. Agar does not distribute uniformLy when melted. A safe way to ensure a uniform distribution for pouring plates or tubes is to drop a magnetic stir bar in the flask or bottle, then gently stir the medium after sterilization, while it cools. Stirring distributes the agar evenly. If screw cap bottles are used, the cap must be loosened prior to sterilization.

Procedure:

- ❖ Cool the media with stirring (30 min) and pour the plates
- ❖ Measure appropriate volume of deionized water into a flask or bottle
- ❖ Drop in a stir bar
- ❖ Layer the powder on the water surface, allow to soak in
- ❖ Do not use mechanical mixing for most complex media; lumps will form that will not go into solution
- ❖ Stir or swirl to mix then heat in a microwave oven to melt the agar (uncapped)
- ❖ Place cap or foil on opening
- ❖ Steam sterilize for minimum of 15 min in appropriate autoclave tray
- ❖ After safely removing the materials, use stir plate to mix sterilized agar and allow it to cool enough to be handled
- ❖ Pour recommended volume (15-20 mL) into each plate in hood (recommended) or with very conscientious aseptic technique, at a bench
- ❖ Allow plates to cool and lose some moisture; best practice is to leave closed in a hood for a day or so
- ❖ Store plates inverted in a closed container
- ❖ Aside to contamination from dust particles due to careless handling, condensation and insect contamination are our worst enemies; usually we do not refrigerate plates; watch for fruit fly larvae.

Tryptic soy agar consists of a pancreatic digest of casein (milk sugar) and a papaic digest of soybean meal, with sodium chloride and agar. It is a general purpose medium for the culture of fastidious and no fastidious microorganisms. Most isolates should grow on tryptic soy agar provided that you inoculate the plate with living material and culture it at an appropriate temperature. Some isolates, though, may struggle on medium that is too rich. Media are purchased as dehydrated granules or powder and are rehydrated by mixing a measured amount of medium per measured volume of deionized water. Instructions for rehydration are usually printed on the container (40 gms/liter for tryptic soy agar). When complex media are required, look first for the pre-mixed powder. Prepare from scratch only if necessary. Some media such as phenol red broth or decarboxylase media require that you add a nutrient component and/or adjust pH before sterilization. Some antibiotics and other heat-labile components must be filter-sterilized and then added to cooled liquid agar. Watch for special instructions on bottles. For example, some analytical media are to be heated to dissolve components, but not steam sterilized.

Agar tubes and Agar slant: Prepare agar for a tube as agar for pouring plates, use an open vessel. Beakers are most appropriate. Medium must be uniformLy distributed after melting the agar. As with broth tubes, it is easiest to use a syringe or some other repeating dispenser to deliver media to individual tubes. Some applications call for a tube that is partially filled with agar to give a level surface. For maintaining stocks of isolates or to prepare material for assays, slant tubes are helpful. A slant is simply a tube placed at an angle during cooling to give a large slanted surface for inoculation. The tube can be tightly capped for relatively long term storage of an isolate with low risk of contamination or drying out of the culture. Some liquid near the bottom of the surface also helps serve that purpose. To prepare an agar slant each tube should be filled sufficiently to allow the agar to flow to just below the neck when the neck is laid over a horizontal 10 mL glass pipette. The tubes are sterilized with caps loose as with all media, laid on their sides using a pipette to keep them tilted up just enough to create a long slanted surface. After cooling, the caps are tightened and the tubes are ready for use.

Experiment 6: Simple Staining.

Staining of Bacteria

We most often use basic stains to examine bacteria. Basic stains, due to their positive charge will bind electrostatically to negatively charged molecules such as many polysaccharides, proteins and nucleic acids. Acid stains bind to positively charged molecules which are much less common, meaning acidic stains are used only for special purposes. Some commonly encountered basic stains are crystal violet, safranin (a red dye) and methylene blue. Basic stains may be used alone (a simple stain) or in combination (differential stain) depending on the experiment involved. Slightly different techniques must be used for preparing bacteria for staining depending on whether the bacteria are growing on agar or in broth. The concentration of bacteria in a colony on an agar plate is extremely high, thus the major problem is having so many bacteria that they form a dense mass in which individual cells stain poorly and whose morphology is hard to distinguish. In broth, the bacteria are relatively dispersed so we have to ensure that we get a sufficient number onto the microscope slide so they are not too hard to find.

Principle: In order to observe most bacterial cells using bright field microscopy the cells must be dark enough to see, that is they must have contrast to the light. To create contrast a simple stain can be used. Simple stains use basic dyes which are positively charged. These positive dyes interact with the slightly negatively charged bacterial cell wall thus lending the colour of the dye to the cell wall.

Requirements:

1. Bacterial culture

2. Microscopic slide

3. Bunsen burner

4. Staining set – Methylene Blue, Crystal violet and Carbol Fuchsin

5. Microscope

Procedure

Step 1.

(i) **Bacteria from colonies:** Clean a glass slide and place a small mark slightly off center using a grease pencil. Using your loop, transfer one small drop of water to the center the slide, being careful to be close to but not overlapping the grease pencil mark. Do not transfer too much water because these drops will have to air dry. Sterilize the loop and touch a single colony and transfer the bacteria to the water droplet on the slide and mix well. Do not scoop up a whole colony.

(ii) Bacteria from broth: Clean a glass slide and place a small mark slightly off center using a grease pencil. Mix the broth containing the bacteria well because the bacteria may sediment to the bottom of the container. Use a sterile loop and transfer one or two droplets of bacteria to the center of a cleaned glass slide, close to but not overlapping the grease pencil mark.

Step 2. Drying: Allow the bacterial slurry (called the smear) to air dry. Do not heat the sample nor blow on it to hasten drying time because that could force bacteria into the air leading to contamination and possible infection.

Step 3. Heat fixation: Holding the slide by one edge, pass it slowly through a bunsen burner flame. Do not move so slowly that the edge of the slide holding heats up to uncomfortable levels. This heat fixation step denatures bacterial proteins causing the cells to stick to the slide while also killing the bacteria making them safe for the following steps.

Step 4. Staining: Place the stain in a staining rack and cover the smear with the stain of choice. Allow the stain to work for 30 seconds. Remove the stain by rinsing with water from the squeeze bottle and gently blot (do not rub) the stain dry using bibulous paper. The slide is now ready to look at under the microscope. Because the bacteria were heat fixed, it will not be necessary to use a cover slip.

Experiment 7: Gram Staining.

The Gram stain is classified as a differential stain because it allows us to distinguish between different types of bacteria. Bacteria can be quickly divided into two distinct morphological and functional groups on the basis of the Gram stain. By this technique, Gram positive bacteria stain purple and gram negative stain red. The bacteria are first stained with crystal violet followed by a brief treatment with Gram's iodine. The iodine functions as a mordant to help the crystal violet bind more firmLy. The bacteria are then rinsed with ethanol. Gram positive bacteria, which have multiple layers of peptidoglycan, retain the crystal violet while it is quickly rinsed out of Gram negative bacteria because their peptidoglycan is a single layer thick. The bacteria are stained a second time (counter stained) with the dye safranin which will not show up on the already purple Gram positive but will stain the decolourized Gram negative bacteria red.

Requirements:

1. Bacterial culture

2. Microscopic slide

3. Bunsen burner

4. Staining set: Crystal violet, Gram's iodine, 95% ethyl alcohol and Safranin

5. Microscope.

Procedure

Step 1. Preparation: Smear and heat fix the bacteria as described above (steps 1 through 3) for the simple stain.

Step 2. Primary stain: Cover the smear with crystal violet and incubate for 30 seconds. Rinse the dye off with distilled water (dH₂O) from the squeeze bottle.

Step 3. Mordant: Cover the smear with grams iodine. After 20 seconds, rinse the slide with dH₂O.

Step 4. Decolourization: Rinse the stain with 95% ethanol. This step must be done very carefully. Hold the slide at a 45° angle over the staining rack and rinse with ethanol one drop at a time. Watch the ethanol as it runs off the slide looking for blue colour. Stop dropping ethanol as soon as no more colour is releases and rinse the slide immediately with water. A few drops of ethanol too many and the gram positive bacteria will also lose their crystal violet.

Step 5. Counter stain. Cover the bacteria with Safranin for 30 seconds. Rinse with dH₂O and and blot the slide dry with bibulous paper.

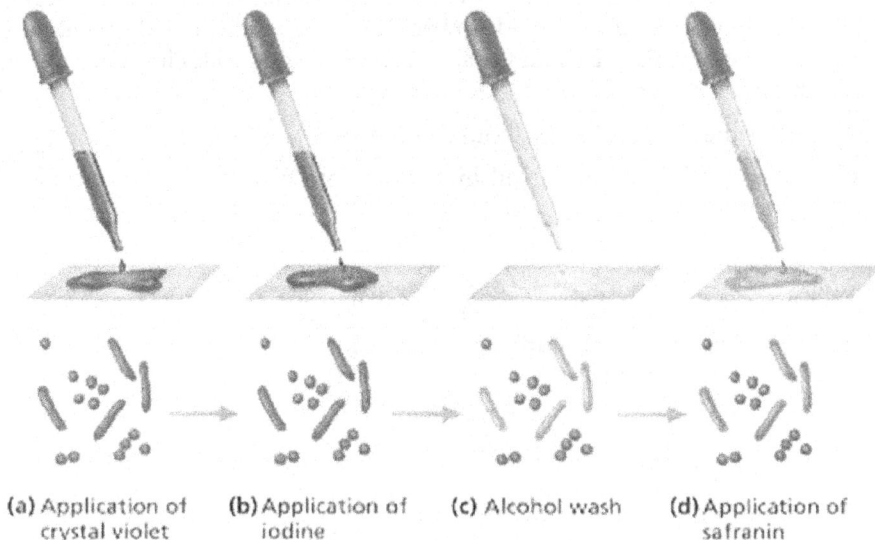

(a) Application of crystal violet (b) Application of iodine (c) Alcohol wash (d) Application of safranin

Gram Staining Process

Experiment 8: Negative staining.

Principle: The negative stain uses the dye nigrosin, which is an acidic dye. By giving up a proton (as an acid) the chromophore of the dye becomes negatively charged. Because the cell wall is also negatively charged only the background around the cells will become stained, leaving the cells unstained.

Requirements

1. Bacterial culture

2. Microscopic slide

3. Bunsen burner

4. Staining set - Nigrosin

5. Microscope

Procedure:

1. Place a very small drop (more than a loop full less than a free falling drop from dropper) of nigrosin near one end of a well cleaned and flamed slide.

2. Remove a small amount of the culture from the slant with an inoculating loop and disperse it in the drop of stain without spreading the drop.

3. Use another clean slide to spread the drop of stain containing the organism using the following technique.

4. Rest one end of the clean slide on the center of the slide with the stain. Tilt the clean slide toward the drop forming an acute angle and draw that slide toward the drop until it touches the drop and causes it to spread along the edge of the spreader slide. Maintaining a small acute angle between the slides, push the spreader slide toward the clean end of the slide being stained dragging the drop behind the spreader slide and producing a broad, even, thin smear.

5. Allow the smear to dry without heating.

6. Focus a thin area under oil immersion and observe the unstained cells surrounded by the gray stain.

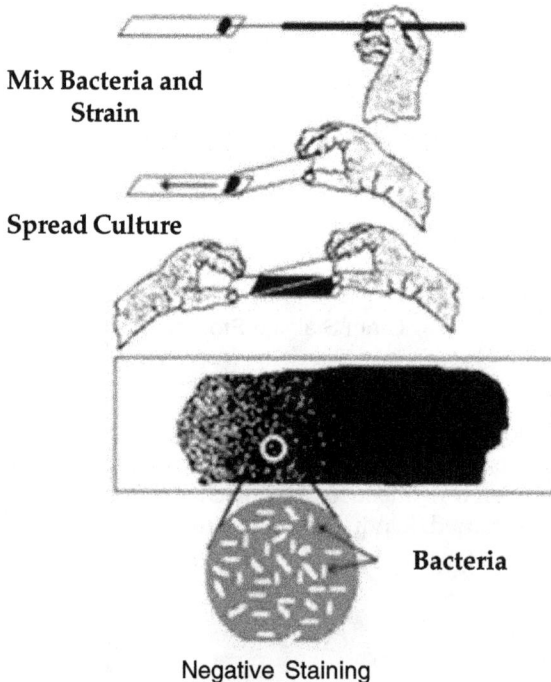

Mix Bacteria and Strain

Spread Culture

Bacteria

Negative Staining

Experiment 9: Biochemical Characterization.

1. IMViC Reactions

IMViC reactions are a set of four useful reactions that are commonly employed in the identification of members of family enterobacteriaceae. The four reactions are Indole test, Methyl Red test, Voges Proskauer test and Citrate utilization test.

Indole Test

Principle: Some bacteria can produce indole from amino acid tryptophan using the enzyme typtophanase.

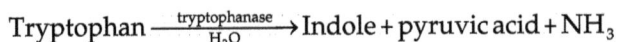

$$\text{Tryptophan} \xrightarrow[\text{H}_2\text{O}]{\text{tryptophanase}} \text{Indole} + \text{pyruvic acid} + NH_3$$

Production of indole is detected using Ehrlich's reagent or Kovac's reagent. Indole reacts with the aldehyde in the reagent to give a red colour. An alcoholic layer concentrates the red colour as a ring at the top.

Requirements

1. Sim (Hydrogen-Sulfide, Indole, Motility) agar
2. Kovac's reagent
3. Bunsen burner
4. Inoculating needle
5. Test tubes and test tube rack

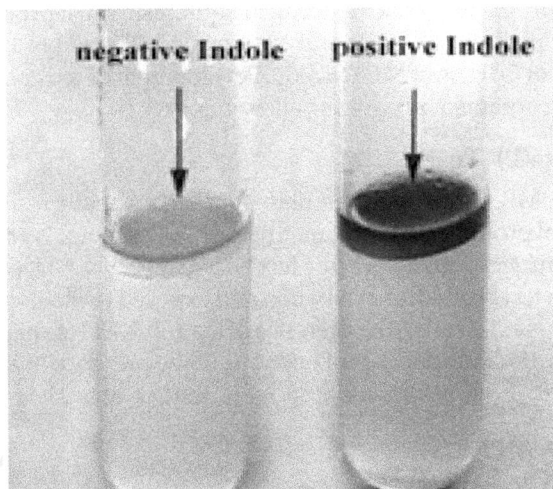

Indole Test

Procedure: Bacterium to be tested is inoculated in peptone water, which contains amino acid tryptophan and incubated overnight at 37°C. Following incubation few drops of Kovac's reagent are added. Kovac's reagent consists of para-dimethyl aminobenzaldehyde, isoamyl alcohol and conc. HCl. Ehrlich's reagent is more sensitive in detecting indole production in anerobes and non-fermenters. Formation of a red or pink coloured ring at the top is taken as positive.

Methyl Red (MR) Test

Principle: This is to detect the ability of an organism to produce and maintain stable acid end products from glucose fermentation. Some bacteria produce large amounts of acids from glucose fermentation that they overcome the buffering action of the system. Methyl Red is a pH indicator, which remains red in colour at a pH of 4.4 or less.

Requirements

1. MR-VP Broth
2. Methyl red indicator
3. Bunsen burner
4. Inoculating needle
5. Test tubes and test tube rack

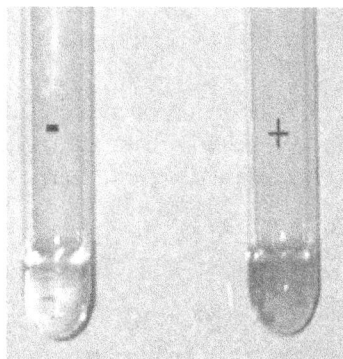

Methyl Red Test

Procedure: The bacterium to be tested in inoculated into glucose phosphate broth, which contains glucose and a phosphate buffer and incubated at 37⁰C for 48 hours. Over the 48 hours the mixed-acid producing organism must produce sufficient acid to overcome the phosphate buffer and remain acid. The pH of the medium is tested by the addition of 5 drops of MR reagent. Development of red colour is taken as positive. MR negative organism produces yellow colour.

Voges Proskauer (VP) Test

Principle: While MR test is useful in detecting mixed acid producers, VP test detects butylene glycol producers. Acetyl-methyl carbnol (acetoin) is an intermediate in the production of butylene glycol. In this test two reagents, 40% KOH and alpha-naphthol are added to test broth after incubation and exposed to atmospheric oxygen. If acetoin is present, it is oxidized in the presence of air and KOH to diacetyl. Diacetyl then reacts with guanidine components of peptone, in the presence of alphanaphthol to produce red colour. Role of alpha-naphthol is that of a catalyst and a colour intensifier.

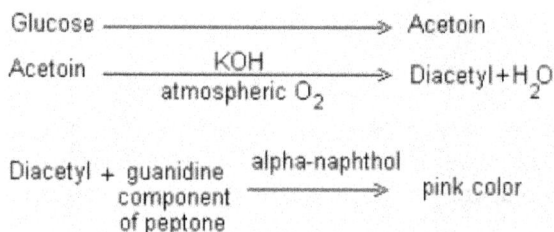

$$\text{Glucose} \longrightarrow \text{Acetoin}$$

$$\text{Acetoin} \xrightarrow[\text{atmospheric } O_2]{\text{KOH}} \text{Diacetyl} + H_2O$$

$$\begin{array}{c}\text{Diacetyl + guanidine}\\ \text{component}\\ \text{of peptone}\end{array} \xrightarrow{\text{alpha-naphthol}} \text{pink color}$$

Requirements

1. MR-VP Broth
2. Barritt's reagents A and B
3. Bunsen burner
4. Inoculating needle
5. Test tubes and test tube rack

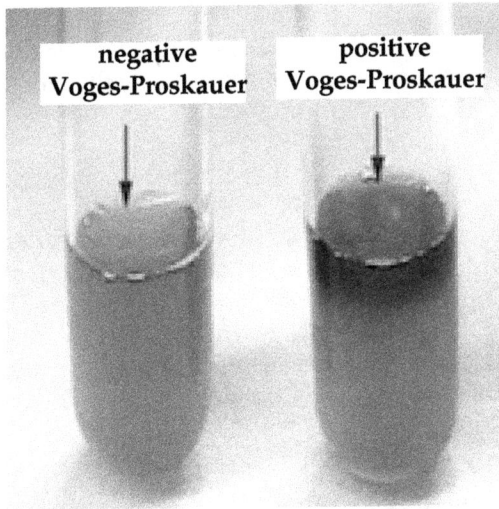

VP Test

Procedure: Bacterium to be tested is inoculated into glucose phosphate broth and incubated for at least 48 hours. 0.6 mL of alpha-naphthol (VP I) is added to the test broth and shaken. 0.2 mL of 40% KOH (VP II) is added to the broth and shaken. The tube is allowed to stand for 15 minutes. Appearance of red colour is taken as a positive test. The negative tubes must be held for one hour, since maximum colour development occurs within one hour after addition of reagents.

Citrate Utilization Test

Principle: This test detects the ability of an organism to utilize citrate as the sole source of carbon and energy. Bacteria are inoculated on a medium containing sodium citrate and a pH indicator bromothymol blue. The medium also contains inorganic ammonium salts, which is utilized as sole source of nitrogen.

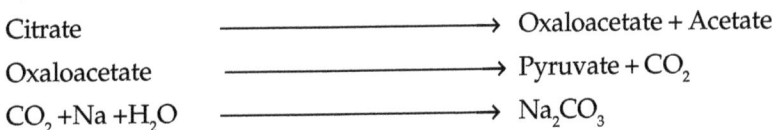

$$\text{Citrate} \longrightarrow \text{Oxaloacetate} + \text{Acetate}$$

$$\text{Oxaloacetate} \longrightarrow \text{Pyruvate} + CO_2$$

$$CO_2 + Na + H_2O \longrightarrow Na_2CO_3$$

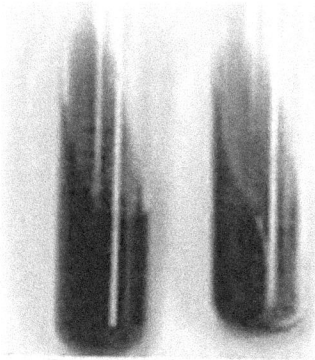

+   –
Citrate Test

Requirements

1. Simmons citrate agar
2. Bunsen burner
3. Inoculating needle
4. Test tubes and test tube rack

Procedure: Bacterial colonies are picked up from a straight wire and inoculated into slope of Simmon's citrate agar and incubated overnight at 37°C. If the organism has the ability to utilize citrate, the medium changes its colour from green to blue.

1. Catalase Test

Principle: The catalase test is most commonly used to differentiate streptococci (catalase negative) from staphylococci (catalase positive). It is also useful in test schemas for other common bacteria in the general Microbiology Laboratory. Catalase is a bacterial enzyme that decomposes hydrogen peroxide into oxygen and water. When the oxygen gas is freed, bubbling or effervescence, occurs.

Requirements

1. Trypticase Soy agar
2. 3% Hydrogen peroxide
3. Bunsen burner
4. Inoculating needle

Test tubes and test tube rack

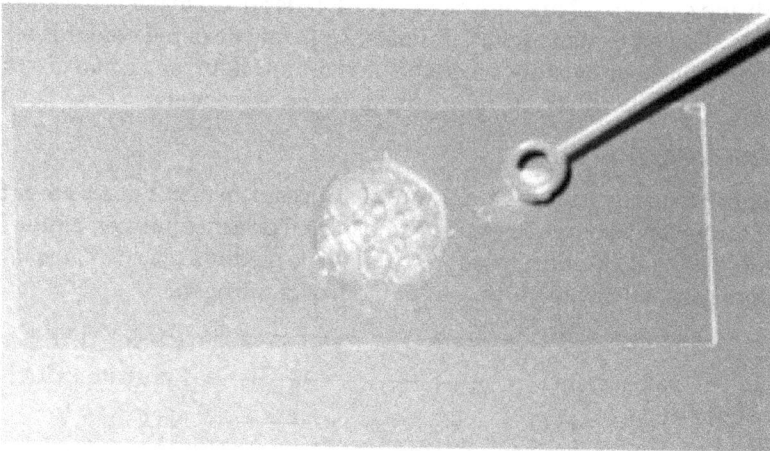

Catalase Test

Procedure

❖ Add 3-4 drops of hydrogen peroxide to an overnight growth on an agar slant.

❖ Look for vigorous bubbling occurring within 10 seconds.

1. Urease Test

Principle: Urea is a nitrogen containing compound that is produced during decarboxylation of the amino acid arginine during the urea cycle. Urea is highly soluble in water and is therefore an efficient way for the human body to expel excess nitrogen. This excess urea is then taken out of the body via the kidneys as a component of urine. Some bacteria produce the enzyme urease as part of its metabolism to break down urea to ammonia and carbon dioxide. While many enteric bacteria have the ability to hydrolyze urea as part of their metabolism, members of the genus Proteus are considered rapid urease producers due their efficiency in carrying out this process. Therefore, this experiment is useful in distinguishing members of Proteus, a urinary tract pathogen, from other enterics based on their ability to rapidly hydrolyze urea. Many enterics can hydrolyze urea; however, only a few can degrade urea rapidly. These are known as rapid urease-positive organisms. Members of the genus Proteus are included among these organisms.

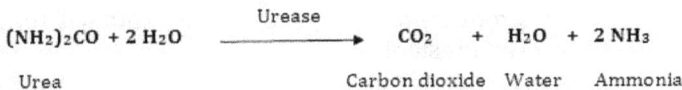

$$(NH_2)_2CO + 2 H_2O \xrightarrow{\text{Urease}} CO_2 + H_2O + 2 NH_3$$

Urea   Carbon dioxide   Water   Ammonia

Requirements:

1. Urea broth
2. Bunsen burner
3. Inoculating needle
4. Test tubes and test tube rack

Procedure:

1. Inoculate slope heavily over the entire surface and stab with loop/nichrome wire.

2. Incubate inoculated slope at 35-37°C in a water bath or on a hot block or in an incubator.

3. Examine slopes after 4 hours and after overnight incubation.

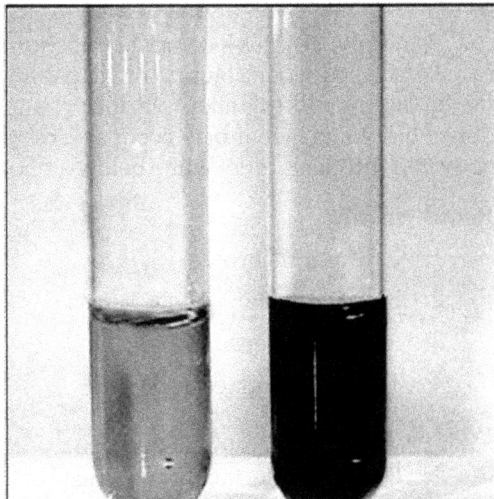

−   +

Urease Test

4. Nitrate Reductase Test

Principle and Interpretation: Nitrate, present in the broth, is reduced to nitrite which may then be reduced to nitric oxide, nitrous oxide or nitrogen. The nitrate reduction test is based on the detection of nitrite and its ability to form a red compound when it reacts with sulfanilic acid (reagent A) to form a complex (nitrite-sulfanilic acid) which then reacts with a á- naphthylamine (Reagent B) to give a red precipitate (prontosil). Zinc powder catalyses the reduction of nitrate to nitrite.

Requirements:

1. Nitrate broth
2. Solution A (sulfanilic acid), solution B (α-Naphthylamine) and Zink powder
3. Bunsen burner
4. Inoculating needle
5. Test tubes and test tube rack

Procedure

i. Inoculate nitrate broth with an isolate and incubate for 48 hours.

ii. Add 10-15 drops each of sulfanilic acid and N, N-dimethyl-1-naphthylamine. If the bacterium produces nitrate reductase, the broth will turn a deep red within 5 minutes at this step.

iii. If no colour change is observed, then the result is inconclusive. Add a small amount of zinc to the broth. If the solution remains colourless, then both nitrate reductase and nitrite reductase are present. If the solution turns red, nitrate reductase is not present.

5. Litmus Milk Test

Principle: Milk is a complex nutritional source that contains proteins (mainly casein) in an aqueous solution of lactose and minerals. Bacterial enzymes alter the media and may bring about various changes. Litmus is added to the medium to detect pH changes that may occur as a result of these enzymatic reactions. The pH above 8.3, litmus is blue, while below a pH of 4.5 litmus is red.

Requirements:

1. Litmus milk broth
2. Bunsen burner
3. Inoculating needle
4. Test tubes and test tube rack

Procedure:

1. Using sterile technique, inoculate each experimental organism into its appropriately labeled deep tube by means of a stab inoculation. The last tube will serve as a control.

2. Incubate tubes for 24 to 48 hours at 37^0C.

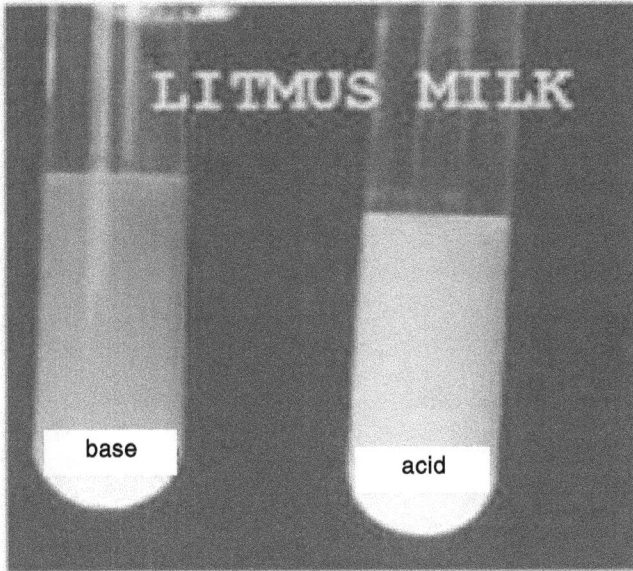

Litmus Test

Experiment 10. Determination of Bacterial Growth by Turbidimetric method.

Most widely used methods for determining bacterial numbers are the standard or viable, plate count method and spectrophotometric (turbidimetric) analysis. Although the two methods are somewhat similar in the results they yield, there are distinct differences e.g., standard plate count method is an indirect measurement of cell density and reveals information related only to live bacteria. The spectrophotometric analysis is based on turbidity and indirectly measures all bacteria (cell biomass), dead and alive. An indirect method for calculating cell mass is turbidimetry. The higher the cell concentration is, the higher the turbidity. Spectrophotometers are electrical appliances that can measure turbidity very accurately. The culture is placed in a translucent cuvette; the cuvette is placed in the machine and the turbidity measured immediately. Simple mathematical formulae help convert the detected turbidity to cell concentration. Using spectrophotometry for measuring the turbidity of cultures is known as turbidometry. Increased turbidity in a culture is another index of bacterial growth and cell numbers (biomass). By using a spectrophotometer, the amount of transmitted light decreases as the cell population increases. The transmitted light is converted to electrical energy, and this is indicated on a galvanometer. The reading, called absorbance or optical density, indirectly reflects the number of bacteria. This method is faster than the standard plate count but is limited because sensitivity is restricted to bacterial suspensions of 10^7 cells or greater.

Requirements:

- ❖ 24-hour 10 mL nutrient broth culture of *Escherichia coli*,
- ❖ 4 sterile 99 mL saline blanks,
- ❖ 1-mL pipettes with pi-pump,
- ❖ 6 petri plates,
- ❖ 6 agar pour tubes of nutrient agar (plate count agar),
- ❖ 48 to 50°C water bath,
- ❖ Boiling water bath,
- ❖ Bunsen burner,
- ❖ 6 micro-cuvettes and rack,
- ❖ 1 micro-cuvette holder,
- ❖ Spectrophotometer,
- ❖ 4 tubes of 5 mL nutrient broths,
- ❖ 4-5mL pipets and pi-pump.

Procedure:

1. Put the original tube of *E. coli* and four tubes of the sterile NB in a test tube rack. Each tube of NB contains 5 mL of sterile broth. Use four of these tubes (tubes 2 to 5) of broth to make four serial dilutions of the culture.

2. Transfer 5 mL of *E. coli* to the first tube of NB, thoroughly mixing the tube afterwards. Transfer 5 mL from that tube to the next tube, and so on until the last of the 4 tubes has 5 mL added to it. These tubes will be ½, 1/4, 1/8, and 1/16 dilutions.

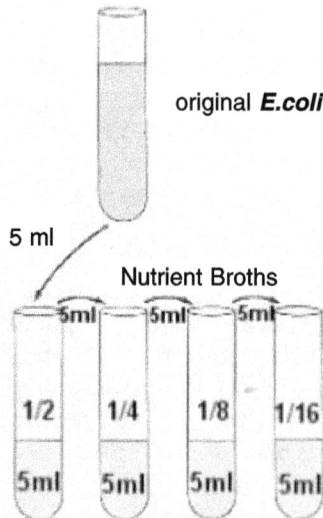

Set spectrophotometer as below.

(a) The wavelength is preset somewhere between 550-600 nm.

(b) Standardize the spectrophotometer as directed.

(c) Obtain 6 micro-cuvettes. The lined or etched sides of the cuvettes face you, with the clear sides facing the light source. The microcuvette must contain 1mL for spectrophotometer to read fluid.

open end

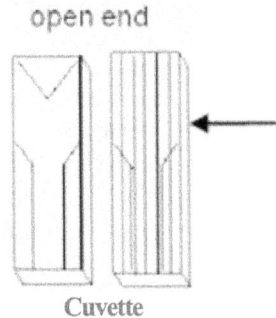

Cuvette

(d) The blank used to standardize the machine is sterile nutrient broth; it is called the blank because it has a sample concentration equal to zero. Pipette 1mL of the sterile NB into one of the micro-cuvettes. Place into the black cuvette holder, close the cover and read. Save blank to re-standardize the machine to infinity absorbance and zero absorbance before each reading because the settings tend to drift.

(e) Pipette 1mL of the original bacterial specimen into a second micro-cuvette. Place in cuvette holder and read. When read, discard micro-cuvette into bleach container on your table. Next pipette the ½ dilution into the third cuvette and read it. Repeat this with the ¼, 1/8, and 1/16 dilutions.

4. Record values, along with the dilutions that they came from. Using the plate count data, calculate the colony forming units per milliliter for each dilution.

Things to remember:

❖ Place micro-cuvette with parallel lines facing you into cuvette holder.

❖ Close the hatch when reading the spectrophotometer so no light enters.

❖ Re-standardize between readings to account for drift.

❖ Mix the dilutions before pipetting into the micro-cuvette to read absorbance.

❖ Read to the nearest thousandth (0.001) on the absorbance digital display.

Observations:

1. Fill absorbance values for 5 tubes in the spectrophotometer.

2. Calculate the number of bacteria in original tube of E. coli and place that value in the observation table.

3. Calculate the approximate numbers of bacteria in the ½, 1/4, 1/8, and 1/16 by halving the number in the cell.

4. Plot these 5 coordinates on a graph, using excel software (MS-Excel).

Dilutions	Absorbance (X)	# Of Bacteria (Y)
Original *E. coli*		
1/2		
1/4		
1/8		
1/16		

Results:

Experiment 11: Preparation of Alcohol from Fruit Juice.

Yeasts, especially strain of *S. cerevisiae* are the main producer of ethanol. They have been used as a major biological tool for the formation of ethanol since the discovery of fermentation process by the time of L. Pasteur. During 1890s fermentation of froth was discovered in sugar solution on addition of yeast extracts obtained by its grinding. This was the first evidence for a biochemcial process of *in vitro* formation of ethanol in the absence of yeast cells. The extract supplied inorganic phosphate (Pi) which is incorporated in fructose-1:6-bisphosphate. Fructose- 1:6-bisphosphate is accumulated due to lack of ATP utilization for energy requiring reactions in the cell free systems. Therefore, an excess of ATP is maintained. The reaction is given below:

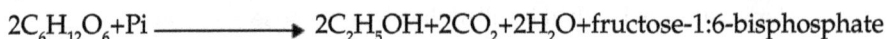

$$2C_6H_{12}O_6 + Pi \longrightarrow 2C_2H_5OH + 2CO_2 + 2H_2O + fructose\text{-}1\text{:}6\text{-}bisphosphate$$

This equation is known as Harden-Young equation after the name of the discoverer. Energetics of EMP pathway reveals that one molecule of glucose yields only 2 molecules of

ATP from 2 molecules of ADP under anaerobic condition in contrast of 38 molecules of ATP through respiration:

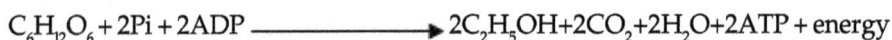

$$C_6H_{12}O_6 + 2Pi + 2ADP \longrightarrow 2C_2H_5OH + 2CO_2 + 2H_2O + 2ATP + energy$$

A total of 15.4 Kcal energy is evolved from one molecule of glucose as about 77 Kcal free energy is obtained from one molecule of ATP. Fermentation of carbohydrate is exothermic where certain amount of energy is lost to the environment as heat. However, temperature of fermenter gets increased. Increase in temperature (11-22°C) depends on size of the fermenter.

Microorganisms Used in Alcohol Production: There is a limited number of micro organisms which ferment carbohydrates (pentose or hexose sugars) into alcohols and yield some by-products. Following are some of alcohol producing microorganisms:

Bacteria: *Clostridium acetobutylicum, Klebsiella pneumoniae, Leuconostoc mesenteroides, Sarcina ventriculi, Zymomonas mobilis,* etc.

Fungi: *Aspergillus oryzae, Endomyces lactis, Kloeckera* sp., *Kluyreromyees fragilis, Mucor* sp., *Neurospora crassa, Rhizopus* sp., *Saccharomyces beticus, S. cerevisiae, S. elltpsoideus, S. oviformis, S. saki, Torula* sp., *Trichosporium cutaneum,* etc.

Requirements:

- ❖ Ripen/rotten Apples
- ❖ Spectrophotometer
- ❖ Claisen condenser apparatus
- ❖ Yeast extract peptone-dextrose agar medium (YEPD)
- ❖ *S. cerevisiae* Culture
- ❖ Erlenmeyer flask
- ❖ Graduated cylinders
- ❖ Test tubes

Procedure:

First clean and dry a 125-mL Erlenmeyer flask. Weigh the flask. To the empty, clean flask add 50 mL of room temperature apple juice using a 50 mL graduated cylinder. Now add several grains of dry wine yeast to the flask; be sure there are at least 5 grains. Using an analytical balance that reads to 200 grams, obtain the mass of the flask containing the juice and yeast. Once this is done, place a 9-inch helium quality balloon over the top of the flask, making sure the balloon stretches approximately 1 inch down the neck of the flask. Now place a bag tie or rubber band tightly around the neck of the flask to seal the balloon on the flask. Let the apparatus set for 1 week undisturbed. After 1 week the fermentation should be complete. The balloon should now be inflated to some extent. This is due to the formation of carbon dioxide in the process of fermentation. A procedure for the determination of the volume of gas collected in the balloon now needs to be devised. Some of the items that can be used in this process are a 600-mL beaker, 50-mL beaker, 50 mL graduated cylinder, and a 6-inch test tube. An inverted vessel, full of water, works well in the collection of small volumes of gas. Once the volume of gas has been collected, the flask which now contains cider needs to be re-weighed. The mass is smaller than the starting mass. One product, carbon dioxide gas was released, thereby causing a decrease in mass of solution. This mass will be used to calculate the % mass of alcohol in the solution. The volume of gas collected through the devised procedure will also be used to calculate a separate % mass alcohol. A comparison of these two measurements will be made and discussed as a group.

1. Weigh a clean 125-mL Erlenmeyer flask.
2. Place 50-mL of apple juice and grains of dry wine yeast in flask.
3. Weigh the flask containing the juice and yeast.
4. Place a helium balloon on top and seal with a rubber band or bag twist.
5. Let sit for one week.
6. Determine the volume of gas collected in the balloon.
7. Weigh the flask containing the cider.
8. Calculate % mass of alcohol in the cider.

The fruits were washed and rinsed many times in distilled water. They were

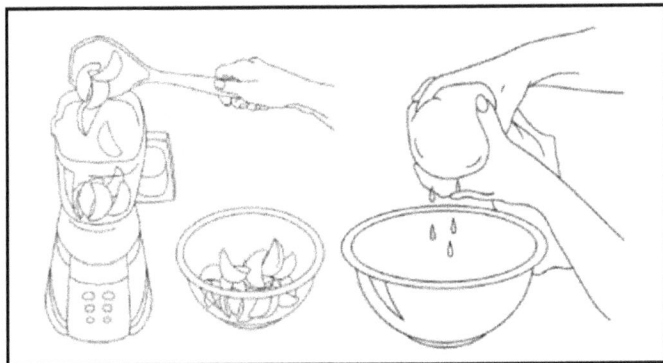

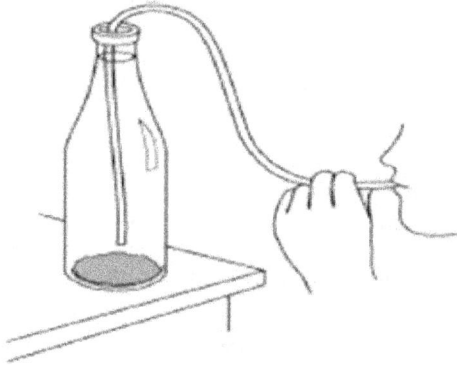

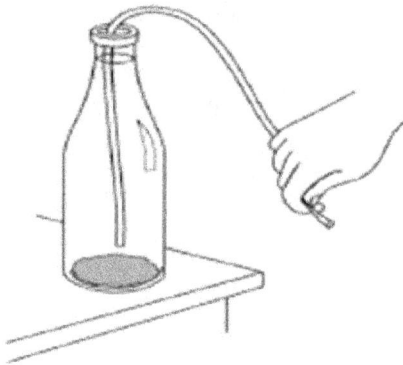

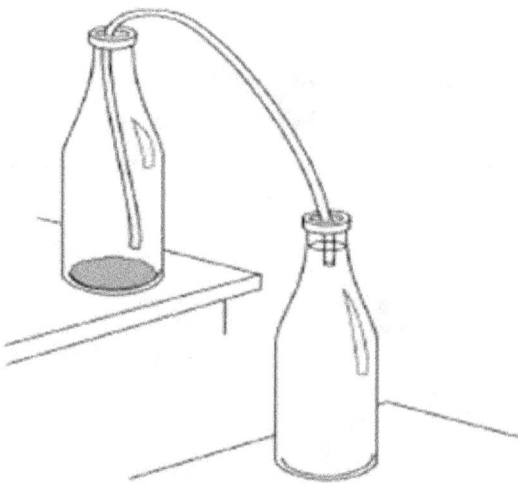

then cut, squeezed and the juice collected in separate sterile flasks.

Samples of the juice were diluted serially and 0.1 mL of diluted and undiluted samples was placed on yeast extract peptone-dextrose agar medium (YEPD) supplemented with 0.1 mg/mL streptomycin sulphate as previously described. The plates were incubated at 30°C for 24 to 48 h. morphologically distinguished colonies were then selected under a dissection microscope. The yeasts were purified by subsequent streaking on YEPD medium. Pure culture of each strain was kept on YEPD agar slants and stored at 40°C until needed.

14% v/v juice was prepared in distilled water. The 100 mL juice was distributed in each flask. Sugar (dextrose) and yeast granules were added as per the table. The flasks were placed at room temperature for 21 days, after which the flasks where checked for alcohol content using Dichromate method of alcohol estimation. The sets were carried out in duplicates.

Distillation

After fermentation the yeast cells were separated by filtration. The liquid part was distilled by Claisen condenser apparatus .The fractions were collected up to 78.5°C. Collected fractions were analyzed for ethanol percentage (v/v) by optical density method using a colourimeter.

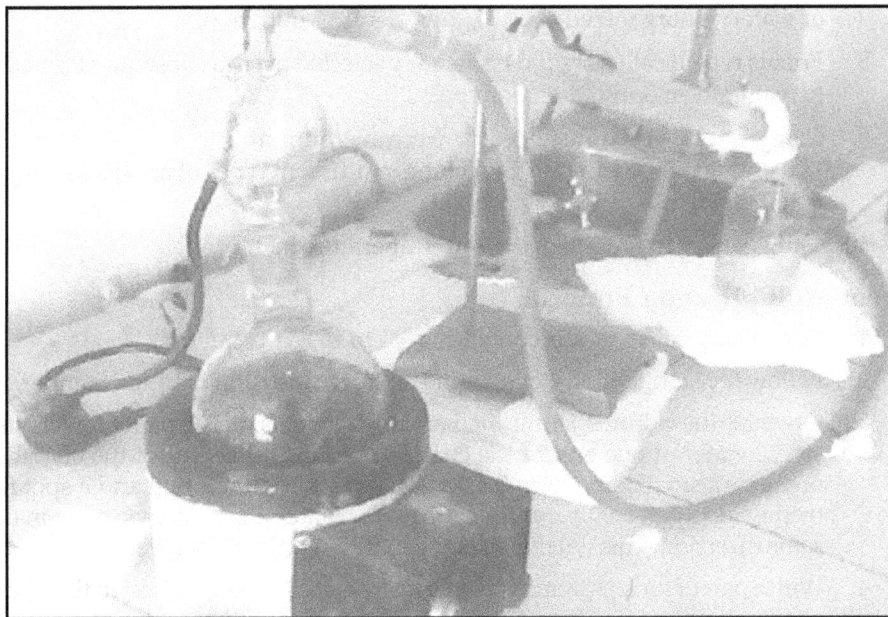

Experiment 12: Sterilizing Plant Materials.

To sterilize all plant material in diluted domestic bleach solution containing 1 drop of detergent as a surfactant. Put plant pieces in a jar containing the bleach for 10–20 minutes. Agitate frequently. Transfer the tissue in the bleach solution to the sterile area. Discard the chlorine solution. Rinse plant pieces twice with sterile water.

Callus Formation Protocol

1. Prepare a batch of basic media without added coconut milk or malt extract.

2. Follow the sterilization steps for the medium, instruments and chamber.

3. Organize the cultures, sterile media, sterilized tools and sterile paper towels and sterile water at one end of the chamber. At the other end of the chamber organize a small paper bag for trash, a jar of bleach solution and a spot for freshly inoculated cultures. The idea is for materials to always move in the same direction. This will help keep you from getting confused. Sterilize your plant tissue, following this protocol.

4. Take a sterilized piece of tissue from the jar with a pair of forceps. Working on a dampened sterile paper towel, use the scalpel or a razor blade to cut the tissue sample into 2 to 3 cm long pieces.

5. Put 1 piece of the tissue into each container (it is important to have only 1 shoot per container at this stage so that if the shoot is contaminated it cannot spread to the others). Shut the lids of the containers.

6. Store jars at room temperature away from direct sunlight. Callus will start to become visible after about 7 days post-initiation.

7. Friable type II callus should be separated from more organized callus and/or watery unorganized callus 2–3 weeks after initiation.

8. Friable type II callus should be visually selected at each subsequent transfer to maintain an optimal phenotype.

9. Callus should be transferred to fresh medium at 2 to 4-week intervals, depending on growth rate. Switching to different types of media also helps maintain vigor.

10. Callus can be maintained at room temperature in the dark.

Shoot Multiplication Protocol

1. Prepare a batch of media containing 5% to 10% coconut milk.

2. Follow the sterilization steps for the medium, instruments and chamber.

3. Organize the cultures, sterile media, sterilized tools, sterile paper towels and sterile water at one end of the chamber. At the other end of the chamber organize a small paper bag for trash, a jar of bleach solution and a spot for freshly inoculated cultures. The idea is for materials to always move in the same direction. This will help keep you from getting confused.

4. With a pair of forceps, remove a culture from its container. Moisten the sterile paper with some sterile water. It is important to do all the manipulation on a damp paper towel, as these plants are very soft and can desiccate readily.

5. Cut stems off the culture and transfer to new jars. At this stage, up to 5 stems may be put inside each jar.

6. Store cultures as explained in the previous stage.

Root Formation Protocol

Once you have established enough shoots, let them grow to at least 2 cm before beginning the rooting process.

1. Prepare a batch of media containing malt extract.

2. Follow the sterilization steps for the medium, instruments and chamber.

3. Organize the cultures, sterile media, sterilized tools, sterile paper towels and sterile water at one end of the chamber. At the other end of the chamber organize a small paper bag for trash, a jar of bleach solution and a spot for freshly inoculated cultures. The idea is for materials to always move in the same direction. This will help keep you from getting confused.

4. With a pair of forceps, remove a stem from its container. Wash all of the media off the culture and transfer to malt media. Malt contains auxins, which promote root formation.

5. Up to 5 shoots may be put in each culture vessel. Store containers in their usual place as before. Roots should form within 2 to 4 weeks.

Acclimatization Protocol

1. Fill plastic vegetable bags with a potting mix that contains no fertilizer.

2. Autoclave for 15 minutes in the pressure cooker.

3. When cool, inoculate with mycorrhizae.

4. Remove the rooted plants from agar medium using a pair of forceps.

5. Wash off the agar thoroughly from the roots using lukewarm water.

6. Poke a hole in the middle of the potting mix, using a sterile instrument; gently insert the roots in that hole.

7. Dampen the potting mix with basic nutrient mix.

8. Spray the foliage with a hand spray containing sterile water.

9. Keep these bags inside larger plastic containers with a glass cover, out of direct sunlight. Gradually remove the glass cover, but watch for signs of desiccation and if needed, use the hand spray to spray water on the foliage. Gradually increase the light intensity for the plants also.

10. When the roots are well established and the plants are acclimatized, they can be given fertilizer and be treated like any other plant.

Flowering Protocol

1. Prepare a batch of jars with per-oxidated media.

2. Follow the sterilization steps for the instruments and chamber.

3. Organize the cultures, sterile media, sterilized tools, sterile paper towels and sterile water at one end of the chamber. At the other end of the chamber organize a small paper bag for trash, a jar of bleach solution and a spot for freshly inoculated cultures. The idea is for materials to always move in the same direction. This will help keep you from getting confused.

4. With a pair of forceps, remove a plantlet from its container. Wash all of the media off the plantlet and transfer it to per-oxidated media.

5. Watch the cultures carefully for growth of flower buds.

Anther/Ovule Culture Protocol (For Producing Haploid Lines)

1. Collect immature flower buds from plants grown either in the field, the greenhouse or in vitro.

2. Pre-culture the flower buds in dry test tubes in the refrigerator for 2 days.

3. Dip the flower buds in 70% ethanol for 30 seconds and then surface sterilize with 0.5%–1.0% sodium hypochlorite for 20 min in your glove box.

4. Rinse the flower buds with sterile distilled water 3 times and aseptically excise the anthers and/or ovules using a scalpel and a needle.

5. Culture the anthers/ovules on semisolid nutrient medium.

6. Incubate the cultures under complete darkness at room temperature.

7. Once calli or embryos are initiated, transfer the cultures to daylight.

8. Culture the developing embryoids on standard propagation medium.

Plant Protoplast Preparation Protocol

1. Buffer Solution: Dissolve 56.94 g of mannitol in 200 mL of distilled water. Add distilled water to bring the final volume to 500 mL.

2. Digestion Solution. Measure 10 mL of buffer solution into a 15-mL test tube or small beaker. Measure 0.1 g pectinase and 0.2 g cellulace onto weighing paper. Drop the premeasured, powdered enzymes into this solution. Swirl the beaker or cap the test tube and shake it back and forth until the enzymes are completely dissolved.

3. Carefully pour all 10 mL of enzyme solution into the bottom of a sterile jar.

4. Use forceps to float each tissue sample on the surface of the enzyme solution.

5. Seal the jar with Saran Wrap or tape and leave it at room temperature (approximately 25°C) overnight. If proper equipment is available, gentle agitation of the dishes will be helpful.

6. The next day, gently swirl and shake the solution in the petri dish. If no protoplasts are observed with the microscope, let the solution stand for another 15–30 minutes, then look again for protoplasts.

7. At the end of the digestion period, gently shake the petri dish to release the protoplasts.

8. Filter the enzyme protoplast suspension through successively smaller filters, starting with the 100-mm sieve. One sieve will trap mostly protoplasts.

Chemical Protoplast Fusion Protocol

1. Mix 2 droplets of protoplasts from 2 genetically different strains, along with

a droplet of PEG (polyethylene glycol) in a test tube.

2. Flood the protoplasts with baking soda dissolved in basic growing mix.

3. After 20 minutes, wash with basic growing mix and centrifuge in the salad spinner centrifuge.

4. Transfer the fused protoplasts onto callus culture medium.

Electrical Protoplast Fusion Protocol

1. Place 2 droplets of protoplasts from 2 genetically different strains, between 2 electrodes.

2. Apply 10 volts per millimeter of electrode separation for 1 minute.

3. Apply a 10- to 20-msec pulse at 100 volts per millimeter. This will require building an electrical pulse apparatus. A 555 timer discharging through an automotive coil might do the trick.

4. Wash with basic growing mix and centrifuge in the salad spinner centrifuge.

5. Transfer the fused protoplasts onto callus culture medium.

Polyploidization Protocol

1. Prepare a batch of media containing 0.001% to 0.01% trifluralin.

2. Follow the sterilization steps for the medium, instruments and chamber.

3. Organize the cultures, sterile media, sterilized tools, sterile paper towels, sterile water and bleach solution in the glove box.

4. Place a clean culture or fused protoplast on trifluralin media.

5. Store containers in a cool, dark location. Within 2 to 4 weeks, polyploid shoots should begin developing.

Sand-Supported Culture Protocol

The purpose of agar in growth media is solely to support the tissue. Instead of agar, use sand to support the culture.

1. Boil sand in water on stovetop.

2. Store the clean sand in a plastic bag.

3. Put ½ inch of sand in a baby food jar.

4. Sterilize jars in your pressure cooker.

5. Place sterilized jars, prepared caps and sterile media solution in your glove box.

6. In the glove box, add enough sterile media solution to just saturate, but not cover, the sand.

7. Close the jar with a prepared cap.

Do not microwave the sand, it will splatter all over. When transferring cultures, make sure they are in good contact with the sand but not swimming in the media.

Experiment 13: Demonstration of *in vitro* Morphogenesis and Totipotency of Seedling.

Explants: A simple exercise demonstrating plant totipotency as well as the nutritional requirements of different plant organs employs shoot tip and root tip explants cut from aseptically germinated seedlings. Each type of explant is transferred to three simple tissue culture media.

Background: During seed formation, the developing embryo and associated tissues tend to exclude pathogens and foreign materials that may be in the parent plant. Contents of the seed, then, are essentially aseptic and the resultant seedlings can be maintained in the aseptic condition if the outer surface of the seed (seed coat) is sterilized with sodium hypochlorite or other surface sterilant prior to germinating the seeds in a sterile Petri dish.

Methods: Week 1

The manipulations that are required for the germination of aseptic seedlings are as below:

Out side of transfer chamber

Chamber Preparation

Be certain that chamber has been aseptically cleaned prior to use. First swab the

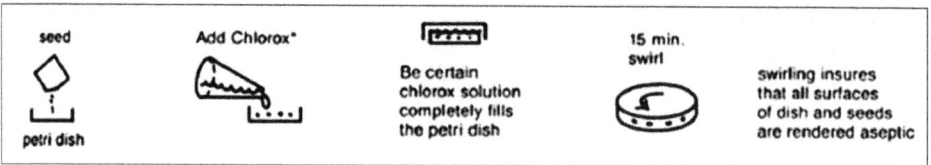

floor and walls of chamber with 70% ethanol. Turn on + run laminar hood for 10-15 minutes. Prioer to the nest aseptic trasfers:

(i)   Roll up sleeves

(ii) Wash hands with soap.

(iii) Wipe external aspects of petri dish with 70% ethanol

(iv) Wipe hands with 70% ethanol.

Inside Transfer Chamber

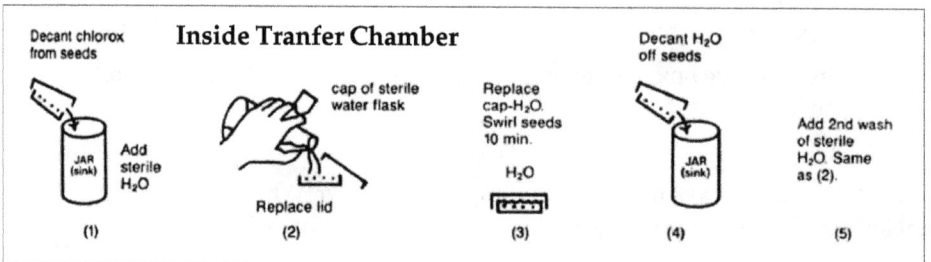

Manipulations Required for Germination of Aseptic seedlings (Week 1)

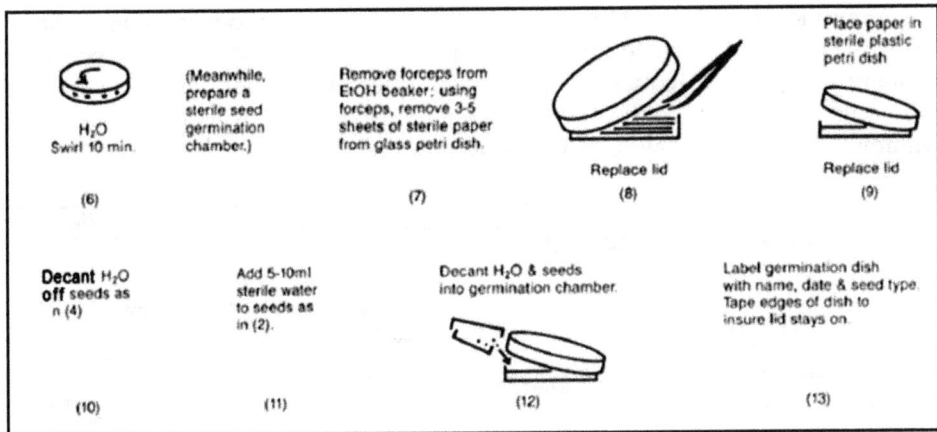

1. Outside Laminar flow hood: Place several (5 to 10) tomato or lettuce seeds in a small petri dish. Fill the petri dish with a 7% chlorox solution to which a drop of wetting agent has been added. The soapy chlorox solution is usually a good surface sterilant. Swirl the seeds intermittently during the 10- or 15-minute chlorox treatment.

2. Preparation for aseptic transfers: Begin by washing your hands and forearms with soap, followed by swabbing with 70% ethyl alcohol (EtOH). Sterilize the laminar flow hood by wiping the inside (top, sides and bottom) with EtOH. Turn on the hood; 10–15 minute operation of the hood before use insures aseptic conditions within the work area of the hood.

Continue to swirl the seeds intermittently during the chlorox treatment. Prior to actual aseptic transfers inside the chamber, swab hands and forearms with EtOH again; also wipe the external surface of the Petri dish before placing it inside the hood. The hood should contain the following: a large jar which can be used as a sink, flasks of sterile water, forceps in a beaker of ethanol, sterile filter paper (5–7 cm diameter filter paper can be sterilized in glass Petri dishes) and sterile petri dishes which can be used as the seed germination dishes.

3. Inside the laminar flow hood: Decant chlorox and replace with sterile H_2O. Rinse this way twice. Each rinse should rest 10 minutes. Prepare the sterile germinating Petri dish by retrieving a forceps from the 70% EtOH beaker. Using the sterile forceps remove three rounds of sterile filter paper from a sterile container and place them in the germinating dish (sterile plastic petri dish). Finally, add 5–10 mL of sterile H_2O to the seeds; decant seeds and water into the sterile germinating dish and incubate at 25°C until the next laboratory. Both tomato and light-insensitive lettuce seeds germinate in the light. Since shoots become green but roots remain white under these conditions, seedling morphology is recognized more easily when light-germinated.

Methods: Week 2

Examine the contents of the aseptic germinating dish without opening the lid. If there is no fungal or bacterial contamination around the seedlings, proceed; if contamination exists, request a dish of aseptic seedlings from the instructor. The manipulation required for the transfer of seedling explants to Mineral Salts (M) and Minimal Organic (O) growth media are outlined below:

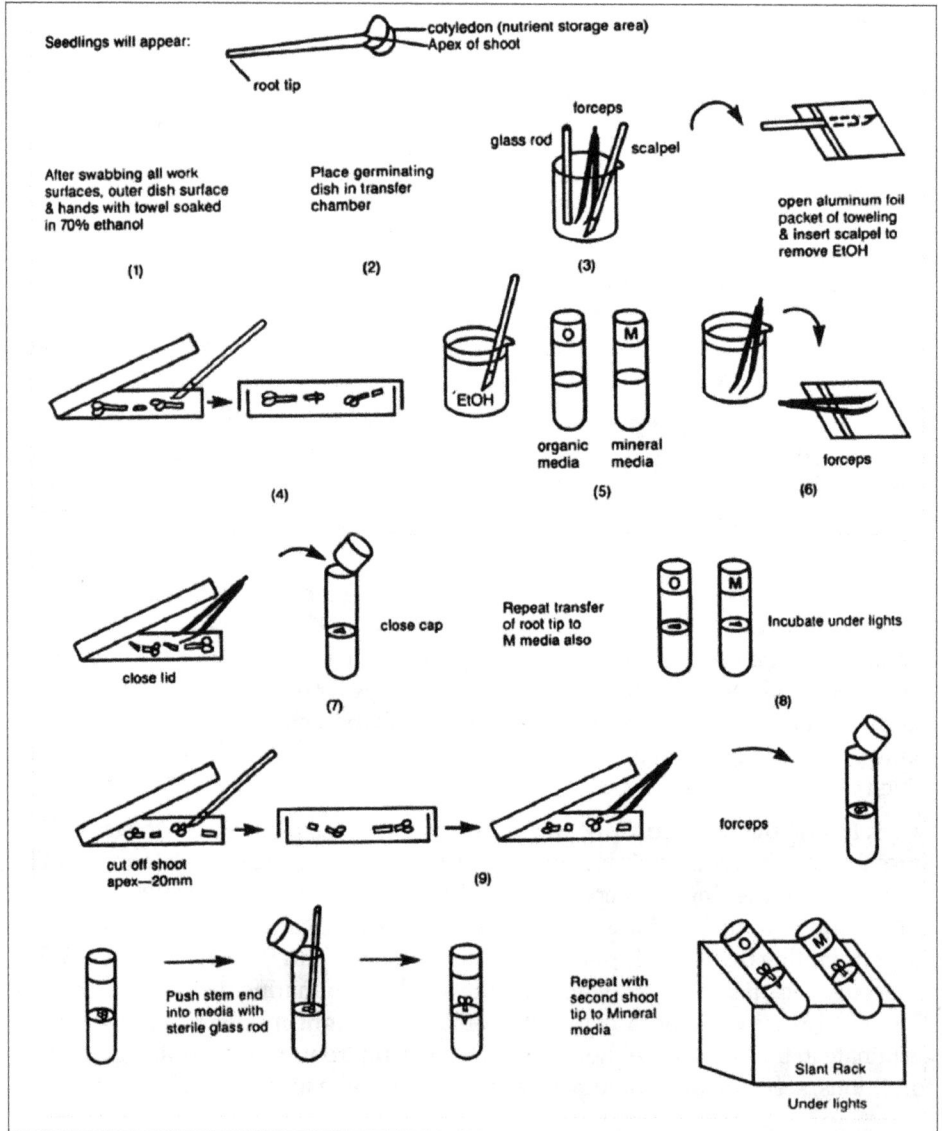

1. Swab chamber, hands and upper/lower surfaces of Petri dish with 70% ethanol.

2. Place germinating dish in transfer chamber.

3. Remove scalpel or scissors from the ETOH beaker already in the hood. Slip instrument between sheets of sterile toweling to remove ETOH (ethanol).

4. Lift one edge of lid and cut off no more than 10 mm of root tip. Excise two root tips. Lower lid. Place scalpel back into ETOH beaker.

5. Place tubes with sterile media into the transfer chamber. Use one tube of Minimal Organic Medium (O) and one of Mineral Salts Medium (M). Loosen these caps.

   The manipulations required for the transfer of seedling explants to Mineral Salts (M) and Minimal Organic (O) growth media (Week 2).

6. Remove forceps or inoculating loop from ETOH. Slip between sterile towelings to remove ETOH.

7. Remove excised root tip from germinating dish and transfer to the surface of the Minimal.

   Organic Medium (O). Transfer second root tip to the surface of the Mineral Salts Medium (M).

   Caution: pick up root tip by the severed end; damage to the apical meristem disrupts mitosis!

   Measure or estimate length of root tips. Record.

8. Using aseptic technique as above, prepare and transfer one shoot tip into each type of media.

   Pick up the shoot tip by the severed end and insert it part way into the medium with an overall vertical orientation of the cotyledons and shoot tip. Record size and shape of shoot tip.

9. Place the four tubes in a slant rack under lights.

10. Examine cultures each week. Record observations on the amount of growth and morphogenesis of both root and shoot cultures.

Observations

As cultures progress it should be possible to correlate size/shape changes with the nutrient content of the medium. A third medium, the B-deficient Medium, contains the same mineral constituents as does the Mineral Salts Medium (M) and the same amount of sucrose as the Minimal Organic Medium (O), but is devoid of B vitamins. Thus, this medium is referred to as B-deficient (-B). Shoot tips and root tips have been transferred to this demonstration medium. Growth on this medium can be evaluated and compared with growth on student experimental media M and O. The Mineral Salts Medium (M) is the basal growth medium, supplying essential mineral nutrients for autotrophic plant growth.

Predict the resultant growth in each circumstance, then monitor the growth and development of root and shoot explants in each medium (M, O and B) and evaluate the following (record Observations table):

1. Effect of B-vitamins on:

   (a) Shoot growth (increase in size) and morphology (change of shape),

   (b) Root growth and morphology.

2. Effect of organic medium containing sucrose on:

   (a) Shoot growth and morphology,

   (b) Root growth and morphology.

   Optional: media M, O and -B are set up with root tip and shoot tip explants in darkness. This set of samples can be observed along with those in the light to evaluate the effect of light as well as media contents on the growth and development of plant organs. A row labeled etiolation would be added to the bottom of Table.

Observation Table

Media	Shoot			Root		
	White	Red	Blue	White	Red	Blue
Cap colour						
Change in length						
Change in Biomass						
Extent of morphogenesis						
Totipontecy						
Primordia						
Number of Branches						

Experiment 14: Effects of Hormone Balance on Explant Growth and Morphogenesis.

Introduction

Plant hormones, like animal hormones, are relatively small molecules that are effective at low tissue concentrations. The two types of plant hormones used in this experiment are cytokinins and auxins. Cytokinins are derived from adenine and produce two immediate effects on undifferentiated cells: the stimulation of DNA synthesis and increased cell division. Cytokinins also produce a delayed response in undifferentiated tissue which is the formation of shoot primordia. Both naturally occurring cytokinins, such as zeatin and synthetic analogs, such as kinetin, demonstrate cytokinin effects. Although low tissue concentrations of cytokinins e.g., 1×10^{-8} M zeatin have noticeable effects, higher concentrations are found in actively dividing tissues such as those of plant embryos and developing fruits. Auxins are indole or indole-like compounds that stimulate cell expansion, particularly cell elongation. Auxins also promote adventitious root development. Indoleacetic acid (IAA), a naturally occurring auxin and napthaleneacetic acid (NAA), a synthetic auxin. Only small amounts of auxin (1×10^{-6} M) are required to demonstrate an IAA response and even smaller amounts of synthetic auxin e.g., NAA are required for a tissue response. The likely reason for potency of synthetic auxins is their stability in plant tissue *i.e.* the enzymes and processes that degrade IAA do not recognize synthetic auxins). Synthetic auxins, then, are more effective hormones that also last for an extended length of time. Furthermore, light influences the physiological activity of IAA while synthetic auxins are not as light sensitive. Plant hormones do not function in isolation within the plant body, but, instead, function in relation to each other. Hormone balance is apparently more important than the absolute concentration of any one hormone. Both cell division and cell expansion occur in actively dividing tissue, therefore cytokinin and auxin balance plays a role in the overall growth of plant tissue. Since hormone balance is presumably important to the overall effect on growth and morphological changes, then the hormone differentials in each of the experimental media (A, B and C) should produce somewhat different effects on the growth and development of excised explants.

Source of Aseptic Explant Material

During seed development the embryos are formed with a placenta-like interface of intervening tissues between parental vascular supply and the embryo proper. This circumstance depresses passive migration of most foreign bodies and microorganisms into the developing embryo. If the embryo which often develops aseptically is released from the seed by aseptic germination procedures, then aseptic seedlings result. Any part of the aseptic seedling can be used as *in vitro* experimental material. In this experiment three explant types will be used hypocotyl (undeveloped lower stem), epicotyl (shoot apex) and cotyledons.

Media Formulae

Media A, B, C, D and E each contain the same complement of minerals, that is, salt base as in Medium D. The effect of minerals alone on explant growth and development constitute basal growth rate against which the effects of other media constituents can be measured. Medium D, then, serves as the base-line control for endogenous growth. Medium E, containing both essential minerals plus sucrose, constitutes the organic and inorganic control which can be used as the base-line indicator of explant growth when both minerals and sucrose are supplied. In addition to the substrate, sucrose, Medium E contains two organic growth factors, inositol and thiamine, which promote sugar metabolism and general anabolic growth processes. Medium E also contains additional phosphate thereby matching the phosphate concentrations of the experimental media (A, B, C). The experimental media contain similar inorganic and organic complements, but differ in hormone content. Since cytokinins are derived from adenine, adenine sulfate has been added to each of the experimental media (A, B, C). In addition, either kinetin or 2iP ([2-isopentenyl]-adenine), both of which are synthetic cytokinins having immediate hormone activity, are supplemental cytokinins in media A, B and C. Of the three experimental media, Medium A contains the highest amount of active cytokinin (30 mg/Liter), while media B and C contain much lower amounts (2 mg/Liter and 1 mg/Liter, respectively). Conversely, Medium A contains only a small amount of auxin (0.3 mg IAA/liter), while Medium B contains a higher amount (2 mgIAA/liter). Medium C contains the lowest absolute concentration of auxin (0.1 mg NAA/liter), but this synthetic auxin is more efficient in promoting cell expansion and root formation than the naturally occurring auxin, IAA. Medium C, then, may actually represent the formula with the highest physiological auxin activity. Since cytokinin/auxin balance is reportedly important to the final overall effect on growth and development, the results for each experimental media may be expected to differ. The balance represented by Medium A is decidedly skewed towards a high cytokinin/low auxin ratio. Medium B represents a more even distribution of cytokinin and auxin, while Medium C may have an effectively higher auxin than cytokinin ratio because of the *in vivo* stability of NAA as well as its effectiveness as an auxin.

Methods: Week 1 (Aseptic Seed Germination)

Materials:

(a) Cucumber or tomato seeds

(b) 95% ethanol sterile jars, sterile water

(c) 25% chlorox, freshly prepared

(d) Sterile forceps or spatula

Procedure:

1. Sterilize seeds (cucumber) for 1 minute with 95% EtOH.

2. Rinse in sterile water

3. Sterilize in 25% bleach for 5 minutes and rinse three times with sterile water.

4. Transfer 10 seeds with a sterile forceps or spatula to a nutrient agar plate.

5. Incubate for 1 week (20–23°C).

Methods: Week 2

Seedling explants (approximately 1 cm in length) of aseptically germinated cucumber (or tomato) can be cut from the seedlings as shown below. Aseptic techniques including the use of the laminar flow hood are necessary to evaluate growth experiments in which nutrient rich media are used. An explant (hypocotyl, epicotyl or cotyledon) should be placed on each of the following experimental media:

(a) Murashige Shoot Multiplication, Medium A,

(b) Murashige Shoot Multiplication, Medium B

(c) Murashige Shoot Multiplication, Medium C, which contain different concentrations of growth hormones.

For comparison, one explant of each type should be placed on each control media:

❖ Murashige and Skoog Salt Base, Medium D and

❖ Murashige Minimal Organic Medium + Sucrose with $NaH_2PO_4 \cdot H_2O$, Medium E.

Seal the petri dishes with parafilm to prevent desiccation and incubate at low light intensity until next week. Record incubation conditions.

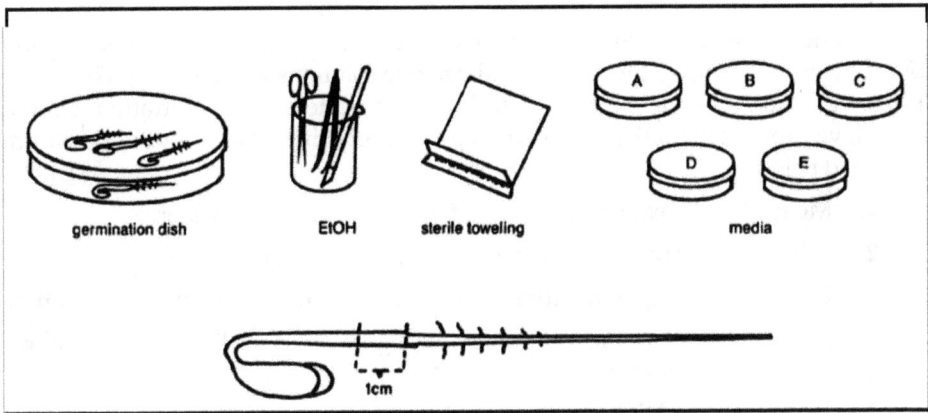

germination dish   EtOH   sterile toweling   media

1cm

1. Remove lid of germination dish and cut explants from 5 seedlings. Cover the dish and replace the instrument in EtOH.

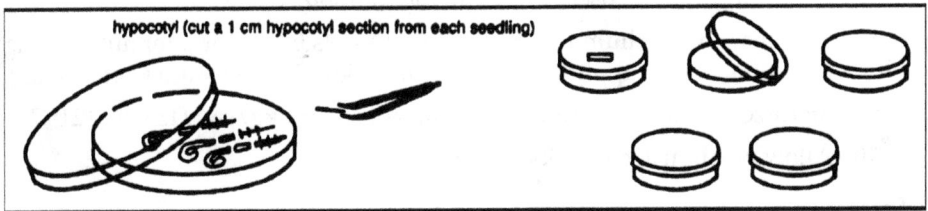

hypocotyl (cut a 1 cm hypocotyl section from each seedling)

2. Remove the forceps from EtOH. Slip between sterile toweling to remove EtOH. Remove each excised hypocotyls from the germination dish to one of 5 meida plates. Slightly depress the hypocotyls into the media for adequate transfer of nutrients into the explants.

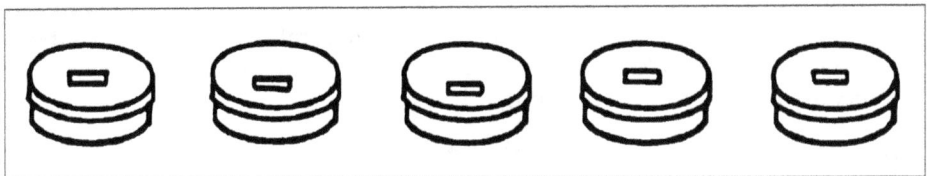

3. Repeat with epicotyls explants using one of 5 media and cotyledon explants using one of each 5 media. A total of 15 plates results for analysis.

4. Seal the plate with parafilm and incubate under low light intensity until next week. Record incubation condition e.g., temperature, light condition, etc.

Transfer of explants to differential growth media using aseptic techniques (Week 2)

Experiment 15: Preparation from Basal Salt Solutions.

Introduction

Liquid 10x solutions are offered for your convenience. To avoid precipitation over long term storage, Sigma has formulated two solutions which when mixed at the proper dilution make a solution with the appropriate salt concentration. Do not autoclave product in bottle. The basic steps for preparing 1 liter of culture medium are listed below.

1. Measure approximately 700 mL of tissue culture grade water.
2. While stirring the water, add 100 mL of macronutrient solution.
3. Continue stirring the mixture while adding 100 mL of micronutrient solution.
4. Add desired heat stable supplements e.g., sucrose, gelling agent, vitamins, auxins, cytokinins, etc.
5. Add additional tissue culture grade water to bring the medium to the final volume.
6. While stirring, adjust medium to desired pH using NaOH, HCl or KOH.
7. If a gelling agent is used, heat until the solution is clear.
8. Dispense the medium into the culture vessels before or after autoclaving according to your application. Add heat labile constituents after autoclaving.
9. Sterilize the medium in a validated autoclave at 1 kg/cm^2 (15 psi), 121°C.
10. Allow medium to cool prior to use.

Materials

❖ Deionized tissue culture grade water

❖ 1 N Hydrochloric Acid

❖ 1 N Sodium Hydroxide

❖ Medium additives as required

Storage: Store basal salt solutions at 0-5 °C. Deterioration of basal salt solutions may be recognized by colour change, pH change and precipitation of components or inability to promote growth when properly used.

Experiment 16: Callus Formation and Multiplication.

Callus is defined as an unorganized tissue mass growing on solid substrate. Callus forms naturally on plants in response to wounding, infestations or at graft unions. Since extensive callus formation can be induced by elevated hormone levels, tissue culture media designed to produce callus contain pharmacological additions of cytokinins and auxins. Callus formation is central to many investigative and applied tissue culture procedures. Callus can be multiplied and later used to clone numerous whole plants. Additionally, various genetic engineering protocols employ callus initiation procedures after DNA has been inserted into cells; transgenic plants are then regenerated from transformed callus. In other protocols callus is generated for use in biotechnological procedures such as the formation of suspension cultures from which valuable plant products can be harvested.

Callus Formation

Explants from several parts of large intact plants can be used to form callus. The most successful explants are often young tissues of one or a few cell types. Pith cells of young stem are usually a good source of explant material. Initially, callus cells proliferate without differentiating, but eventually differentiation occurs within the tissue mass. Actively dividing cells are those uppermost and peripheral in the callus. The extent of overall differentiation usually depends on the hormone balance of the support medium and the physiological state of the tissue.

Callus Multiplication

Actively growing callus can be initiated on culture media with an even physiological balance of cytokinin and auxin. After callus biomass increases two to four times (after 2–4 weeks of growth), callus can be divided and placed on fresh Tobacco Callus Initiation Medium for callus multiplication. Multiplication procedures can be repeated several times (up to eight sequential transfers) before gross chromosome instability or contamination occurs.

Differentiation and Plant Regeneration

Multiplied callus can be stimulated to form shoots by increasing the cytokinin concentration and decreasing auxin content of culture media. Shoot masses can be cut apart and transferred to rooting medium. Once rooted, regenerated plants can be acclimatized to natural rather than in vitro growth conditions. Regenerated plants are especially valuable if the parent plant was itself unique or if the plants were genetically engineered. If, for example, multiplied callus was first used to form suspension cultures on which genetic engineering or cell selection was accomplished, resultant regenerated plants via tissue culture could possess special traits or capabilities.

Materials and Methods

Callus Formation

1. Obtain a 5 cm section of tobacco stem.
2. Cut off all leaves.
3. Immerse it in a beaker of 95% ethanol for 15 seconds.
4. In the laminar flow hood, expose the pith by cutting away epidermis, cortex and vascular tissue with a sterile scalpel.
5. Slice the exposed length of pith into a sterile petri dish.
6. Cover the dish to keep pith sterile.
7. Aseptically slice 5-mm cross-sections of pith.
8. Transfer one cross-section to each plate of Tobacco Callus Initiation Medium.
9. Cover the dishes, seal with parafilm and place in an incubator at 22–25°C.

Callus Multiplication

1. Obtain a plate of tobacco callus.

2. Aseptically divide the callus into smaller pieces.

3. Transfer divided callus pieces to fresh Tobacco Callus Initiation Medium.

By using pith explant and plating procedures, callus can be generated from pith cells placed on Tobacco Callus Initiation Medium.

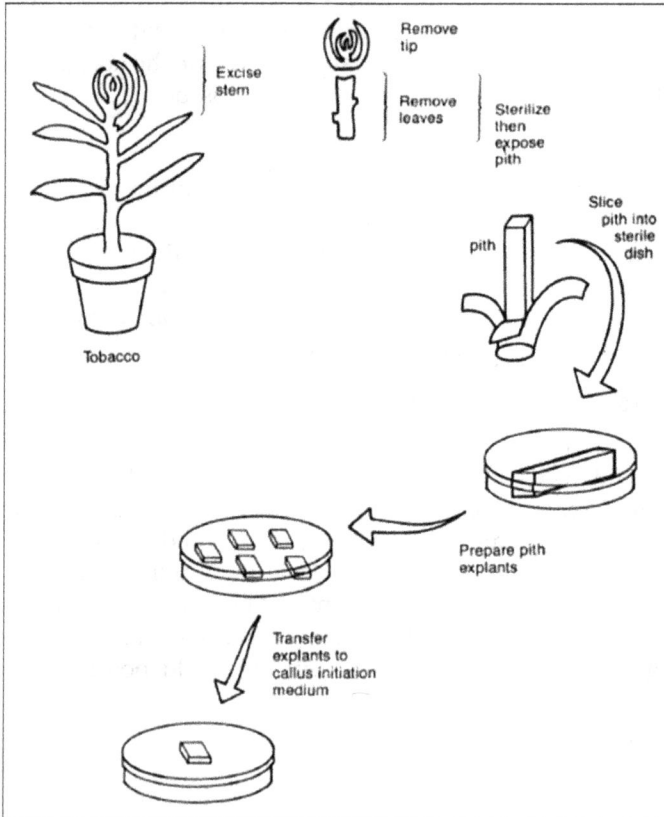

Experiment 17: Establishment of Suspension Cultures.

Introduction

Suspension cultures are suspensions of individual plant cells and small cell clusters (microcalli) grown in liquid media. Suspension cultures are established by transferring small pieces of callus to liquid medium which is subsequently placed on a gyratory shaker. Within a few days individual plant cells and microcalli should be detached from the original inoculum and growing in the constantly agitated medium. Suspension cultures grow best if the larger pieces of callus are removed after the culture has been initiated.

Methods

1. Break up tobacco callus into small pieces and transfer to liquid medium (Tobacco Callus Initiation Medium, without the agar). Use 25–50 mL medium in 250-mL flask for adequate aeration for the swirling culture.

2. A thick suspension of callus should continue to proliferate within the next week on a gyratory shaker.

3. Remove large pieces of callus from suspension culture by passing through a sterile sieve. Large pieces of callus are usually detrimental to the maintenance of a suspension culture.

4. Suspension cultures can be multiplied by diluting 5 mL of the original strained suspension culture to 50 mL total volume (1:10 dilution, vol:vol) of fresh medium. The growth rate and cell generation time can be determined.

Usefulness of Suspension Cultures

Suspension cultures are used in a number of biotechnological procedures such as inoculum for plant bioreactors, which resemble biofermentors. Valuable plant products can be extracted from bioreactors during the growth of plant cells as cell suspensions. This type of biotechnology is still in the initial stages of development and industrial scale-up. Suspension cultures treated with enzymes that degrade cell walls produce protoplast cultures which can be used in DNA transformation experiments as well as in protoplast fusion (somatic hybridization) experiments.

Experiment 18: Anther Culture.

Introduction

The purpose of anther and pollen culture is the production of haploid plants by the induction of embryogenesis from repeated divisions of microspores or immature pollen grains. The chromosome complement of these haploids can be doubled by colchicines treatment or other techniques to yield fertile homozygous diploids. The resultant diploids can be used in plant breeding to improve crop plants The haploid nature of embryoids should be determined by standard chromosome staining procedures (acetocarmine or Feulgen reaction) prior to colchicine treatment. Similarly, the effect of colchicine on chromosome doubling needs to be monitored by chromosome staining.

Materials

- ❖ Tobacco buds,
- ❖ Sharp pointed forceps, surgical scissors,
- ❖ 95% ethanol,
- ❖ Petri dishes of culture medium (1/2 strength MS, 2% sucrose 0.8% agar, glutamine [800 mg/Liter], serine [100 mg/Liter]).

Methods

1. Obtain two buds at the appropriate stage. This occurs in tobacco when the sepals and the petals in the bud are the same length.

2. Holding the bud by the pedicel between the thumb and first finger, dip the entire bud in 95% ethanol for 15 seconds.

3. Remove bud and allow excess alcohol to drip off.

4. With a pair of sterile forceps, remove the outer layer of tissue, the sepals.

5. Next, remove the inner layer of tissue, the petals, exposing the anthers.

6. Open the petri dish containing the medium for the induction of haploids. Remove each anther from the bud and drop it onto the medium. Do not damage the anther or include any filament tissue.

7. Repeat for another bud.

8. When finished, seal the plates and place in incubator (25°C).

9. In 2–3 weeks examine for somatic embryo initiation. Embryoid-forming cells are characterized by dense cytoplasmic contents, large starch grains and a relatively large nucleus. Embryoids appear opaque among translucent cells. Embryoids also exhibit high dehydrogenase activity and can be detected by tetrazolium staining.

Experiment 19: Culture of Primary Chick Embryo Fibroblasts (CEF).

The avian embryo, especially the chicken embryo, is a valuable and widely used medium for the initial isolation and subsequent passage of many viruses for stock cultures and the production of vaccines. Chicken embryos are used almost exclusively because of their availability, economy, convenient size, relative freedom from latent infection and extraneous contamination, and lack of production of antibodies against the viral inoculum. Eggs only from healthy, disease-free flocks should be used. It is desirable to have one source of supply for reasons of uniformity of production and management of the breeder flock.

Material Required

❖ 10- to 12-day-old embryonated eggs,

❖ Forceps and scissors,

❖ Sterile petri dishes,

❖ Sterile 125 mL Erlenmeyer flask with magnetic stir bar,

❖ Sterile 25 cm^2 flasks containing MEM plus 10% fetal calf serum,

❖ Sterile 0.5% trypsin in Saline A,

❖ Sterile 15 mL centrifuge tubes containing 0.5 mL of serum,

❖ Hemacytometers,

❖ 1 mL and 10 mL pipettes,

❖ Sterile Saline A,

Procedure

1.   Disinfect the surface of the egg over the air sac. With scissors or the blunt-end of a forceps, break the shell over the air sac. Sterilize forceps by dipping in alcohol and flaming. Cool forceps, then peel away the shell over the air sac, sterilize forceps again and pull back the shell membrane and chorioallantoic membrane to expose the embryo.

2.   Resterilize the forceps, grasp the embryo loosely around the neck and remove the entire embryo from the egg to a sterile Petridish.

3.   Using two forceps or a scissors plus a forceps, decapitate and eviscerate the embryo. Mince the embryo carcass into very small fragments with a scissors.

4.   Add about 10 mL of sterile Saline A to tissue fragments in the Petri dish, swirl gently for 1 to 2 minutes to resuspend and wash fragments and carefully pour entire contents into a 125 mL Erlenmeyer flask. Tilt flask, allow fragments to settle and gently decant saline. Discard saline.

5.   Add 10 mL of sterile warm trypsin solution to fragments in flask cover and stir slowly with magnetic bar for 5 to 10 minutes. Tilt flask, allow fragments to settle and pour the trypsin-cell suspension into a 15 mL centrifuge tube containing 0.5 mL of serum. The serum contains a trypsin inhibitor that will prevent further damage to cell membranes by the enzyme.

6.   Add 10 mL of sterile warm trypsin to fragments and repeat step 5. At the end of this second treatment, the size of tissue fragments will be greatly reduced and a large number of single cells should be suspended in trypsin.

7.   Visually balance volume in centrifuge tubes (transfer liquid) and centrifuge at 1,500 rpm for 10 minutes. Carefully decant and discard supernatant, resuspend pooled cell pellets in a total of 5 mL of MEM. (Resuspend the pellet in one tube, then transfer the suspension to the second tube and resuspend that pellet.) Mix well for counting in a hemacytometer.

8.   In most hemacytometers, each heavily etched square surrounded by double or triple lines and containing either 16 or 25 smaller squares is 1 mm on each side and 0.1 mm deep. Therefore, the area is 1 mm^2 and the volume is 0.1 mm^3. After centrifugation, the cells should be packed in a tight pellet at the bottom of each tube.

9.   Place the cover slip on top of the hemacytometer, bridged on the two glass arms beside the etched pattern. Add one drop of evenly suspended cell suspension to the groove in the hemacytometer stage and allow it to fill the chamber under the cover slip. Examine with 10× objective. If there are too many cells to count (>200), make a 1:10 dilution of the cell suspension in MEM (0.1 mL of cell suspension plus 0.9 mL of MEM) for counting.

     The following example shows how to convert your cell count to the concentration of cells in your original suspension. Assume you made a 1:10 dilution and then counted a total of 168 cells in one 16-square grid:

$$168 \times 10^4 \times 10 = 1.68 \times 10^7 \text{ cells/cm}^3$$

10. Calculate what volume of the original cell suspension you will need to add

to the growth medium in the flask to give between 2×10^5 and 8×10^5 cells/mL ($\sim 5 \times 10^5$ cells/mL).

Note: If you have 5 mL of growth medium in the flask, you need a total of 5 mL $\times 5 \times 10^5$ cells/mL = 2.5×10^6 cells. Add the appropriate volume of original cell suspension to the medium in flask.

11. Be sure to examine cell cultures both macroscopically and microscopically each day. Actively growing cells produce acidic metabolic by-products and their medium becomes yellow and thus the pH of the medium may need to be adjusted by the addition of a drop or two of 7.5% $NaHCO_3$. If floating (dead) cells and debris are present or the colour of the medium indicates a basic pH, the medium should be changed.

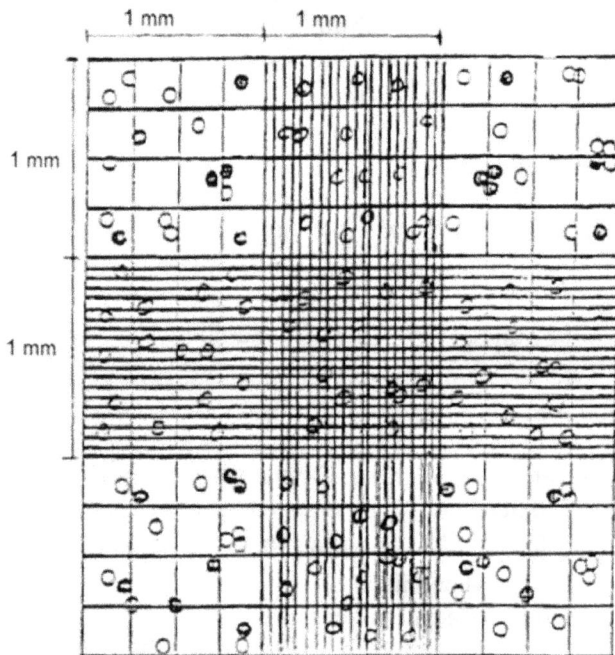

Hemacytometer (improved Neubauer counting chamber).

Experiment 20: Transfer of Cell Cultures

Introduction: After cultured cells have formed a confluent monolayer on the surface of their culture vessel, they may be removed from the surface, diluted and seeded into new vessels. If the initial culture was primary, the new cultures are called secondary and are likely to consist of fewer cell types. Removal of cells from glass or plastic surfaces may be by either physical methods scraping with a sterile rubber policeman or chemical methods, proteolytic enzymes or chelating agents or a combination of the two. After removal, cells are pipetted up and down against the bottom of the flask to break up clumps, diluted and counted. Primary cultures can usually be diluted 1:2 or 1:3 for secondary culturing and after one becomes familiar with the growth characteristics of a certain cell type, counting can usually be dispensed with. The same procedure can be used to transfer both primary cells and a continuous cell line, removing the cells from flasks with a mixture of trypsin and EDTA in physiological saline (STE stands for saline, trypsin, EDTA).

Procedure:

1. Examine the cells growing in a 25-cm² flask with an inverted microscope to see if they have formed a confluent cell monolayer. If there are sufficient cells, pour off the medium.

2. Wash the monolayer with 2 mL of Saline A. Rinse well without shaking (shaking produces bubbles) and pour off. Repeat.

3. Add 1.0 mL of STE to the flask and incubate at 37°C for 2 to 10 minutes with STE covering the cells. Observe periodically to determine when cells are loosened from plastic.

4. When cells are seen to detach from the surface upon shaking or jarring against the heel of hand check in the microscope), add 4 mL of fresh growth medium with 10% serum and suspend cells by pipetting up and down a few times. Count cells in a hemacytometer, calculate the volume of additional medium needed to bring the cell concentration to $\sim 5 \times 10^5$cells/mL and add this volume to the cell suspension.

5. Seed an appropriate volume for the size of flask or 1 mL of cell suspension into each well of a 24-well cluster dish or 5 mL of cell suspension into a new 25-cm² plastic flask.

Experiment 21: Preservation of Cultured Cells by Freezing.

Principle: Viability of viruses and bacteria is preserved during freezing, but original attempts to preserve animal cells by freezing resulted in cell death. This was first thought to be due to laceration of cell plasma membranes by ice crystals, but more recent evidence suggests the cause may be osmotic changes during freezing which give rise to irreversible changes in lipoprotein complexes in intracellular membranes. In any event, the answer to animal cell preservation has proved to be the addition of glycerol, ethylene glycol or dimethyl sulfoxide (DMSO) to the medium and slow freezing, ideally at a cooling rate of one Celsius degree per minute. Cells must be stored at -70°C or lower (ideally in liquid nitrogen at -196°C) and when they are recovered, thawing must be rapid. With careful technique, 50 to 80% of the cells of a healthy culture will survive freezing.

Procedure:

1. Remove the confluent cell monolayer from the culture flask by the method described in the cell transfer procedure. Suspend cells in added MEM, transfer to tubes containing fetal bovine serum and centrifuge at 1,500 rpm for 5 to 10 minutes. After centrifugation, resuspend cells in 0.5 mL of cold medium containing 10% serum and 10% DMSO and place in a small cryotube.

2. Immediately place tubes in an ice bath. They will then be transferred to an insulated container and cooled to 20°C at a rate of -1°C per minute after a few days these cells can be moved from -70°C to liquid nitrogen for permanent storage. Cells stored at - 70°C will not remain viable as long as cells stored in liquid nitrogen. If cells are to be stored in liquid nitrogen, they must be placed in sealed ampules or cryotubes.

3. To recover cells, remove tubes from -70°C or liquid nitrogen and place directly in 37°C water bath.

Note: liquid nitrogen can cause burns, therefore, care should be taken when handling liquid nitrogen and tubes should be held in your fingers for as brief a period of time as is possible. When thawing is barely complete, add contents of the tube to a 25-cm² flask containing 5 mL of medium with 10% serum. The culture medium should be changed approximately 4 hours later to minimize the time of exposure to DMSO at 37°C.

Experiment 22: Isolation of DNA from Animal Tissue (Blood).

Centrifugation process: Centrifugation produces a centripetal force that can be many hundreds or thousands of times the force of gravity, thus speeding up the process considerably. Greater the number of revolutions per minute (RPM), greater the force of gravity. The usefulness of centrifugation in cell fractionation would be limited if all we could do is drive suspended particles to the bottom of a tube. However, investigators are able to control the size of particles that are brought down, thanks to the physics of particles in suspension. In a suspension of round particles of equal density but different diameters, the force that drives a given particle to the bottom is equal to its mass times the applied acceleration. The volume of the particle is a function of its radius and its mass is equal to its volume times its density coefficient, which is a constant. The volume of a sphere is equal to 4/3 times pi (constant) times the cube of the radius. For a suspension of spherical particles of equal densities under a specific set of conditions, the only variable that determines the force on a given particle is its radius. The resistance to movement through a solution is proportional to that part of the surface area that pushes through the medium. For particles of similar shape, smaller particles encounter less resistance than larger ones. Since the surface area of a sphere is 4 times pi times the square of the radius and 4 times pi is a constant, then for spherical particles of equal composition, the only variable that determines resistance under a given set of conditions is the radius of the particle. Driving force increases proportionally to the cube of the radius. Resistance to movement increases proportionally to the square of the radius. It isn't difficult to see that as the radius of particle increases, its tendency to approach the bottom increases as well. Add a significant amount of' drag and the gravity experiment that has been attributed to Galileo doesn't work so well, after all. Since large particles sediment more rapidly than small particles, an investigator can separate large from small organelles, cells, etc., simply by controlling the time and rpm of a centrifuge run.

Fractionation by Differential Centrifugation: For a typical cell homogenate, a 10 min. spin at low speed (400-500 x g) yields a pellet consisting of unbroken tissue, whole cells, cell nuclei and large debris. The low speed pellet is traditionally called the nuclear pellet. A 10 min. spin at a moderately fast speed, yielding forces of 10,000 to 20,000 x g brings down mitochondria along with lysosomes and peroxisomes. Therefore the second pellet in the traditional cell fractionation scheme is called the mitochondrial pellet. Further cell fractionation by differential centrifugation requires the use of an ultracentrifuge. Such an instrument is designed to spin rotors at high angular velocities, to generate very high g forces. The air must be pumped out of the chamber in order to avoid heat buildup due to air friction. In fact, many rotors that are designed for an ultracentrifuge are not even built aerodynamically, since they are spun in a vacuum. A one hour high speed ultracentrifuge run that generates a force on the order of 80,000 x g yields a microsomal pellet. Microsomes include fragments of membrane, including cell membrane and endoplasmic reticulum. Membrane fragments form vesicles when disrupted in an aqueous medium, so examination would reveal numerous membrane vesicles of various sizes. The vesicles themselves can be separated on the basis of density, due to varying protein content. But that's a subject for another document. Spin for several hours at 150,000 x g or so and you can bring down ribosomes and even the largest of macromolecules. The supernatant that remains consists of soluble components of the cytoplasm, including salts, small macromolecules and precursor molecules and dissolved gases.

Principle: Blood is colloidal solution which contains a numbers of cells, platelets and other components. It is also a good source of DNA preparation because it is available and can be stored for long time. Blood lymphocytes serve as the source of DNA. The principle for isolation of genomic DNA is similar to that of bacterial cells, except that here a detergent that is SDS ifs used to lyses cells and these are devoid of cell wall. Blood cells are first collected by centrifugation and washed with high T.E buffer as to completely wash off contaminating proteins and other factors. Since blood cells do not have cell wall they are always kept in buffers that maintain isotonic condition till further lysis. Lysis is achieved by the treatment of blood cells with SDS and proteinase K which completely disrupt the cell membrane. After the genomic DNA is extracted with phenol chloroform and then concentrate by using isopropanol precipitation. After isolating the gnomic DNA it should be checked by running on to 1% agarose gel and then quantities after words to find out the yield of DNA.

Requirement

Trisbase, EDTA, NaCl, Protinase K, Phenol, Chloroform, Isoamyl alcohol, Ethanol.

Stock Solutions:

1. 1M TrisCl buffer (pH 8.0) [100 mL]: Dissolve 12.114 g of Tris buffer in 80 mL water, Adjust the pH 8.0 by 6N HCl and finally make the volume upto 100 mL. Autoclave and store at room temperature.

2. 0.5M EDTA (pH 8.0) [100 mL]: Dissolve 18.612 g of EDTA Na, in 80 mL of double distilled water (add 10 N NaoH to make the pH 8.0, so that EDTA dissolves completely). Make up the final volume to 100 mL. Autoclave and keep it at room temperature.

3. 10N NaOH [50 mL]: Dissolve 2.0 g NaOH in 30 mL autoclave double distilled water and makes the final volume 50 mL and store at room temperature.

4. 1M NaCl [100 mL]: Dissolve 5.85 g NaCl in 80 mL water and finally make the volume upto 100 mL. Autoclave and store at room temperature.

5. 10% SDS: Dissolve 10 g SDS in 100 mL Autoclaved distilled water and store at room temperature.

Working solutions:

1. High TE (Ph 8.0), 100 mL: 100 m M Tris 10 mL(1M stock) 40 Mm EDTA 8 mL (0.5 M Stock) Make the final volume upto 100 mL with autoclaved double distilled water.

2. Lysis buffer (pH 8.0), 100 mL:-

10 mM	1 mL (1M stock)
1 mM	200 µl (0.5 M stock)
0.4M NaCl	40 mL (1M stock)

Make the final volume upto 100 mL with autoclaved double distilled water.

3. Incubation buffer, 100mL: 10 mM Tris 1mL (1M stock) 1 mM EDTA 20µL (0.5M stock)

0.4 M Nacl 40 mL (1M stock) 1% SDS 10µl (10% stock)

4. Protinase K: Dissolve 10 mg of proteinase K in 1mL of double distilled water and store in aliquots of 50 µL at -20°C.

Procedure:

1. Collection of blood: Take 1 mL of fresh blood in a test tube containing 200 µL of ACD solution. Composition of ACD solution (Acid citrate dextrose solution)

2. Dissolve it in 100 mL of double distilled water. Autoclave and store at 4°C.

3. Take 1 mL of fresh blood and spin at 10000 rpm at 4°C for 20 mintue.

4. Decant the supernatant and suspended the palette in 1 mL of high T.E.

5. Centrifuge and decant supernatant.

6. Wash the pellet again with high T.E.

7. Suspend the pellet in 0.5 mL of incubation buffer and proteinase K to the final concentration.

8. At the concentration of 250µg/mL and incubated at 37°C overnight.

9. Add 1.5 mL of lysis buffer in each tube mixed by inverting the tube gently. Add equal volume of phenol: chloroform: isoamyl alcohol (25:24:1).

10. Mix gently by inverting and centrifuged at 1000 rpm at 20°C for 10 mintues. Took aqueous phase in fresh tube added equal volume of chloroform:amyl alcohol (24:1)

Citric acid	0.48 g
Sodium citrate	1.32 g
Glucose	1.47 g

11. Mix gently by inverting, centrifuged at 1000 rpm for 4°C for 10 mintues.

12. Take aqueous in fresh tube and fadeed 1/10 volume of 3 M sodium acetate (pH 5.2) and volume of chilled ethanol.

13. Mix thoroughly until DNA is precipitated.

14. Keep at 20°C overnight, centrifuged 10,000 rpm for 10 mintue at 4°C.

15. Wash the DNA with cold 75:1 ethanol. Air dried DNA, dissolve in it minimum amount of T.E.

Experiment 23: Isolation of DNA from Plant Leaves (C-TAB Method).

Introduction:

The principle is essential for bacterial genomic DNA except that various steps differ considerably cells is usually ruptured by mechanical force following several methods. The most commonly used method is grinding the plant tissues in mortar and pestle in the presence of liquid nitrogen. Liquid nitrogen freezes the tissue rapidly and allows fine grinding in mortar and pestle. Sometimes plant tissues are ground by using glass, steel or tungsten carbide beads in pestle n mortar. The disrupted plant cell are lysed and extracted with a suitable buffer which contains detergent such as CTAB (acetyl trimethyl ammonium bromide). Heat treatment is often given at this stage to completely lyse the cell and after that it is extracted once with chloroform which dissolves most of the impurities like protein, carbohydrates, cell debries etc. Nucleic acids come in aqueous phase which is then separated by centrifugation. DNA can be spooled out using a glass rod. Spooled DNA can be taken into fresh tube and then it is dissolved in TE buffer and quantified.

Requirements: CTAB, Tris buffer, NaCl, EDTA, β-mercaptoethanol (BME), Iso-propanol, Ethanol, Chloroform, Iso-Amyl Alcohol.

Stock solution:

(i) **Tris-Cl Buffer (pH 8.0) [10 0mL]:** Dissolve 12.114 g of tris-base in 80 mL of ddw. Adjust the pH to 8.0 with 6N HCl. Now make the volume up to 100 mL by ddw. Autoclave and store at 4°C.

(ii) **0.5M EDTA (pH 8.0), [50 mL]:** Dissolve 9.3 g of EDTA in 300 mL of water (add 10N NaOH to make the pH 8.0). Make the final volume up to 50 mL. Autoclave and store at 40°C.

Working stock:

(i) Extraction buffer: 25 mL.

2% (w/v) CTAB: 0.5 gm.

100 MM Tris-Cl: 2.5 mL.

1.4 M NaCl : 2.0475 gm

20mm EDTA: 1mL (0.5 M stock)

0.2% BME: 50 microliters.

(ii) TE buffer (pH 8.0): 25 mL.

10 mm Tris-cl: 250 micro litres (1M stock) 1 mm

EDTA: 50 micro litres (0.5 M stock)

Procedure

1. Wash the leaf material with autoclaved ddw and then with absolute alcohol.

2. Grind 0.5 gm leaf material in liquid nitrogen to fine powder using pre-chilled pestle and mortar.

3. Transfer the powder to 15 mL. Polypropylene tubes containing 3.0 mL of pre-warmed extraction buffer. Use spatula to dispose the material completely.

4. Incubate samples at 60°C for 30 minutes with occasional mixing by gentle swirling.

5. Add 3 mL chloroform; isoamyl alcohol (24:1) and mix the inversion to emulsify.

6. Spin at 15,000 rpm at RT for 10 minutes.

7. Remove the aqueous phase with a wide bore pipette, transfer to a clean tube, add double volume of isopropanol and mix by quick gentle inversion.

8. Spool DNA using a bent pasture, transfer to another tube or spin at 10,000 rpm for 10 min to precipitate the DNA.

9. Wash the DNA pellet in 70% ethanol for 20 minutes.

10. Dry the pellet and dissolve in 50 microlitre TE buffer stored at 20 degree Celsius.

11. Quantitative determination of DNA of the sample and check the quality by agarose gel electrophoresis.

Observation Table:

Amount of Bacterial cell	OD at 260 nm.	OD at 280 nm.	Ratio OD_{260}/OD_{280}	Yield (µg/ml.)

Results:

Experiment 24: Isolation of High Molecular Weight Genomic DNA from Bacteria.

Introduction

Preparation of total cell DNA from bacteria of following steps:

1. Growth of bacterial cell: The bacterial cells are multiplied in synthetic or undefined liquid medium. *E.coli.* for example are grown in LB medium Bacterial cells are separated by centrifugation and re-suspended in into a volume 1% of the initial volume.

2. Rupture or lysis of cells to obtain cell extract: Cell extract is either obtained by rupturing them mechanically or by laying them chemically. All bacterial cells are surrounded by plasma membrane which itself is encoded in a rigid cell wall. Mechanical lysis involves crusting the bacterial mass in pestle and mortar in presences of liquid nitrogen. Chemical lysis is most commonly used method; it employs Lysozyme , EDTA or a combination of both to lysed bacteria and related organisms Lysozyme digests the polymeric compounds that impart the rigidity to cell wall . EDTA on the other hand cheats magnesium ions which are responsible for maintained of cell envelope integrity. In case bacterial cells do not lyze following Lysozyme or EDTA treatment, a detergent like SDS is also added. Detergent solubilizing the liquid molecules of cell membranes therefore disrupts it completely. Sometimes a combination of mechanical and chemical lysis is also employed for bacterial cell lysis. Following cell lysis, cell debris is removed by centrifugation.

3. Purification of DNA: The genomic DNA is purified by treating it with phenol, chloroform mixture that removes the protein. In case it has heavy load of proteins, it is treated with RNase using silica/glass beads.

4. Concentration of DNA: DNA can be precipitated by treatment with isopropanol/ethanol. Upon its treatment, if DNA conc. is high DNA can be seen at interface of alcohol and DNA solution. At this stage, it can be collected by using a glass rod .This is known as spooling of DNA. If DNA conc. is low; it can be precipitated by keeping it at 20°C. After precipitation of DNA, it is sedimented and dissolves in suitable buffer such as TE buffer and afterwards it is quantitated.

Requirements: Tris base, EDTA, NaCl, Liquid Nitrogen, Tris saturated phenol, absolute alcohol, sodium acetate.

Stock Solutions:

❖ **1M Tris-Cl Buffer (ph-8.0), 100 mL:** Dissolve 12.114g of tris base in 80 mL water, adjust pH to 8.0 with 6N HCl and finally make volume 100 mL. Autoclave and store at RT.

❖ **0.5 M EDTA (ph-8.0), 100 mL:** Dissolve 18.612 g of EDTA Na_2 in 80 mL H_2O (add 10 N NaOH to adjust the pH 8.0. So that EDTA dissolves), make final volume 100 mL. Autoclave and store at room temperature.

❖ **10N NaOH, 50 mL:** Dissolve 20g NaOH IN 30 mL H_2O. Make the final volume 50mL autoclave and keep at room temp.

❖ **1M NaCl, 100 mL:** Dissolve 5.85 g of NaCl 80 mL of double distilled water. Make final volume upto 100 mL. Autoclave and store at room temperature.

❖ **10% SDS, 50 mL:** Autoclave 50 mL of double distilled water, dissolve 5 g of SDS in 50 mL. Keep it at 37°C or at 60°C water bath for complete dissolution.

Working Solutions:

❖ **Saline EDTA Solution: 100 mM NaCl:** 5 mL (1M NaCl) 1mM EDTA: 50μL (0.5 M EDTA) Make volume upto 500 mL, autoclaved double distilled water.

❖ **3M Na Sodium acetate (pH 7.0)- 25 mL:** Dissolve 10.20g of sodium acetate in 15 mL of ddw. Adjust ph to 7.0 with dil. acetic acid. Finally make the volume upto 20 mL with ddw. Autoclave and store at 4°C.

❖ **70% Alcohol;** 100mL

❖ **TE (pH 8.0)- 20 mL 100 mM tris-Cl:** 200ìl (1M tris-Cl) 1mM EDTA: 40 mL (0.5M EDTA)

Procedure:

1. Took 0.5 g of harvested cells and wash with them saline EDTA solution.

2. Freezed the pellet with liquid nitrogen .The frozen pellet is then crushed in a pre-cooled, autoclaved pestle and mortor in the presence of liquid nitrogen and incinerated cover slips.

3. Cells were crushed for about 15 mins till the powder like consistency is reached.

4. The fine powder was transfer to 50 mL sterile Oakridge tube.

5. The mortar was allowed to warm at RT and then 10 mL of saline EDTA was used to wash any residual cell out of mortar into the tube.

6. Egg white Lysozyme is added to a final concentration of 200 μg/mL and tube was incubated at 37°C with gentle swirling for 1hour.

7. Added proteinase K to the final conc. of 250 μg/mL and incubate at 60-65°C for 15 minutes.

8. Added SDS to the final conc. of 3.5% (v/v) and further incubate the tubes at 60-65°C for additional 15 mints with occasional swirling.

9. Cooled the tubes to room temperature and added equal volume of phenol (tris saturated pH 7.0) shaked gently till on emulsion is formed.

10. Centrifuged at 5000 rpm for 15 minutes at 10°C. Remove the top aqueous layer with cut tips and transferred to a fresh centrifuged tube.

11. Repeat this step till a clear interface is observed.

12. Repeated the same treatment with chloroform isoamyl alcohol (24:1) twice. Add two volumes of chilled ethanol.

13. Mix the two phases with a sterile tip. The DNA starts spooling around the tip.

14. Took out the tip with the adhered DNA on it and dipped in 70% ethanol.

15. The DNA is air dried and dissolved in TE. This DNS is left at 4°C until it dissolves completely.

Experiment 25: Isolation of Plasmid DNA from *E. Coli* Bacteria.

Introduction: Plasmids are commonly isolated by alkaline lysis method. First bacterial cells containing the desired plasmids are grown in a broth medium. The cell pellet is resuspended in a solution that contains glucose/ sucrose, EDTA/Lysozyme and tris-buffer. This cause disintegration of cell wall and weakening of bacterial cell membrane as osmotic pressure till increases. Next cells are lysed by plasmid then in solution that contains alkali (NaOH), SDS. SDS detergent denatures partial proteins and causes dissolution of biochemical cell membrane and NaOH denatures the plasmid and chromosomal DNA and began hydrolysis of DNA. The preparation is then neutralized by using concentrated solution of sodium acetate or potassium acetate upon neutralization, plasmid DNA renatures rapidly because of its small size and covalent confirmation while chromosomal DNA cannot renatures and it forms an entangled complex in which and denatured proteins are trapped. Most of the chromosomal DNA and bacteria proteins precipitate along with the SDS complex and are removed by centrifugation. The reannealed plasmid DNA present along with RNA in the supernatant is then concentrated by isopropanol precipitation. Centrifugation will precipitate the plasmid DNA which then can be dissolved in TE buffer.

Requirements: Centrifuge, tips, eppendrof tubes and tips.

Material and Reagents

Stock Solutions: Solution I: 15% sucrose or glucose 25 mM Tris (pH 8.0) 10 mM EDTA Autoclave and store at 4°C. Do not autoclave if glucose is being used.

Solution II: 0.2 N NaOH and 1% SDS. Dilute it from the stock of NaOH and SDS and prepare it fresh before use.

Solution III: 5M Potassium Acetate (pH 5.2). Take 60 mL. 5 M Potassium acetate. Add 11.5 mL. glacial acetic acid. Make it up to 100 mL. Autoclave and store it at 4°C.

Solution IV: Isopropanol TE buffer: - TE Buffer contains 100 mM Tris and 1 mM EDTA. TE buffer composition for 100 mL:- 10 mM Tris HCl (pH-8.0)- Take 1 mL. from stock 1mL. Tris HCl (pH-8.0) 1mM EDTA: - Take 0.5 mL. from stock 0.5 M EDTA (pH-8.0) Add distilled water to 100 mL.and autoclave it.

Procedure:

1. Pick single colony and inoculate into 10 mL. LB broth containing ampicillin (50µg/mL). Incubate using shaker at 37^0 C O/N.

2. Spin for 8-10 minute at 6,000 rpm. Discard the supernatant. Invert the viable on blotting paper to chain left over supernant. Place on ice.

3. Resuspend cell pellet in 100 µl of ice-cold solution I, vortex gently. Place on ice for 5 minute and shift to room temperature.

4. Thaw and add 200 µL of sol. I at RT. Mix gently by inverting the tube five times. Do not vortex.

5. Add 15 µL of sol.III. Mix gently by inverting the tubes. Place on ice for 5 minute. Place on ice for 5 minute.

6. Spin for 10 minute at 6-8000 rpm.

7. Transfer immediately the supernatant to a fresh eppendrof tube and add 900 µL of ice cold isopropanol. Mix by inverting to precipitate the DNA. Allow to stand 10-15 minute at room temperature.

8. Spin for 20 minute at 10,000 rpm for 30 minute, at 6,000 rpm. Decant the supernatant, invert the vial on blotting paper to drain left over supernant DNA will be seen as white ppt. sticking to the side. Dry for 10-15 minute at 37⁰C till there is no trace of solution IV.

9. Re-suspend the pellet in 20 µL of 1x TAE (add along sides), mix by tapping tubes with fingers so that DNA goes into solution. Be sure mixing is complete with intermittent tapping for 20 minute.

10. Add RNase A at the concentration of 50 µg/mL. (to remove RNA) and incubate for 30 minute at 37°C.

11. Add 3 µL of gel loading buffer to prepare DNA and 20 µL of control DNA.

12. Load prepared DNA and control DNA samples in separate wells and electrophoresis in 0.8% or1% agarose gel.

Experiment 26: Purification of DNA.

Introduction: Purification of DNA from a complex mixture of cellular molecules is most readily accomplished by removal of proteins and other molecules into an organic solvent. This extraction procedure takes advantage of properties of phenol and chloroform that lead to denaturation of proteins. DNA and RNA are not soluble in the organic solvents and thereby remain associated with aqueous phases of mixtures that contain solvents for protein extraction.

Reagents:

❖ Chloroform- mixture of chloroform: isoamyl alcohol in 24: 1 (v/v)

❖ DNA sample, mini-prep

❖ Ethanol (100%; store at 20°C)

❖ Gloves

❖ Ice

❖ Microcentrifuge tubes (1.5 mL)

❖ Micropipettors

❖ Phenol

❖ TE buffer (pH 8.0)

Equipment: Microcentrifuge at 4°C microcentrifuge at room temperature

Procedure:

1. Mix 50 µL of mini-prep DNA sample in 1.5 mL microcentrifuge tube with 50mL of TE buffer (pH 8.0) to obtain a workable volume.

2. To this mixture add 100 µL of phenol. This organic solvent serves to denature and extract protein.

3. Mix the contents by inverting the tube gently several times, until an emulsion forms. This avoids breakage of DNA that occurs by shear forces generated in vortexing and violent stirring.

4. Centrifuge in the microcentrifuge for 20 seconds at top speed at room temperature (about 14,000 rpm).

5. With a micropippettor, transfer the upper aqueous phase to a clean 1.5 mL microcentrifuge tube.

6. Repeat the extraction of the remaining lower organic phase and interphase in the original tube by adding 100 mL of TE buffer. Mix by inversion. Centrifuge as in Step 4. Collect the aqueous phase and combine with the first aqueous phase collected.

7. Extract the combined aqueous phases by adding about 100 mL of phenol and 100 mL of chloroform. The chloroform also serves to extract and denature protein.

    Mix by inversion, centrifuge as in Step 4 and transfer the upper phase to a clean 1.5 mL microcentrifuge tube.

8. Extract the upper, aqueous phase from Step 7 with 200 µL chloroform only.

This final chloroform extraction serves to remove residual phenol from the DNA-containing aqueous phase. Mix, centrifuge as in Step 4 and collect the upper phase that contains purified DNA, which should be stored at 4°C.

Experiment 27: Quantitative Estimation of DNA by Spectrophotometric Method.

Introduction:

DNA exhibit strong absorption of ultraviolet light due to the presence of conjugated double bands of the constituent purine and pyrimidine base. These have a characteristics absorbance mixture of 269 nm which is linearly related with the concentration of DNA in solution upto on OD value of 20. This Spectrophotometric method can also be employed for judging purity of DNA preparation. Proteins are usually the major contaminates in nucleic acid extracts and these absorption maxima at 280 nm. The ratio of absorption at 260-280 nm, hence provides a rough idea about the extent of contaminants in the preparation. A ratio between 1.8 to 2.0 is indicative of fairly pure DNA preparation but values less than is signify the presence of proteins as impurities.

Materials and Reagents

1. UV Spectrophotometer.

2. Saline Sodium Citrate (SSC) solution: Prepare 0.015M solution of Sodium Citrate (pH 7.0) and dissolve NaCl so that its final concentration in solution is 0.15 M.

Procedure:

1. Switch on the spectrophotometer and allow it to warm up for about 10 min. Adjust the wavelength at 260 nm and put on; the UV lamp.

2. Set the instrument at zero absorbance with SSC solution.

3. Read absorbance of solution of provided sample. If OD is too high, appropriately dilute the sample solution with SSC and again take the reading.

4. Calculate concentration of DNA in the sample from following formula:

For dsDNA:

$$\text{Concentration of DNA} = \frac{50 \ x \ \text{OD at 260} \ x \ \text{DF}}{1000}$$

where   DF= Dilution Factor in sample solution

Calculation: Conc. of DNA $= \dfrac{50 \ x \ \text{OD at 260} \ x \ \text{DF}}{1000}$

Dilution factor = 100

Observation Table:

DNA sample	OD at 260nm	OD at 280nm	Ratio OD260/OD280	DNA conc.
B_1				
B_2				
B_3				

Average=B_1+B_2+B_3/3 = ...µg/µL

Results: Quantity of DNA (conc.) by spectrophotometric method = µg/µl.

Experiment 28: Agarose Gel Electrophoresis (Age) for Separation of DNA.

Gel-Loading Buffers: Gel-loading buffers are mixed with the samples before loading into the slots of the gel. These buffers serve three purposes. They increase the density of the sample, ensuring that the DNA sinks evenly into the well; they add colour to the sample, thereby simplifying the loading process; and they contain dyes that, in an electric field, move toward the anode at predictable rates. Bromophenol blue migrates through agarose gels -2.2-fold faster than xylene cyanol FF, independent of the agarose concentration. Bromophenol blue migrates through agarose gels run in 0.5× TBE at approximately the same rate as linear double stranded DNA 300 bp in length, where-as xylene cyanol migrates at approximately the same rate as linear double-stranded DNA 4 kb in length. These relationships are not significantly affected by the concentration of agarose in the gel over the range of 0.5- 1.4%.

6X Gel-loading Buffers

Buffer type	Buffer type 6X Buffer	Storage Temperature
I.	0.25% bromophenol blue	4°C
	0.25% xylene cyanol FF	
	40% (w/v) sucrose in H_2O	
II.	0.25% bromophenol blue	Room temp
	0.25% xylene cyanol FF	
	15% Ficoll	
III.	0.25% bromophenol blue	4°C
	0.25% xylene cyanol FF	
	30% glycerol in H_2O	
IV.	0.25% bromophenol blue	4°C
	40% (w/v) sucrose in H_2O	

Materials:

Buffers and Solutions

(i) **Agarose solutions:** Agarose gels are cast by melting the agarose in the presence of the desired buffer until a clear, transparent solution is achieved. The melted solution is then poured into a mold and allowed to harden. Upon hardening, the agarose forms a matrix, the density of which is determined by the concentration of the agarose.

(ii) **Electrophoresis buffer** (1× TAE or 0.5× TBE)

(iii) **Ethidium bromide** or SYBR Gold staining solution

(iv) 6× Gel-loading buffer.

Nucleic Acids and Oligonucleotides

❖ DNA samples

❖ DNA size standards

Samples of DNAs of known size are typically generated by restriction enzyme digestion of a plasmid or bacteriophage DNA of known sequence. Alternatively, they are produced by ligating a monomer DNA fragment of known size into a ladder of polymeric forms. Size standards for both agarose and polyacrylamide gel electrophoresis may be purchased from commercial sources or they can be prepared easily in the laboratory. It is a good idea to have two size ranges of standards, including a high-molecular-weight range from I kb to >20 kb and a low-molecular weight range from 100 bp to 1000 bp. A stock solution of size standards can be prepared by dilution with a gel-loading buffer and then used as needed in individual electrophoresis experiments.

Equipment:

❖ Equipment for agarose gel electrophoresis

❖ Clean, dry horizontal electrophoresis apparatus with chamber and comb or clean dry glass plates with appropriate comb.

❖ Gel-sealing tape.

❖ Common types of lab tape, such as Time tape or VWR lab tape, are appropriate for sealing the ends of the agarose gel during pouring.

❖ Microwave oven or Boiling water bath.

❖ Power supply device capable of up to 500 V and 200 mA. Water bath preset to 55°C.

Procedure:

1. Seal the edges of a clean, dry glass plate or the open ends of the plastic tray supplied with the electrophoresis apparatus with tape to form a mold. Set the mold on a horizontal section of the bench.

2. Prepare sufficient electrophoresis buffer (1x TAE or 0.5x TBE) to fill the electrophoresis tank and to cast the gel.

3. Prepare a solution of agarose in electrophoresis buffer at a concentration appropriate for separating the particular size fragments expected in the DNA sample. Add the correct amount of powdered agarose to a measured quantity of electrophoresis buffer in an Erlenmeyer flask or a glass bottle. The buffer should occupy less than 50% of the volume of the flask or bottle.

4. Loosely plug the neck of Erlenmeyer flask with Kim wipes. If using a glass bottle, make certain the cap is loose. Heat the slurry in a boiling-water bath or a microwave oven until the agarose dissolves.

5. Use insulated gloves or tongs to transfer the flask/bottle into a water bath at 55°C. When the molten gel has cooled, add ethidium bromide to a final concentration of 0.5 µg/mL.

   Mix the gel solution thoroughly by gentle swirling.

6. While the agarose solution is cooling, choose an appropriate comb for forming the sample slots in the gel. Position the comb 0.5-1.0 mm above the plate so that a complete well is formed when the agarose is added to the mold.

7. Pour the warm agarose solution into the mold. The gel should be between 3 mm and 5 mm thick. Check that no air bubbles are under or between the teeth of the comb. Air bubbles present in the molten gel can be removed easily by poking them with the corner of a Kirnwipe.

8. Allow the gel to set completely (30-45 minutes at room temperature), then pour a small amount of electrophoresis buffer on the top of the gel and carefully remove the comb. Pour off the electrophoresis buffer and carefully remove the tape. Mount the gel in the electrophoresis tank.

9. Add just enough electrophoresis buffers to cover the gel to a depth of 1 mm. It is not necessary to pre-run an agarose gel before the samples are loaded.

10. Mix the samples of DNA with 0.20 volumes of the desired 6x gel-loading buffer.

11. Slowly load the sample mixture into the slots of the submerged gel using a disposable micropipette, an automatic micropipettor or a drawn-out Pasteur pipette or glass capillary tube. Load size standards into slots on both the right and left sides of the gel.

12. Close the lid of the gel tank and attach the electrical leads so that DNA will migrate toward the positive anode (red lead). Apply a voltage of 1-5 V/cm measured as the distance between the positive and negative electrodes. If the leads have been attached correctly, bubbles should be generated at the anode and cathode (due to electrolysis) and within a few minutes, the bromophenol blue should migrate from the wells into the body of the gel. Run the gel until the bromophenol blue and xylene cyanol have migrated an appropriate distance through the gel.

13. When the DNA samples or dyes have migrated a sufficient distance through the gel, turn off the electric current and remove the leads and lid from the gel tank. If ethidium bromide is present in the gel and electrophoresis buffer, examine the gel by UV light and photograph the gel. Otherwise, stain the gel by immersing it in electrophoresis buffer or H_2O containing ethidium bromide (0.5 pg/mL) for 30-45 minutes at room temperature or by soaking in a 1:10,000-fold dilution of SYBR Gold stock solution in electrophoresis buffer.

Range of seperation of standard Low-EEO Agarose

Agarose concentration in gel (% w/v)	Range of separation of linear DNA molecules (kb)
0.3	5
0.6	1
0.7	0.8-10
0.9	0
1.2	0
1.5	0
2.0	0

Precautions

1. The maximum amount of DNA that can be applied to a slot depends on the number of fragments in the sample and their sizes. The minimum amount of DNA that can be detected by photography of ethidium-bromide stained gels is 2 ng in a 0.5 cm wide band. More sensitive dyes such as SYBR Gold can detect as little as 20 pg of DNA in a band. If there is more than 500 ng of DNA in a band of 0.5 cm, the slot will be overloaded, resulting in trailing, smiling and smearing - problems that become more severe as the size of the DNA increases. When simple populations of DNA molecules e.g., bacteriophage or plasmid DNAs are to be analyzed, 100-500 ng of DNA should be loaded per 0.5 cm slot. When the sample consists of a very large

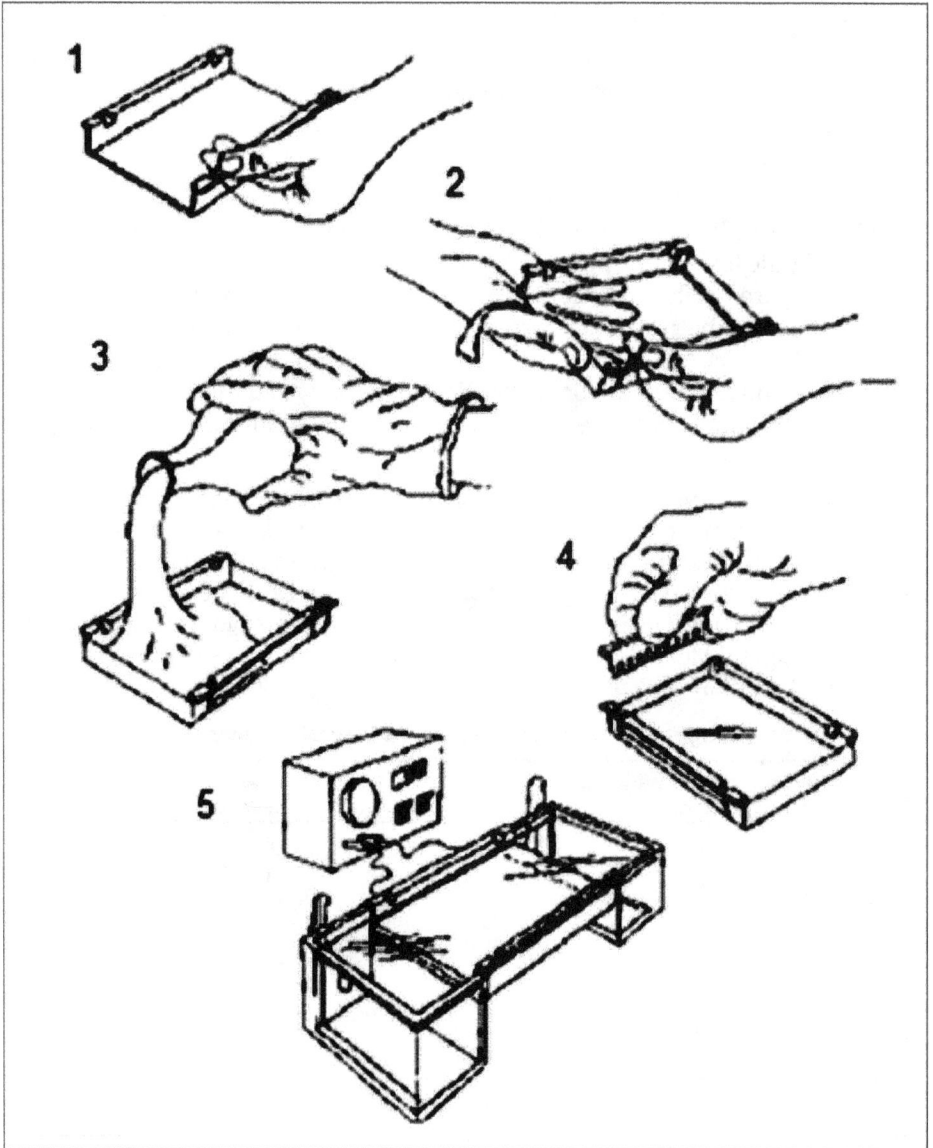

Range of Separation of standard Low-EEO Agarose

number of DNA fragments of different sizes e.g., restriction digests of mammalian DNA, it is possible to load 20-30 pg of DNA per slot without significant loss of resolution.

2.   When preparing gels that contain low concentrations of agarose (<0.5%), first pour a supporting gel (1% agarose) without wells. Allow this gel to harden at room temperature on the glass plate or plastic tray and then pour the lower-percentage gel directly on top of the supporting gel. Stacking the gels in this way reduces the chance that the lower percentage gel will fracture during subsequent manipulations e.g., photography and processing for Southern hybridization. Make sure that both gels are made from the same batch of buffer and contain the same concentration of ethidium bromide. Gels cast with low-melting-temperature agarose and gels that contain less than 0.5% agarose can also be chilled to 4°C and run in a cold room to reduce the chance of fracture.

3.   The maximum volume of solution that can be loaded is determined by the dimensions of the slot. A typical slot [0.5 x 0.5 x 0.15 cm] will hold about 40 μL. Do not overfill a slot with a DNA sample solution. To reduce the possibility of contaminating neighboring samples, it is best to make the gel a little thicker or to concentrate the DNA by ethanol precipitation rather than to fill the slot completely.

4.   The presence of ethidium bromide allows the gel to be examined by UV illumination at any stage during electrophoresis. The gel tray may be removed and placed directly on a transilluminator. Alternatively, the gel may be examined using a hand-held source of UV light. In either case, turn off the power supply before examining the gel.

5.   During electrophoresis, the ethidium bromide migrates toward the cathode (in the direction opposite to that of the DNA). Electrophoresis for protracted periods of time can result in the loss of significant amounts of ethidium bromide from the gel, making detection of small fragments difficult. In this case, re-stain the gel by soaking it for 30-45 minutes in a solution of ethidium bromide.

Glossary

Abiotic element: A physical or chemical feature of an environment or ecosystem.

Abiotic: Non-biological.

Absolute temperature: Temperature measured from absolute zero.

Absorption: The process by which one substance is taken into the body of another substance.

Abundance: The number or amount of something.

Acclimation: The process during which an individual organism undergoes morphological and/or physiological adaptation to one or more abiotic elements.

Acclimatization: The adaptation of a living organism (plant, animal or microorganism) to a changed environment that subjects it to physiological stress. Acclimatization should not be confused with adaptation.

Acellular: Describing tissues or organisms that are not made up of separate cells but often have more than one nucleus.

Acid precipitation: Acidic rain, snow or dry particles deposited from the air due to increased acids released by anthropogenic or natural resources.

Acid rain: Generally, precipitation in any form or dry deposition, with a pH lower than would be expected from natural and artificial causes.

Acid: A substance which releases hydrogen ions when dissolved in water. A strong acid will release a large proportion of hydrogen ions whereas a weak acid will release a small proportion of hydrogen ions.

Acidity: The ability of a water solution to neutralize an alkali or base.

Acrylamide gels: A polymer gel used for electrophoresis of DNA or protein to measure their sizes (in daltons for proteins or in base pairs for DNA). Acrylamide gels are especially useful for high resolution separations of DNA in the range of tens to hundreds of nucleotides in length.

Actinomycetes: Filamentous bacteria, many of which are valuable in the production of antibiotics.

Activated carbon: A material that has a very porous structure and is an adsorbent for organic matter and certain dissolved gases.

Activated sludge method: A method of sewage treatment in which wastes are degraded by complex populations of aerobic microorganisms.

Activated sludge: The active material, consisting largely bacteria and protozoa used to purify sewage.

Active solar system: A mechanical system that actively collects, concentrates and stores solar energy.

Active transport: The energy-requiring process by which molecules are carried across cell boundaries. Molecules are often concentrated inside cells as a result.

Acute poverty: Insufficient income or access to resources needed to provide the basic necessities for life such as food, shelter, sanitation, clean water, medical care and education.

Adaptation: The fitness of a structure, function or entire organism for life in a particular environment, the process, brought about by natural selection, of becoming so fitted.

Adiabatic: A thermal process occuring without any exchange of heat.

Advanced waste treatment: The removal of noncarbonaceous materials such as excess phosphorus and nitrogen. The term implies treatment beyond secondary treatment and advanced treatment is most effective after the organic matter has been removed.

Aerobes: Organisms that can only existt with free oxygen, *i.e.* that have aerobing breathing.

Aerobic organisms: Organisms that can utilize oxygen as the final electron acceptor during metabolism.

Aerodynamics: The science dealing with the motion of gases and bodies in gases.

Aerosols: Gaseous, solid or liquid materials distributed very finely in the air.

Aerotaxis: Responding to oxygen.

Aflatoxin: Any of several toxins produced by molds such as *Aspergillus flavus*; some are suspected of being carcinogenic.

Agar: A gelatinous polysaccharide, extracted from Ceylon moss that is used to prepare solid media for cultivating bacteria.

Agrobacterium tumefaciens*:* A gram-negative, rod-shaped flagellated bacterium responsible for crown gall tumor in plants. Following infection, the TI plasmid from the bacterium becomes integrated into the host plant's DNA and the presence of the bacterium is no longer necessary for the continued growth of the cell. This bacterium is now used to deliberately transfer genetic material into plants through biotechnology.

Agroecosystem: A community of microorganisms, plants and animals, together with their abiotic environment, that occurs on farmed land and including the crop species.

Algae: A group of simple aquatic plants capable of photosynthesis.

Alternative energy: Energy derived from sources other than the burning of coal petroleum or natural gas or from nuclear fusion or nuclear fission. Examples of alternative energy installations are biogas, solar power, hydroelectric power or wind power.

Alum: A common name for aluminum sulfate, used as a coagulant.

Amalgam: A solution of a metal in mercury.

Ammonia fertilizer: A material with a high concentration of nitrogen compounds put on soil to stimulate plant growth.

Ammonification: The reduction of nitrates and nitrites to ammonium compounds by soil saprobes.

Anabolism: The synthesis of complex molecules from simpler ones.

Anaerobes: Organisms that can exist without free oxygen *e.g.*, intestial bacteria, tape worms, in contrast to aerobes. See also denitrifikation.

Anaerobic biological treatment: Any treatment that utilizes anaerobic organisms to reduce organic matter in wastes.

Antagonism: Opposing effects produced by drugs, hormones etc., on living systems.

Anthropogenic: Produced as aresult of human activities.

Anthropogenous: A concept based on Greek word *anthropos* (=Man). An anthropogenous factor is a factor which is caused or created by Man.

Antibiotic resistance: Plasmids generally contain genes which confer on the host bacterium the ability to survive a given antibiotic. If the plasmid pBR322 is present in a host, that host will not be killed by ampicillin or tetracycline. By using plasmids containing antibiotic resistance genes, the researcher can kill off all the bacteria which have not taken up his plasmid, thus ensuring that the plasmid will be propagated as the surviving cells divide.

Antibiotic: A secondary biotic substance secreted by an organism which inhibits growth in other organisms.

Antigen: A substance that can incite the production of specific antibodies and can combine with those antibodies.

Antiseptic: A substance that inhibits or kills microbes.

Antitoxin: An antibody that neutralizes a toxin.

Aquatic: Occurring in water, existing in water, in contrast to terrestrial.

Aquifer: A body of rock or a zone within a body of rock, those contain sufficient saturated permeable material to yield economically significant quantities of ground water to wells and springs.

Artesian aquifer: An aquifer bounded above and below by impermeable beds or beds of distinctly lower permeability than that of the aquifer itself, causing the water to be under a hydrostatic pressure.

Artificial recharge: The practice of increasing, by artificial means, the amount of water that enters a ground water reservoir.

Asbestos: The fibrous form of several silicate minerals, at one time widely used for electrical and thermal insulation and fire protection and as a strong, durable and cheap construction material.

Asbestosis: A dust disease caused by the inhalation of asbestos fibers.

Assimilation capacity: The ability of a body of water that receives waste components to permit the aerobic metabolism of waste to proceed without elimination due to oxygen supply.

Association: A conceptual grouping of populations in a community characterized by particular dominant species.

Autecology: The study of the relationships between a single species and its environment.

Autoclave: A sterilizing device employing steam under pressure.

Autolysis: The decomposition of a dead microorganism by its own enzymes.

Autoradiography: A process to detect radioactively labeled molecules which usually have been separated in an SDS-PAGE or agarose gel based on their ability to create an image on photographic or X-ray film. This process does not result in a linear relationship between the intensity of the signal and the amount of radioactivity unless special steps are taken. There is now increasing use of phosphor imagers and other modern devices to detect and quantitate radioactive molecules which have been separated in gels.

Autotrophic nutrition: The process by which an organism manufactures its own food from inorganic compounds.

Autotrophic: Applied to organisms which synthesize organic from inorganic substances.

Axial-flow pump: A pump in which the fluid is forced along parallel to the axis.

B cells: An important class of white blood cells that mature in bone marrow and produce antibodies. They are largely responsible for the antibody-mediated or humoral immune response; they give rise to the antibody-producing plasma cells and some other cells of the immune system.

BAC: Bacterial Artificial Chromosome, a cloning vector capable of carrying between 100 and 300 kilobases of target sequence. They are propagated as a mini-chromosome in a bacterial host. The size of the typical BAC is ideal for use as an intermediate in large-scale genome sequencing projects. Entire genomes can be cloned into BAC libraries and entire BAC clones can be shotgun-sequenced fairly rapidly.

Bacillus thuringiensis (Bt): A naturally occurring bacterium present in soil and used successfully by home gardeners and organic farmers to control certain insects for more than 30 years. When ingested by a target insect, the protein produced by *Bt.* controls the insect by disturbing the digestive system. The *Bt.* protein is harmLess to other insects, people and animals.

Backwash: The process in which beds of filter or ion-exchange media are subjected to flow opposite to the service flow direction to loosen the bed and to flush suspended matter, collected during the service run, to waste.

Bactericide: An agent capable of killing bacteria.

Bacteriophage lambda: A virus which infects *E. coli* and which is often used in molecular genetics experiments as a vector or cloning vehicle. Recombinant phages can be made in which certain non-essential lambda DNA is removed and replaced with the DNA of interest. The phage can accommodate a DNA insert of about 15-20 kb. Replication of that virus will thus replicate the investigator's DNA.

Bacteriophage: A virus that infects bacteria.

Bacteriostat: An agent that prevents bacterial growth by interfering with reproductive and metabolic process.

Bacterium: A class of single cell organisms.

Balance of nature: Ecological balance.

Base: A component of DNA made up of nitrogen and carbon atoms in a ring structure. There are two classes of bases: purines (adenine and guanine) and pyrimidines (cytosine and thymine). The bases pair in the DNA double helix.

Batch culture = batch system: Culture technique in which the nutrients are not renewed or the waste prducts removed during the process. A system that is not fed continuously.

Batch fermentation: A process in which cells or micro-organisms are grown for a limited time. At the beginning of the fermentation, an inoculum is introduced into fresh medium, with no addition or removal of medium for the duration of the process.

Benthic: Applied to organism living close to the bottom of a lake or sea.

Benthos: The bottom of a sea or lake anywhere from the high water mark down to the deepest level; the organisms living there.

Bentonite: A very fine clay formed by the alteration of volcanic ash deposits.

Binding site: A place on cellular DNA to which a protein (such as a transcription factor) can bind. Typically, binding sites might be found in the vicinity of genes and would be involved in activating transcription of that gene (promoter elements), in enhancing the transcription of that gene (enhancer elements) or in reducing the transcription of that gene (silencers).

Binomial system: The system of naming organisms by two Latin words.

Bioassay: The quantitative measurement, under standardized conditions of the effects of a substance on an organism or part of an organism.

Biobased products: Fuels, chemicals, building materials or electric power or heat produced from biological material. The term may include any energy, commercial or industrial products, other than food or feed that uses biological products or renewable domestic agricultural (plant, animal and marine) or forestry materials.

Biocenosis: The community of different life forms regularly occurring in a biotope.

Biochemical oxygen demand (BOD): The amount of oxygen used for biochemical oxidation by a unit volume of water at a given temperature and for a given time.

Biocides: Agents that kill living organism. Sometimes the term is used as a synonym for pesticides.

Biodegradation: The breakdown of substances by microorganisms.

Bioenergetics: Considerations of energy flow in living systems.

Biogeochemical cycling: The pathways of nutrients through ecosystems.

Biological-biochemical degradation: The breakdown of a material (sewage, refuse, etc.) by the action of organisms, bacteria and weathering.

Biological boundaries: A concept that differentiates one organism from another and suggests that organisms cannot or should not exchange genetic material. An alternative concept is that genes are defined not by the organism from which they came, but by their function. As scientists have identified genes in seemingly non-related organisms such as plants and humans, they have found identical genes in each.

Biological control: The control of pests by the use of the other living organisms.

Biological indicator: A species or organism that is used to grade environmental quality or change.

Biological magnification or biomagnification: The phenomenon in which the concentration of a chemical substance such as a pesticide increases in the organism the higher the organism is on the food chain.

Biological monitoring: The direct measurement of changes in the biological status of a habitat, based on evaluations of the number and distribution of individuals or species before and after a change.

Biological process: A process which involves a reaction normally carried out in a living cell or organism.

Biomass fuel: A carbon based fuel derived from plants that were living recently as opposed to a fossil fuel.

Biomass: The total weight of the organism's continuing a given tropic level or inhabiting a defined area. The standing crop that is the total amount of living organic material in a given ecosystem. The total weight of all organisms in any particular environment.

Biopharming: The production of biopharmaceuticals in plants or domestic animals.

Bioseston: All the living matter floating or swimming in water.

Biosphere: That part of the Earth and its atmosphere in which organisms live. The portion of the earth in which living systems are encountered.

Biosystematics: The study of biology of population especially in regard to their breeding systems and reproductive behaviour.

Biota: The flora and fauna of an area.

Biotechnology: A set of biological techniques developed through basic research and now applied to research and product development. Biotechnology refers to the use of recombinant DNA, cell fusion and new bioprocessing techniques.

Biotechnology: The application of living organisms to develop new products.

Biotechnology-derived: The use of molecular biology and/or recombinant DNA technology or *in vitro* gene transfer, to develop products or to impart specific capabilities in plants or other living organisms.

Biotic element: The organisms, populations and communities of an ecosystem.

Biotic factors: Influences on the environment that result from the activities of living organisms.

Biotic potential: An estimate of the maximum rate of increase of a species in the absence of competition from predators, parasites, etc.

Biotic: Living or biological in origin.

Biotope: A habitat that is uniform in its main climatic, soil and biotic conditions.

Biowastes (wetwastes): Biowastes are organic wastes such as food, vegetables and fruits which are sent to compost factory and converted into humus matter (stabilized organic matter).

Box: Refers to a short nucleic acid consensus sequence or motif that is universal within kingdoms of organisms. Examples of DNA boxes are the Pribow box (TATAAT) for RNA polymerase, the Hogness box (TATA) that has a similar function in eukaryotic organisms and the homeo box. RNA boxes have also been described, such as Pilipenko's Box-A motif that may be involved in ribosome binding in some viral RNAs.

Bt **corn:** A corn plant that has been developed though biotechnology so that the plant tissues express a protein derived from a bacterium, Bacillus thuringiensis, which is toxic to some insects but non-toxic to humans and other mammals.

Buffer: A substance in a solution capable of neutralizing both acids and bases.

Calorie: The amount of heat required to raise the temperature of 1 gram of water from 15 to 16°C; 1 joule = 4,182 calories.

Calorific value: The number of units of heat obtained by the complete combustion of a unit mass of a substance.

Cap site: Two usages: In eukaryotes, the cap site is the position in the gene at which transcription starts and really should be called the transcription initiation site. The first nucleotide is transcribed from this site to start the nascent RNA chain. That nucleotide becomes the 5' end of the chain and thus the nucleotide to which the cap structure is attached. In bacteria, the CAP site (note the capital letters) is a site on the DNA to which a protein factor (the Catabolite Activated Protein) binds.

Cap: All eukaryotes have at the 5' end of their messages a structure called a cap, consisting of a 7-methylguanosine in 5'-5' tri-phosphate linkage with the first nucleotide of the mRNA. It is added post-transcriptionally and is not encoded in the DNA.

Capsid: Protein coat that surrounds the nucleic acid of a virus.

Capsule: A gelatinous structure that surrounds some bacteria.

Carburetor: A device which mixes air and gasoline for firing in an internal combustion engine.

Carcinogen: Cancer causing agent.

Carcinogenity: The characteristics of triggering off cancer, cancer can be triggered off amongst other things by various chemicals, physical cause or viruses.

Carrying capacity: The steady state population density of a given habitat for a particular species.

CAT assay: An enzyme assay. CAT stands for chloramphenicol acetyl transferase, a bacterial enzyme which inactivates chloramphenicol by acetylating it. CAT assays are often performed to test the function of a promoter. The gene coding for CAT is linked onto a promoter (transcription control region) from another gene and the construct is transfected into cultured cells. The amount of CAT enzyme produced is taken to indicate the transcriptional activity of the promoter (relative to other promoters which must be tested in parallel). It is easier to perform a CAT assay than it is to do a Northern blot, so CAT assays were a common method for testing the effects of sequence changes on promoter function. Largely supplanted by the reporter gene luciferase.

Catabolism: The breaking down by organisms of complex molecules into simpler ones with the liberation of energy.

Catabolite repression: The inhibition of gene activity by an efficiently degraded catabolite.

Catabolite: A compound that is capable of being degraded.

Catalyst: A substance that speeds up the rate of a chemical reaction without being altered or depleted in the process.

CCAAT box: (CAT box, CAAT box and other variants) A sequence found in the 5' flanking region of certain genes which is necessary for efficient expression. A transcription factor (CCAAT-binding protein, CBP) binds to this site.

Cell recycle: The return of a concentrated biomass to a continuous flow reactor.

Cell: The lowest denomination of life thought to be possible. Most organisms consist of more than one cell which becomes specialized into particular functions to enable the whole organism to function properly. Cells contain DNA and many other elements to enable the cell to function.

Cell: Volumetric elements of solid waste which is covered with natural soil or covering material and compacted in the sanitary landfill area.

Cellulase: Enzyme that degrades cellulose into glucose units.

Cellulose: A polymer of glucose subunits, principal structural component of plant cell walls.

Centrifugal pump: A pump in which the fluid is caused to flow by centrifugal force.

Centrifugation: A process wherein gravitational force in excess of natural gravity is maintained due to rotary motion.

Chain: Four or more bacteria attached end-to-end.

Chelate: A five or six membered ring in which a central metallic ion is bound in a coordination complex.

Chemical-feed pump: A mechanical device designed to introduce chemicals into a water system at a rate proportional to the water flow. Also called a chemical feeder.

Chemical oxygen demand (COD): The weight of oxygen taken up by the organic matter in a sample of water, expressed as parts per million of oxygen taken up from a solution of boiling potassium dichromate in two hours. The test is used to assess the strength of sewage and trade wastes.

Chemoautotrophic: Applied to organisms that produce organic material from inorganic compounds using simple inorganic reactions as a source of energy.

Chemoheterotrophs: Organisms that use chemical energy and an organic sorce of carbon.

Chemolithotrophs: Organisms that grow in strictly mineral medium.

Chemostat: A device used to grow bacteria in the laboratory that allows nutrients to be added and waste products removed continuously.

Chemotaxis, Chemotactic: Movement of an organism in response to chemicals in the environment.

Chemotrophic: Applied to organism that obtains energy from any source other than light.

Chlorinated hydrocarbons: Organic compounds in which one or several of the hydrogen atoms have been replaced by chlorine atoms (as, for example, in solvents, pesticides, plastics).

Chlorination: The use of chlorine gas or solutions of its compounds to disinfect water or as an oxidizing agent.

Chlorine demand: A measure of the amount of chlorine which can be consumed by organic matter and other oxidizable substances in water without chlorine residual.

Chlorophyll: A green pigment, present in algae and higher plants that absorbs light energy and thus plays a vital role in photosynthsis.

Chloroplasts: A plastid in eukaryotes that contains chlorophyll and is the site of photosynthesis and starch formation.

Chromosome walking: A technique for cloning everything in the genome around a known piece of DNA (the starting probe).

Chromosome: The array of genes responsible for the determination and transmission of hereditary characteristics.

Chromosomes: The self-replicating genetic structure of cells containing the cellular DNA. Humans have 23 pairs of chromosomes.

Ciliates: Microorganisms covered with short, whip like extensions called cilia.

Cilium: A short, projecting hair like organelle of locomotion, similar to a flagellum.

Cistron: A nucleic acid segment corresponding to a polypeptide chain, including the relevant translational start (initiation) and stop (termination) codons.

City climate: The climate produced within a city which often differs from the climate in the surrounding countryside.

Clarification: The process of making water clear and free of suspended impurities.

Clarifier: A settling tank.

Climate: The long-term or integrated manifestation of weather.

Clone: Describes a large number of cells, viruses or molecules which are identical and which are derived from a single ancestral cell, virus or molecule. The term can be used to refer to the process of isolating single cells or viruses and letting them proliferate (as in a hybridoma clone, which is a biological clone) or the process of isolating and replicating a piece of DNA by recombinant DNA techniques (molecular clone). The use of the word as a verb is acceptable for the former meaning, but not necessarily the latter meaning.

Coagulase: An enzyme that clots plasma.

Coagulation: The process in which very small, finely divided solid particles, often colloidal in nature, are agglomerated into larger particles.

Coccus: Spherical bacteria.

Coding sequence: The portion of a gene or an mRNA which actually codes for a protein. Introns are not coding sequences; nor are 5' or 3' untranslated regions or the flanking regions, for that matter, they are not even transcribed into mRNA. The coding sequence in a cDNA or mature mRNA includes everything from the AUG (or ATG) initiation codon through to the stop codon, inclusive.

Coding strand: an ambiguous term intended to refer to one specific strand in a double-stranded gene.

Codon Bias: The tendency for an organism or virus to use certain codons more than others to encode a particular amino acid. An important detrminant of codon bias is the guanosine-cytosine (GC) content of the genome. An organism that has a relatively low G+C content of 30% will be less likely to have a G or C at the third position of a codon (wobble position) than an A or T to specify an amino acid that can be represented by more than one codon.

Codon: In an mRNA, a codon is a sequence of three nucleotides which codes for the incorporation of a specific amino acid into the growing protein. The sequence of codons in the mRNA unambiguously defines the primary structure of the final protein. Of course, the codons in the mRNA were also present in the genomic DNA, but the sequence may be interrupted by introns.

Coenzyme: A small organic molecule that transfers small molecules from one enzyme to another.

Coliform bacteria: A group of bacteria that are normally abundant in the intestinal tracts of humans and other warm blooded animals and are used as indicators when testing the sanitary quality of water.

Colloid: A phase so highly dispersed that surface forces are an important factor in determining its properties.

Colonization: Establishment of a site of reproduction of microbes on a material, animal or person without necessarily resulting in tissue invasion or damage.

Colony: A group of bacteria in a culture derived from the multiplication of single cell; usually visible to the unaided eye.

Combustion: The reaction of a substance with oxygen at high temperature with the production of heat.

Community: Any naturally occurring group of organisms that occupy a common environment. The term is a general one, covering groups of various sizes. A grouping of interacting populations in a particular habitat.

Competent: A condition in which a bacterial cell is capable of taking up and integrating high molecular weight DNA into its chromosome.

Competition: The struggle for existence that results when two or more species have requirements which exceed the available supply.

Competitive inhibition: The inhibition of enzyme activity caused by the competition between the inhibitor and the substrate for the active (catalytic) site on the enzyme.

Complex: The meeting of several communities, in which each community is characterized by its own dominants, subdominants etc.

Compost: A soil conditioner made by mixing organic wastes in a container in order to accelerate their decomposition. A matter which is suitable for the soil. It is produced by aerobic stabilization of organic solid wastes.

Compound: A chemical combination of two or more elements in definite ratios by weight in which the set of characteristics of each element is lost.

Compressor: An engine in which a fluid is placed under high pressure.

Conductivity: The quality or power of a medium to transmit electrical charges, in water, the conductivity is related to the concentration of ions capable of holding electrical charges.

Conformational Epitope: An epitope which is dependent upon folding of a protein; amino acid residues present in the antibody binding site are often located at sites in the primary sequence of the protein which are at some distance from each other. The vast majority of B-cell (antibody binding) epitopes are conformational.

Consensus Sequence: A linear series of nucleotides, commonly with gaps and some degeneracy that define common features of homologous sequences or recognition sites for proteins that act on or bind to nucleic acids.

Consensus sequence: A nominal sequence inferred from multiple, imperfect examples. Multiple lanes of shotgun sequence can be merged to show a consensus sequence. The optimal sequence of nucleotides recognized by some factor. A DNA binding site for a protein may vary substantially, but one can infer the consensus sequence for the binding site by comparing numerous examples. For example, the (fictitious) transcription factor ZQ1 usually binds to the sequences AAAGTT, AAGGTT or AAGATT. The consensus sequence for that factor is said to be AARRTT where R is any purine, *i.e.*, A or G. ZQ1 may also be able to weakly bind to ACAGTT which differs by one base from the consensus.

Conservation: The preservation or protection from decay or destruction of anything whose loss it is desirable to prevent.

Conservative Substitution: A nucleotide mutation which alters the amino acid sequence of the protein, but which causes the substitution of one amino acid with another which has a side chain with similar charge/polarity characteristics. The size of the side chain may also be an important consideration. Conservative mutations are generally considered unlikely to profoundly alter the structure or function of a protein, but there are many exceptions.

Consolidation: Squeezing together; making smaller and denser.

Consumer: A heterotophic population in an ecosystem which is utilizing dead or living organic matter as a source of food.

Consumptive use: The difference between the total quantity of water withdrawn from the source for use and the quantity of water, in liquid form, returned to the source. It includes mainly water transpired by plants and evaporated from the soil.

Contact stabilization: A modification of the activated sludge process in which the wastewater is held in contact with a very high concentration of activated sludge for a short period of time. This is followed by quiescent settling and re-aeration of a portion of the sludge prior to its recycling.

Contaminated Soils: The term contaminated soils is applied to former waste disposal sites or storage places of toxic materials and top areas of land polluted by former industrial plants which have not been sealed according to the state of the art and thus represent a danger to the environment, especially to ground water.

Contamination: The introduction to the water or foodstuffs of substances containing toxins or live pathogens which constitute a hazard to human health.

Contig: A series of two or more individual DNA sequence determinations that overlap. In a sequencing project the contigs get larger and larger until the gaps between the contigs are filled in.

Continuous flow system: A biological system in which the feed substrates are fed to the reactor continuously. Usually the system is operated at a constant volume so that the rate of outflow is equal to the rate of inflow.

Control elements: DNA sequences in genes that interact with regulatory proteins (such as transcription factors) to determine the rate and timing of expression of the genes as well as the beginning and end of the transcript.

Control parameters: Factors used in the design and operation of a process to control the rate of the process. For example, mean hydraulic retention time, hydraulic recycle ratio and concentration sludge in the recycle to an activated sludge process are control parameters for the system.

Control: That part of an experimental procedure which is like the treated part in every respect except that it is not subjected to the test conditions.

Convection: The process by which heat is transferred through the movement of gases.

Correlation: The relationship between two variables, according to a specific range of values.

Corrosion: The conversion of iron and other metals to oxides and carbonates by the action of air and water.

Cosmid: A genetically-engineered plasmid containing bacteriophage lambda packaging signals and potentially very large pieces of inserted foreign DNA (up to 50 kb) which can be replicated in bacterial cells. Cosmid cloning allows for isolation of DNA fragments which are larger than those which can be cloned in conventional plasmids.

Cost-benefit analysis: An economic technique for estimating the desirability of a proposed course of action, in which the advantages and disadvantages are listed, expressed in monetary terms and the totals compared.

Cost-benefit ratio: The ratio of the gross costs of a proposed activity to the gross benefits, both costs and benefits being discounted over the life of the project at an annual rate of interest.

Cover glass: A thin glass slip used to cover an object mounted on a glass microscope slide.

Covering material: Soil or another material which covers the compacted solid wastes in the sanitary landfill area.

Cracking: A process that uses heat to decompose complex substances.

Creutzfeldt-Jakob disease (CJD): A disease of humans hypothesized to be caused by a prion or a small protein, which alters the structure of a normal brain protein, resulting in destruction of brain neural tissue. The most common form is thought to have genetic origins. There is strong epidemiologic and laboratory evidence for a causal association between new variant CJD and BSE.

Cross section: A view of a structure cut through at right angles to its axis.

Cry1A: A protein derived from the bacterium *Bacillus thuringiensis* that is toxic to some insects when ingested. This bacterium occurs widely in nature and has been used for decades as an insecticide although it constitutes less than 2% of the overall insecticides used.

Cultivar: Synonymous with variety; the international equivalent of variety.

Culture medium: A preparation containing nutrients and growth factors suitable for the cultivation of microorganisms.

Culture: A growth of microorganisms.

Cyanides: A class of very toxic compounds, ingestion or inhalation of which may cause death to mammals.

Cyanobacteria: Blue-green algae.

Cytolysis: Cell destruction, especially when brought about by the destruction of the plasma memrane.

Cytotype: A sample member of population composed of individuals whose karyotype is identical and different from that of other populations.

Dark field microscopy: A microscopic technique in which objects appear brightly illuminated against a dark background.

Database Search: Once an open reading frame or a partial amino acid sequence has been determined, the investigator compares the sequence with others in the databases using a computer and a search algorithm. This is usually done in a protein database such as PIR or Swiss-Prot. Nucleic acid sequences are in GenBank and EMBL databases. The search algorithms most commonly used are BLAST and FASTA.

Death phase: The stage in which the number of viable bacteria in a population decreases at an exponential rate.

Dechlorination: The removal of excess chlorine residual.

Decibel (dB) : A unit used to measure the intensity of sound on a logarithmic scale based on measurements of sound intensity in watts per square meter and related to a reference 10^{-12} W/m², which is the intensity of the quietest sound perceptible to the human ear.

Decomposer: Heterotropic organisms in an ecosystem which obtain energy from the breakdown of dead organic matter to more simple substances.

Decomposition: The separation of complex organic substances into simpler compounds.

Decontamination: Destruction of pathogenic microorganisms and viruses and their toxic products.

Deep well pump: A pump which operates beneath the surface of the fluid.

Deflation: The picking up and removal of loose material by the wind.

Deformation: Any change in the original form or volume of a rock body produced by any kind of forces.

Degeneracy: Refers to the fact that multiple different codons in mRNA can specify the same amino acid in an encoded protein.

Demography: The study of the age and sex structure, geographical distribution, rate of change of size, etc., of human populations.

Denaturation: With respect to nucleic acids, refers to the conversion from double-stranded to the single-stranded state, often achieved by heating or alkaline conditions. This is also called melting DNA. With respect to proteins, refers to the disruption of tertiary and secondary structure, often achieved by heat, detergents, chaotropes and sulfhydryl-reducing agents.

Denaturing Gel: An agarose or acrylamide gel run under conditions which destroy secondary or tertiary protein or RNA structure. For protein, this usually means the inclusion of 2-ME (which reduces disulfide bonds between cysteine residues) and SDS and/or urea in an acrylamide gel. For RNA, this usually means the inclusion of formaldehyde or glyoxal to destroy higher ordered RNA structures. In DNA sequencing gels, urea is included to denature dsDNA to ssDNA strands. In denaturing gels, macromolecules tend to be separated on the basis of size and charge, while shape and oligomerization of molecules are not important.

Denitrification: A biological process in which nitrite are reduced to nitrogen gas. Denitrification plays a vital role in the nitrogen cycle and it is an important engineering process for the removal of nitrogen from wastewaters. The metabolic process by which nitrate is reduced to nitrogen gas.

Density: The mass of a unit volume of a substance.

Density-dependent: Applied to a limiting factor in the growth of a population that is dependent upon the existing population density (*e.g.*, disease, reproductive rate, access to food).

Density-independent: Applied to a situation in which the percentage mortality or survival of a species varies independently of population density.

Detention period: The average length of time for which a unit volume of fluid is retained in a tank during a flow process.

Detergent: A surface active agent used to remove dirt and grease from a surface. Soap is a detergent.

Diatoms: Single celled alga whose cell walls are composed of polymerized ortho silicic acid.

Dideoxy Sequencing: Enzymatic determination of DNA or RNA sequence by the method of Sanger and colleagues, based on the incorporation of chain terminating di-deoxynucleotides in a growing nucleic acid strand copied by DNA polymerase or reverse transcriptase from a DNA or RNA template. Separate reactions include di-deoxynucleotides containing A, C, G or T bases. The reaction products represent a collection of new. Labeled DNA strands of varying lengths, all terminating with a di-deoxynucleotide at the 3' end (at the site of a complementary base in the template nucleic acid) and are separated in a polyacrylamide/urea gel to generate a sequence ladder. This method is more commonly used than Maxam-Gilbert (chemical) sequencing.

Digestion: The breaking down of complex food substances into simpler compounds, which can then be used in metabolism.

Dilute: Describes a solution which contains a relatively small quantity of solute.

Dilution: The dispersal of a fluid within a much large receiving volume of another fluid.

Dioxin: TCDD (2, 3, 7, 8-tetrachlorodibenzo-p-di-oxin; $C_{12}H_4Cl_4O_2$), A byproduct formed during the preparation of the herbicide 2, 4, 5-T and sometime produced by the incineration of chlorinated organic compounds.

Direct Repeats: Identical or related sequences present in two or more copies in the same orientation in the same molecule of DNA; they are not necessarily adjacent.

Discarded batteries: Used batteries of various types, such as mercury, cadmium, nickel and lead-acid, may be sold for the recovery of reusable materials.

Discharge: The volume of water flowing past a given point in a stream channel in a given period of time.

Disinfection: The destruction of pathogens by applying agents (disinfectants) such as chlorine.

Disposal well: A well used to dispose of waste by injection into a deep aquifer.

Disposal: Procedures which are related with some activities such as temporarily gathering at houses and places, collecting from these places, transporting to final station and appraising for saving of matter and energy. The last procedure includes recycling, recovery and reuse. Sanitary landfill and incineration are also disposal alternatives.

Dissolved oxygen: Oxygen molecules that are dissolved in water, usually expressed in parts per million (ppm).

Dissolved solids: The weight of matter in true solution in a stated volume of water, including both inorganic and organic matter.

Distributor: A device or system designed to produce even flow through all sections of an ion exchange or filter bed and to retain the filter medium in the tank or vessel.

District heating: A system that uses hot water from a single source to heat buildings nearby.

DNA (deoxyribonucleic acid): The genetic material of all cells and many viruses. The molecule that encodes genetic information. DNA is a double-stranded molecule held together by weak bonds between base pairs of nucleotides. The four nucleotides in DNA contain the bases adenine (A), guanine (G), cytosine (C) and thymine (T). In nature, base pairs form only between A and T and between G and C; thus the base sequence of each single strand can be deduced from that of its partner.

DNA Ligase: An enzyme (usually from the T_4 bacteriophage) which catalyzes formation of a phosphodiester bond between two adjacent bases from double-stranded DNA fragments. RNA ligases also exist, but are rarely used in molecular biology.

DNase: Deoxyribonuclease, a class of enzymes which digest DNA. The most common is DNase I, an endonuclease which digests both single and double-stranded DNA.

Domestic solid waste: They are wasted from the houses, which are not stated on the list of hazardous waste. Also, wastes which are originated from the large green areas such as park, garden, picnic area, are classified into this category.

Domestic: A term applying to a household or private residence.

Dominance (clique): A group of individuals in a population which has established itself in the highest position in the social hierarchy.

Dominance (ecological): The phenomena in which energy flowing through an ecosystem is directed especially through a limited number of populations.

Dominance (social): The psychological imposition of a hierarchical order in a population which determines the priority of access of individuals to essential requirements.

Dominant: The characteristic and often the tallest, species in a particular plant community. The dominant species is the one that exerts the greatest influence on the character of the community and may give it its name.

Dormancy: A resting condition in which the growth of an organism is halted and its metabolic rate slowed.

Dot blot: A technique for measuring the amount of one specific DNA or RNA in a complex mixture. The samples are spotted onto a hybridization membrane such as nitrocellulose or activated nylon, etc., fixed and hybridized with a radioactive probe. The extent of labelling as determined by autoradiography and densitometry is proportional to the concentration of the target molecule in the sample. Standards provide a means of calibrating the results.

Double helix: The twisted-ladder shape that two linear strands of DNA assume when complementary nucleotides on opposing strands bond together.

Doubling time: Used in a demograpic sense to indicate the period which is estimated will pass before population density doubles.

Downstream: Identifies sequences proceeding farther in the direction of expression; for example, the coding region is downstream from the initiation codon, toward the 3' end of an mRNA molecule. Sometimes used to refer to a position within a protein sequence, in which case downstream is toward the carboxyl end which is synthesized after the amino end during translation.

Dried matter: Amount of remainder after drying of a sample into an oven at 103°C for 24 hours until it reaches to constant weight, which is taken from solid wastes or composts.

Dry wastes: It can be collected by the containers for valuable materials such as glass, paper, cardboard, plastics, metals and similar recyclable wastes.

Duplex: A nucleic acid molecule in which two strands are base paired with each other.

Dust: Solid particles (1-1100 micrometres in diameter) that are carried into the atmosphere, from which they settle by gravity.

Dynamic stability: In the atmosphere, in the presence of factors that induce turbulence, a condition in which small perturbations of the flow do not tend to grow.

Earthquake: A shaking of the surface of the earth due to a shifting of material beneath the surface.

Ecological balance: Balance of nature. The condition of equilibrium among the components of a natural community such that their relative numbers remain fairly constant and their ecosystem is stable.

Ecological capacity: Carrying capacity.

Ecological equivalent: A population with similar adaptations but different origins which has evolved under comparable environmental selections pressures.

Ecological factor: Any environmental factor that influences living organisms.

Ecological niche: A total expression of the environmental factors to which a particular population is exposed. The particular role that an organism plays in the activities of the ecosystem.

Ecological pyramid: A grouping of the successively diminishing tropic levels of an ecosystem.

Ecology: The study of the relationships among living organisms and between those organisms and their non-living environment.

Economic conservation: The management of natural resources or the environment, so as to sustain a regular yield of a commodity at the highest level feasible.

Ecosphere: The biosphere, together with all the ecological factors that act upon organisms. That portion of the earth which includes the biosphere and all the ecological factors which operate on the living organisms it contains.

Ecosystem: A community of interdependent organism's together with the environment they inhabit and with which they interact and which is distinct from adjacent communities and environments. A conceptual unit formed from a defined series of interacting communities and all the environmental factors which operate upon them.

Ecotoxicology: The science of the effects of toxic substances on ecosystems or their parts.

Ecotype: A sub specific group that is adapted genetically to a particular habitat but which can interbreed with other ecotypes of the same species or coenospecies without loss of fertility.

Edaphic factors: Those chemical, physical and biological characteristics of the soil which affect an ecosystem.

Effluent charge: A charge levied against a polluter for each unit of effluent discharged into public water.

Effluent standard: The maximum amount of a specified pollutant an effluent is permitted to contain.

Effluent: Generally, any fluid emitted by a source. More specifically, a waste fluid (usually liquid) produced by an agricultural or industrial process.

Elasticity: The tendency of a material to return to its original shape after it has been placed under stress.

Electron acceptor: A chemical entity that accepts electrons transferred to it from another compound. It is an oxidizing agent that, by virtue of its accepting electrons, is itself reduced in the process. Oxygen is the terminal electron acceptor in aerobic metabolism.

Electron carrier: A molecule that accepts electrons (is reduced) and passes them to another carrier or to a final electron acceptor.

Electron donor: A compound or element that furnishes electrons for reductive reactions.

Electroporation: A method for introducing foreign nucleic acid into bacterial or eukaryotic cells that uses a brief, high voltage DC charge which renders the cells permeable to the nucleic acid. Also useful for introducing synthetic peptides into eukaryotic cells.

Electrostatic filter: A device in which the application of a static electric charge to a filter improves the efficiency with which it collects small particles.

Embryo: An organism in the process of developing from a fertilized or parthogenetically activated ovum.

Embryonic stem (ES) cells: Cell lines derived from early embryos that have the potential to differentiate into all types of somatic cells as well as to form germ line cells and hence whole animals, when injected into early embryos.

Emigration: The movement of individuals out of the population.

Emission: (Immission): The reception of a substance from a remote source of emission, the opposite of emission.

Emission standards: The maximum amount of a specified pollutant an effluent is permitted to contain.

Emulsifier: A material used to help mix an oily substance with water.

End Labeling: The technique of adding a radioactively labeled group to one end (5' or 3' end) of a DNA strand.

End product inhibition: The inhibition of the first enzyme of a biosynthetic pathway by the end product of the pathway.

Endemic: Confined to a given region and having originated there.

Endogenous: Growing inside a plant or animal.

Endogenous phase: The period of declining growth of a microorganism when stored food is being consumed and respiration is slowed.

Endogenous respiration: The oxidation of internal carbon resources in a cell. The term is also used to describe the process of auto digestion in a microbial population.

Endogenous retrovirus: Integrated retrovirus DNA (provirus) derived from infection of the germLine of an ancestral animal. All animals are thought to carry numerous endogenous (but nonfunctional) retroviruses, some of which were inserted many millions of years ago.

Endonuclease: Cleaves bonds within a nucleic acid chain; they may be specific for RNA or for single-stranded or double-stranded DNA. A restriction enzyme is a type of endonuclease.

Endoplasmic reticulum: Internal membrane of a eukaryotic cell to which ribosomes are attached.

Endospore: A very resistant form of a resting bacterial cell.

Endotoxin: A poisonous substance present in the cell walls of Gram negative bacteria.

Energy budget: A record of the flow of energy through a system.

Energy flow: The passage of energy through the trophic levels of a food chain.

Energy source: Ligth or an oxidizable compound or element utilized by the cell in the synthesis of ATP.

Engine curves: Graphs showing the performance of an engine.

Enhancer: A eukaryotic transcriptional control element which is a DNA sequence which acts at some distance to enhance the activity of a specific promoter sequence. Unlike promoter sequences, the position and orientation of the enhancer sequence is generally not important to its activity.

Enhancer: An enhancer is a nucleotide sequence to which transcription factors bind and which increases the transcription of a gene. It is not part of a promoter; the basic difference being that an enhancer can be moved around anywhere in the general vicinity of the gene (within several thousand nucleotides on either side or even within an intron) and it will still function. It can even be clipped out and spliced back in backwards and will still operate. A promoter, on the other hand, is position and orientation dependent. Some enhancers are conditional, in other words, they enhance transcription only under certain conditions, for example in the presence of a hormone.

Enrichment culture: A technique used for isolating an organs from a mixed culture by manipulating conditions that favor growth of the organism sought and minimize growth of the other organisms present.

Enthalpy : The heat content of a body or system, usually given by the formula $H = U + pV$; where H is the hat content, U the internal energy , p the pressure and V the volume.

Entropy: A measure of the degree of disorder within a system. The term is derived from thermodynamics; heat passes from warmer to cooler bodies, thus becoming dispersed more generally with time, so that within a closed system eventually all heat will be distributed evenly.

Enucleated oocyte (cytoplast): An egg cell from which the nucleus has been removed mechanically.

Environment: It is an outer media in which human or another living being sustain own interactions during their life. The physical elements of this media are air, water and soil; the biological elements are producers (plants), consumers (animals) and decomposers (bacteria and fungus); the economical environmental elements are the activities of human, which are related with utilization and operation of natural, human, economical and materialistic sources; the social elements are demographic structure and historical and cultural infrastructure of human and the type of life with respect to accommodation, health, education and culture demands. The physical, chemical and biotic conditions surrounding a living organism.

Environmental Impact Assessment (EIA): The identification and evaluation of the environmental consequences of a proposed development and of the measures intended to minimize adverse effects. There are five definitions for EIA, given below:

1. Studies which are done for determining the effect of legal procedures, policies, programs, projects and operation conditions on the biogeophysical environment and human health, finding out the magnitude of these effects, conclusion and printing studies of the results.

2. Studies which are done for determining and forecasting of advantages and disadvantages of a planned activity. Environmental impact assessment must be clear and understandable enough for the people and authoritative deciders and supported by the regulations which become effective in whole country.

3. Studies which are done for investigation of environmental, social and economical effects of projects, plans, policies and programs, systematically. The main goal of environmental impact assessment is to define the results of different alternatives for authoritative deciders before the final decision step.

4. Studies which are done for forecasting of the effects of an activity on the environmental quality.

5. Studies which are done for evaluating of the environmental and social effects, which are meaningful, which could be raised after an activity.

Environmental Impact Statement (EIS): A written report, based on detailed studies carried out in the course of an environment impact assessment that describes the environmental consequences of a course of action in order to assist in decision-making.

Environmental Protection Agency (EPA): The federal agency of the US government, established in 1970, that is responsible for dealing with the pollution of air and water by solid waste, pesticides and radiation and with nuisances caused by noise.

Environmental protection: That part of resource management which is concerned with the discharge into the environment of substances that might be harmful or that might have harmful physical effects and with safeguarding beneficial uses.

Environmental quality standards: The maximum limits or concentrations of pollutants that are permitted in specific media.

Environmental resistance: The restriction of population growth by the interaction of ecological factors.

Enzyme: A protein catalyst.

Epilimnion: The warmer uppermost layer of water, which lies above the thermocline in a lake and which are subject to disturbance by wind.

Epitope: As related to protein antigens, B-cell epitopes consist of the amino acid residues of a protein molecule which interact directly through noncovalent bonds with the amino acid residues of a particular antibody molecule (complementarity determining region). The average epitope probably involves about 15-20 contact amino acid residues, but one or two of these may be critical to the epitope's specificity and the avidity of the antibody-antigen reaction. B-cell epitopes may be either linear or conformational in nature. T-cell epitopes represent the small, processed peptides which bind to MHC class I and II molecules on the surface of T cells.

Equilibrium: The state in which the action of multiple forces produces a steady balance, resulting in no change over time.

Equivalent weight : The weight, in grams, of an element, compound or ion which would react with or replace one gram of hydrogen, the molecular weight in grams divided by the valence.

Erosion: The breakdown of solid rock into smalller particles and its removal by wind, water or ice.

Ethidium Bromide: Intercalates within the structure of nucleic acids in such a way that they fluoresce under UV light. Ethidium bromide staining is commonly used to visualize RNA or DNA in agarose gels placed on UV light boxes. Proper precautions are required, because the ethidium bromide is highly mutagenic and the UV light damaging to the eyes. Ethidium bromide is also included in cesium chloride gradients during ultracentrifugation, to separate super coiled circular DNA from linear and relaxed circular DNA.

Etiology: The science of the causes of disease aand the complete range of factors which can lead to disease.

Eukaryote: Organism whose cells has chromosomes with nucleosomal structure and separated from the cytoplasm by a two-membrane nuclear envelope and compartmentalization of functions in distinct cytoplasmic organelles.

Eukaryotic: Complex cells characterized by a nuclear membrane, mitochondria and chromosomes; distinct from prokaryotic.

Euphotic zone: The upper zone of a sea or lake into which sufficient light can penetrate for active photosynthesis to take place.

Eutrophic: Applied to the waters that are rich in plant nutrients and therefore highly productive, the large number of planktonic organisms sometimes rendering them cloudy.

Eutrophication: The enrichment of a water body with plant nutrients.

Evaporating: Changing from a liquid into a vapor form.

Evaporation: The change of phase from liquid to gas, the energy being supplied as latent heat from the surrounding medium.

Evaporation pond: A body of seawater that is enclosed to allow the water to evaporate and so leave behind a deposit of salt.

Evaporimeter: An instrument for measuring the rate of evaporation of water from a surface.

Evaporite: A mineral precipitated as a result of evaporation.

Evapotranspiration: The combined evaporation of water from the soil surface and transpiration from plants. The total loss of water from a land surface, including both that lost from living organisms and from surface evaporation.

Evergreen: Applied to a plant that bears leaves throughout the year.

Evolution: The process of cumulative change, usually gradual.

Excretion: The process by which an organism rids itself of the waste products of metabolism.

Exonuclease: An enzyme which hydroylzes DNA beginning at one end of a strand, releasing nucleotides one at a time, there are 3' or 5' exonucleases.

Exothermic: Applied to animals which achieve any temperature regulation they to possess through behavioral adjustment to external environmental conditions, rather than depending on internal physiological controls.

Exotic: Applied to a specific found in region to which it is not native.

Exponential growth: The increase in a value over a period by a fixed percentage of the original value, such that the increase in each period is equal to the original value plus the interest accumulated in the preceding period.

Exposure: The concentration of environmental factors, for example chemicals, which a particular object is exposed to.

Expression clone: This is a clone (plasmid in bacteria or maybe ë phage in bacteria) which is designed to produce a protein from the DNA insert. Mammalian genes do not function in bacteria, so to get bacterial expression from your mammalian cDNA, you would place its coding region *i.e.* no introns, immediately adjacent to bacterial transcription/translation control sequences. That artificial construct (expression clone) will produce a pseudo-mammalian protein if put back into bacteria. Often, that protein can be recognized by antibodies raised against the authentic mammalian protein and vice versa.

Expression Vector: A plasmid or phage designed for production of a polypeptide from inserted foreign DNA under specific controls. Often an inducer is used.

The vector always provides a promoter and often the transcriptional start site, ribosomal binding sequence and initiation codon. In some cases the product is a fusion protein.

Expression: Usually used to refer to the entire process of producing a protein from a gene, which includes transcription, translation, post-translational modification and possibly transport reactions.

Extended aeration process: A modification of the activated sludge process in which all of the sludge from the secondary clarifier is returned to the aeration chamber. The process is intended to achieve total oxidation of both the inflowing waste and the biomass produced in the process.

Extinction: The disappearance of a population as a result of the total failure of any individuals within it to reproduce the unique genotypes which it contained.

Extracellular: Outside of the cell wall.

Facultative: Used to describe organisms that are able to grow in either the absence or presence of a specific environmental factor.

Facultative anaerobe: An organism that can grow in the presence or absence of oxygen.

Family: Applied in taxonomic sense, a commonly utilized classificatory category which incorporates a range of genera possessing a number of characteristics in common.

Fauna: The animals of a particular region or period of time.

Faunal regions: Regions of the world with distinct natural faunas.

Fecal coliform: Matter containing or derived from animal or human waste containing one or more of the coli form groups of bacteria.

Fecal streptococcus: Matter containing or derived from animal or human waste containing one or more of the streptococcus groups of bacteria.

Feral: Refers to an individual or population that has returned to the wild after a history of domestication.

Fermentation: The breakdown of organic substances by organisms with the release of energy; especially the anaerobic breakdown of carbohydrates by yeasts and bacteria to form carbon dioxide and ethanol or other organic compounds.

Fertilizer: Any substance that is applied to land as a source of nutrients for plant growth. It may be a waste that is being recycled (*e.g.*, farmyard manure, crop residues or compost) or produced industrially.

Fibroblast: A type of relatively undifferentiated cell found in many parts of the body involved primarily in wound healing. Fibroblasts are relatively easy to grow in cell culture and often are used for this purpose.

Filament: A threadlike structure.

Filter: As used here, a device of porous material that removes dirt from air that is forced through it.

Filtration: Passage of an aqueous or gaseous carrier, water or air through a porous medium (sand, charcoal, etc.) for the purpose of trapping undesirable materials, usually in suspension, in the water or air.

Final covering: Covering material which acts like daily covering material on the top of the landfill area.

First trophic level: Food chain. A number of organisms that form a series through which energy is passed.

Fitness: The ability to survive to reproductive age and produce viable offspring. Fitness also describes the frequency distribution of reproductive success for a population of sexually mature adults.

Flagelatta: A class of protozoa whose adult members swim by means of flagella.

Flocculation: A process of contact and adhesion whereby the particles of a dispersed substance form large clusters or the aggregation of particles in a colloid to form small lumps, which then settle out.

Flora: The plants of a particular region or period of time.

Flotation : The process in which immiscible liquid particles , such as grease and oil or particulate solid, such as clays or bacteria, are separated from aqueous suspension due to a density difference.

Flow: As used here, air or gas which is involved in the movement of a body through it.

Fly ash: Finely divided particles of ash that are entrained in flue gases resulting from the combustion of fuel or other material.

Food chain: The succession of populations through which energy flow in an ecosystem as a result of consumer - consumed relationships.

Food web: A complex scheme incorporating food chain relationships between populations at various trophic levels in an ecosystem.

Foot printing: A technique by which one identifies a protein binding site on cellular DNA. The presence of a bound protein prevents DNase from nicking that region, which can be detected by an appropriately designed gel.

Formation: Term used for a classificatory category of vegetation characterized by dominants of a specific life form.

Fossil fuel: A fuel derived from ancient organic remains.

Fragmentation: A form of asexual reproduction in which a filament composed of a string of cells breaks up and forms new organisms.

Free-swimming: Not attached; capable of independent movement.

Frequency: The number of occurrences or cycles per second.

Friction: The resistance to the motion of two surfaces against each other.

Fumigation: A rapid increase in air pollution close to ground level, which sometimes leads to very high concentrations of pollutants for an hour or more.

Fungicide: An agent that kills fungi.

Gel electrophoresis: A method to analyze the size of DNA (or RNA) fragments. In the presence of an electric field, larger fragments of DNA move through a gel slower than smaller ones. If a sample contains fragments at four different discrete sizes, those four size classes will, when subjected to electrophoresis, all migrate in groups, producing four migrating bands. Usually, these are visualized by soaking the gel in a dye (ethidium bromide) which makes the DNA fluoresce under UV light.

Gel shift assay: A method by which one can determine whether a particular protein preparation contains factors which bind to a particular DNA fragment. When a radio labeled DNA fragment is run on a gel, it shows a characteristic mobility. If it is first incubated with a cellular extract of proteins or with purified protein, any protein-DNA complexes will migrate slower than the naked DNA- a shifted band.

Gene: An element of deoxyribonucleic acid that transmits a hereditary characteristic.

Gene flow: The exchange of genetic traits between populations by movement of individuals, gametes or spores. It involves the spread of new variants among different populations through dispersal.

Gene frequency: The ratio of the occurrence of one allele of a gene in the population in a relation to other alleles of this same gene.

Gene gun: A device invented at Cornell University that allows genetic material to be introduced into a new organism. The genetic material from the donor is shot into cells of the recipient and the material is incorporated into its DNA.

Gene splicing: The isolation of a gene from one organism and then the introduction of that gene into another organism using techniques of biotechnology.

Gene: The fundamental physical and functional unit of heredity. A gene is an ordered sequence of nucleotides located in a particular position on a particular chromosome that encodes a specific functional product such as a protein or RNA molecule.

A unit of DNA which performs one functions. Usually, this is equated with the production of one RNA or one protein. A gene contains coding regions, introns, untranslated regions and control regions.

General waste: No special treatment is necessary for this waste which can be disposed of with municipal waste. Food waste from tuberculosis or similar category treatment areas should be autoclaved before disposal.

Generation time: The time required for one cell to divide into two.

Genetic engineering: The technique of removing, modifying or adding genes to a DNA molecule to change the information it contains. By changing this information, genetic engineering changes the type or amount of proteins an organism is capable of producing, thus enabling it to make new substances or perform new functions.

Genetic marker: A known site on the chromosome. It might for example be the site of a locus with some recognizable phenotype or it may be the site of a polymorphism that can be experimentally discerned.

Genetically modified organism (GMO): Often, the label GMO and the term transgenic are used to refer to organisms that have acquired novel genes from other organisms by laboratory gene transfer methods.

Genetics: The study of the patterns of inheritance of specific traits.

Genome: All the genetic material in the chromosomes of a particular organism; its size is generally given as its total number of base pairs.

Genomic blot: A type of Southern blot specifically used to analyze a mixture of DNA fragments derived from total genomic DNA. Because genomic DNA is very complicated, when it has been digested with restriction enzymes, it produces a complex set of fragments ranging from tens of bp to tens of thousands of bp. However, any specific gene will be reproducibly found on only one or a few specific fragments. A million identical cells will produce a million identical restriction fragments for any given gene, so probing a genomic Southern with a gene-specific probe will produce a pattern of perhaps one or just a few bands.

Genomic clone: A piece of DNA taken from the genome of a cell or animal and spliced into a bacteriophage or other cloning vector. A genomic clone may contain coding regions, exons, introns, 5' flanking regions, 5' untranslated regions, 3' flanking regions, 3' untranslated regions or it may contain none of these, it may only contain intergenic DNA, usually not a desired outcome of a cloning experiment.

Genomics: It is the mapping and sequencing of all the genetic material in the **DNA** of a particular organism as well as the use of information derived from genome sequence data to further elucidate what genes do, how they are controlled and how they work together.

Genotype: The genetic identity of an individual. Genotype often is evident by outward characteristics.

Genotypic: Applied to variation which arises in an individual as the result of its possession of a specific genome.

Geotropism: A growth response of plants in which the stimulus is gravity.

GermLine cells: Cells that contain inherited material that comes from the eggs and sperm and that are passed on to offspring.

Glycolysis: The anaerobic first stage in the liberation of energy from food during respiration.

Gravity: The force that tends to pull all bodies toward the center of the earth.

GRE (Glucocorticoid Response Element): A binding site in a promoter to which the activated glucocorticoid receptor can bind. The glucocorticoid receptor is essentially a transcription factor which is activated only in the presence of glucocorticoids. The activated receptor will bind to a GRE and transcription of the adjacent gene will be altered. See also Response element.

Gross productivity: The rate which energy is procured by a particular tropic level or levels in an ecosystem.

Ground water: Water in the saturated zone found under hydrostatic pressure.

Growth factor: An organic compound other than the carbon and energy source that an organism requires and cannot synthesize - for example, a vitamin or an amino acid.

Habitat: A physical portion of the environment over which a particular population is dispersed. The dwelling place of a species or community.

Halocline: The boundary between two masses of water whose salinities differ.

Halogen: Halogens are the most reactive nonmetallic elements. The halogens include fluorine, chlorine, bromine, iodine and astatine.

Halogenate: The incorporation of one of the halogens fluorine, chlorine, bromine or iodine in an organic compound.

Halophile: An organism that prefers or requires a high salt medium.

Hardness: A measure of soap-neutralizing ions present in water; predominantly magnesium and calcium, but other alkali metal ions contribute to the effect.

Harmful and hazardous waste (HaHW) : Materials which are explosive, flammable, oxidable, toxic and eco-toxic, corrosive organic or inorganic, which produce toxic and flammable gaseous matter when contact with water.

Heat labile: Destroyed by heating at 100°C for 20 minutes.

Heat stable: Resistant to destruction by heating; heat stable toxin of *E. coli* resists boiling for 30 minutes.

Helix-loop-helix: A protein structural motif characteristic of certain DNA-binding proteins.

Herbicides: Chemical agents for combating weeds.

Herbicide-tolerant crop: Crop plants that have been developed to survive application(s) of one or more commercially available herbicides by the incorporation of certain gene(s) via biotechnology methods such as genetic engineering or traditional breeding methods (such as natural, chemical or radiation mutation).

Herbivore: A heteretroph which obtains energy from the consumption of usually living plants.

Heteroduplex DNA: Generated by base pairing between complementary single strands derived from different parental duplex molecules; heteroduplex DNA molecules occur during genetic recombination *in vivo* and during hybridization of different but related DNA strands in vitro. Since the sequences of the two strands in a heteroduplex differ, the molecule is not perfectly base-paired; the melting temperature of a heteroduplex DNA is dependent upon the number of mismatched base pairs.

Heterogeneous microbial population : A microbial population, for which the initial seed was obtained from some natural source expected to contain a diversity of microorganisms, developed in a system in which no attempt is made to control the species present other than the selection imparted by the environmental or operational conditions under which the cells are being grown.

Heterotrophic: An organism who obtains energy from the breakdown of complex organic substances.

High density polyethylene (PEHD = HDPE): High density plastic material used at bottom parts of non-alcoholic beverage containers, flower pots, drainage pipes and geo-membranes etc.

Holding structure: Any excavation, pond or closed embankment used to contain water or another solution until needed.

Home range: the area over which an animal generally moves in obtaining its food.

Homeostasis: The balanced condition of a biological process in which there is no change in the final products of a particular reaction.

Homolog: In diploid organisms, one member of a pair of matching chromosomes.

Homologous Recombination: The exchange of sequence between two related but different DNA or RNA molecules, with the result that a new chimeric molecule is created. Several mechanisms may result in recombination, but an essential requirement is the existence of a region of homology in the recombination partners. In DNA recombination, breakage of single strands of DNA in the two recombination partners is followed by joining of strands present in opposing molecules and may involve specific enzymes. Recombination of RNA molecules may occur by other mechanisms.

Horizontal gene transfer: Transmission of DNA between species, involving close contact between the donor's DNA and the recipient, uptake of DNA by the recipient and stable incorporation of the DNA into the recipient's genome.

Household dangerous wastes: They are such as batteries, drugs, cans of paint, cans of pesticid etc.

Huge solid waste: They are consisted of domestic materials such as refrigerator, wash machine and armchair, which could not be used and have huge volume.

Humidifier: A mechanical device for increasing the amount of water vapor in the air.

Humification: The microbial breakdown of dead organic matter in the soil to form the largely inert product humus.

Humus: The more or less decomposed organic matter in the soil.

Hybrid: Seed or plants produced as the result of controlled cross pollination as opposed to seed produced as the result of natural pollination. Hybrid seeds are selected to have higher quality traits, for example, yield or pest tolerance.

Hybridization: The process of base pairing leading to formation of duplex RNA or DNA or RNA-DNA molecules.

Hybridoma: A clone of plasmacytoma cells which secrete a monoclonal antibody; usually produced by fusion of peripheral or splenic plasma cells taken from an immunized mouse with an immortalized murine plasmacytoma cell line (fusion partner), followed by cloning and selection of appropriate antibody-producing cells.

Hydration: The chemical addition of water to a compound.

Hydraulic gradient: The change in static head per unit of distance in a given direction. If not specified, the direction generally is understood to be that of the maximum rate of decrease in head.

Hydrogen cyanide: A poisonous gas that has been implicated in industrial accidents.

Hydrological cycle: The circulation of water through the drainage basins on which precipitation falls and eventually back to the atmospher.

Hydrolysis: The chemical decomposition or splitting of a compound by reaction with water.

Hydrophilic: Compounds to which water molecules adhere.

Hydrosphere: Water covering of the Earth (seas, inland waters, ground water, water bound in air and ice).

Hydrostatic head: The height of a vertical column of water.

Hypolimnion: The colder, non-circulating layer of water in a lake lying below the thermocline.

Imhoff tank : A tank in which sedimentation treatment for sewage is combined with anaerobic biological treatment, sewage entering into an upper chamber, solids settling through slots into a lower digestion chamber and sludge removal being automatic.

Immigration: The migration of individuals into a population.

Immission: The reception of a substance from a remote source of emission, the opposite of emission.

Immune system: The system of cells and organs involved in the production and functioning of antibodies.

Immunity: The ability of an organism to combat infection by parasites.

Immunoprecipitation: A process whereby a particular protein of interest is isolated by the addition of a specific antibody, followed by centrifugation to pellet the resulting immune complexes. Often, staphylococcal proteins A or G, bound to sepharose or some other type of macroscopic particle, is added to the reaction mix to increase the size and ease collection of the complexes. Usually, the precipitated protein is subsequently examined by SDS-PAGE.

Impact: It is a change which is caused by an activity which affects the natural, economical and social elements of the environment, directly or indirectly, for a long or short period, permanently or temporarily, positively or negatively.

In vitro: In a test tube or other container as opposed to a plant or animal.

In vivo: In a living plant or animal as opposed to in a test tube or other container.

Incineration: Burning of garbage in special facilities utilizing inherent thermal values of solid wastes.

Incinerator: A device in which solid, semi-solid, liquid or gaseous combustible material is burnt as a means of disposal. If the material does not support combusting auxiliary fuel is added. Many types of industrial and domestic wastes are incinerated and there are many types of incinerator to deal with different wastes.

Incubation period: The time between the infection of the individual by a microorganisms and the first manifestation of the disease.

Indicator agar: Agar medium containing a component that is changed in a unique way a particular species of microorganisms.

Indicator species: Species whose presence indicates certain environmental conditions.

Indicator: A substance that changes from one colour to another in response to a specific chemical reaction.

Inducer: A substance responsible for activating certain genes.

Industrial waste: Solid material that is discarded from trading, commercial and industrial premises and requires disposal. It can be divided roughly into five categories: a) general factory rubbish, uncontaminated by factory process waste, b) relatively inert process waste, c) flammable process waste, d) acid or caustic wastes e) indisputably toxic wastes.

Infection: Invasion of tissues by microorganisms or viruses with or without the production of disease.

Infectious wastes: They could be categorized into three groups. The first group includes tools which carry the illness and are wasted from the clinics and wanted to insulate by the authorized hospital person. The second group includes pathogenic wastes such as tissue, blood organ, guinea pig organisms, etc., which are originated from the laboratories. The third group includes pathogenic samples which are wasted from operating room and emergency room.

Infiltration: The penetration of a permeable solid body or mass by a fluid that fills spaces within it. It is the process by which water seeps into the soil.

Infiltration rate: The speed with which water penetrates the soil. It is governed by the texture of the soil, the amount and type of vegetation cover and the slope of the ground.

Initiation Codon: The codon at which translation of a polypeptide chain is initiated. This is usually the first AUG triplet in the mRNA molecule from the 5' end, where the ribosome binds to the cap and begins to scan in a 3' direction. However, the surrounding sequence context is important and may lead to the first AUG being bypassed by the scanning ribosome in favor of an alternative, downstream AUG. Also called a start codon. Occasionally other codons may serve as initiation codons *e.g.,* UUG.

Insert: Foreign DNA placed within a vector molecule.

Insert: In a complete plasmid clone, there are two types of DNA — the vector sequences and the insert. The vector sequences are those regions necessary for propagation, antibiotic resistance and all those mudane functions necessary for useful cloning. In contrast, however, the insert is the piece of DNA in which you are really intereseted.

Insertion Sequence: A small bacterial transposon carrying only the genetic functions involved in transposition. There are usually inverted repeats at the ends of the insertion sequence.

Interaction: The phenomena which occurs when individual's sympatric populations encounter one another.

Interference: An interaction detrimental to one or more competing sympatric populations.

Intergenic: Between two genes; *e.g.,* intergenic DNA is the DNA found between two genes. The term is often used to mean non-functional DNA (or at least DNA with no known importance to the two genes flanking it). Alternatively, one might speak of the intergenic distance between two genes as the number of base pairs from the polyA site of the first gene to the cap site of the second. This usage might therefore include the promoter region of the second gene.

Intermediates: Compounds in a biochemical pathway that are metabolized further.

Intron: Introns are portions of genomic DNA which ARE transcribed but which are later spliced out. They thus are not present in the mature mRNA. Note that although the 3' flanking region is often transcribed, it is removed by endonucleolytic cleavage and not by splicing. It is not an intron.

Inverted Repeats: Two copies of the same or related sequence of DNA repeated in opposite orientation on the same molecule. Adjacent inverted repeats constitute a palindrome.

Ion exchange: A reversible replacement of certain ions by others; the direction of the exchange depends upon the affinities of the ion exchange for the ions present and the concentrations of the ions in the solution.

Ion exchange capacity: The quantity of a particular ion that can be replaced by ion exchange.

Ionic environment: A collection of all the charged atoms or groups of atoms in a particular environment.

Irrigation: The artificial watering of land.

Irritability: The response of living systems to external stimuli.

Karyotype: The chromosome complement of the nuclei of individual organisms within a population.

KB: Abbreviation for kilobase, one thousand bases.

Kinase: A kinase is in general an enzyme that catalyzes the transfer of a phosphate group from ATP to something else. In molecular biology, it has acquired the more specific verbal usage for the transfer onto DNA of a radio labeled phosphate group. This would be done in order to use the resultant hot DNA as a probe.

Knock In: Replacement of a gene by a mutant version of the same gene using homologous recombination.

Knock Out: Inactivation of a gene by homologous recombination following transfection with a suitable DNA construct.

Labeling of foods: The process of developing a list of ingredients contained in foods. Labels imply that the list of ingredients can be verified. The U S Food and Drug Administration has jurisdiction over what is stated on food labels.

Lagoon: An earthen holding pond for wastewater, usually used for biological treatment of the waste. Lagoons may be mechanically aerated (aerated lagoons), they may be designed to enchance anaerobic metabolism (anaerobic lagoons).

Land reclamation: The treatment of any unusable land *e.g.,* slag heaps, quarries, gravel pits, etc. usually by filling with refuse or leveling, until the land can be brought into productive use.

Land use: The deployment of land for any use. Competition for limited areas of land requires the establishment of priorities among claims, which is the object of land use planning.

Landfill: The disposal of refuse by tipping it on land. Often the refuse is used to fill in old mine workings or low-lying land, to reclaim land from water or to create a feature on flat land. If the refuse is deposited in prepared trenches or holes, over which earth can be heaped at the end of each day, this is called controlled tipping in UK and Sanitary Land-Fill in USA.

Latent: Currently inactive but capable of becoming active.

Leach field: Area where septic tank effluent is distributed for natural leaching.

Leachate: Water that has percolated through soil or a filter material, containing soluble substance and that, therefore, contain amounts of these substances in solution. Liquid which percolate through solid wastes.

Leaching: The removal of the soluble constituents of a rock, soil or ore (that which is leached being known as the leachate) by the action of percolating waters. Leaching is a major process in the development of porosity in limestone in the secondary enrichment of ores and in the formation of soils.

Legumes, leguminous plants: Plants that often have symbiotic nitrogen-fixing bacteria associated with them, such as peas, beans clover, alfalfa and so on.

Library: A library might be either a genomic library or a cDNA library.

Ligase: An enzyme, T4 DNA ligase, which can link pieces of DNA together. The pieces must have compatible ends (both of them blunt or else mutually compatible sticky ends) and the ligation reaction requires ATP.

Ligation: The process of splicing two pieces of DNA together. In practice, a pool of DNA fragments are treated with ligase in the presence of ATP and all possible splicing products are produced, including circularized forms and end-to-end ligation of 2, 3 or more pieces. Usually, only some of these products are useful and the investigator must have some way of selecting the desirable ones.

Lime: The common name for calcium oxide (CaO).

Limestone: A sedimentary rock consisting chiefly of calcium carbonate, primarily in the form of the mineral calcite.

Limnology: The study of the physical, chemical and biological components of fresh water.

Linker: A small piece of synthetic double stranded DNA which contains something useful, such as a restriction site. A linker might be ligated onto the end of another piece of DNA to provide a desired restriction site.

Lipid: A diverse group of organic substances that is relatively insoluble in water, but soluble in alcohol ether chloroform or other fat solvents.

Lithosphere: he uninhabited and, under normal conditions, solid materials of the Earth's crust.

Lithotroph: An organism that uses an inorganic electron donor.

Log phase: The period of growth following the lag phase during which very rapid growth occurs.

Logarithmic growth: The phase of growth in which the time required for doubling of the cell mass is constant.

Logistic curve: As applied to populations, an S-shaped curve of population growth which is initially slow steepens and then flattens out at an asymptote determined by the carrying capacity.

M13: A bacteriophage which infects certain strains of *E. coli*. The salient feature of this phage is that it packages only a single strand of DNA into its capsid. If the investigator has inserted some heterologous DNA into the M13 genome, copious quantities of single stranded DNA can subsequently be isolated from the phage capsids. M13 is often used to generate templates for DNA sequencing.

Macronutrient: An element or compound that is needed in relatively large quantities by an organism. Crop plants require amounts ranging from a few kilograms to a few hundred kilograms per hectare of carbon, hydrogen and oxygen supplied from carbon dioxide and water, as well as nitrogen, potassium and phosphorus supplied from the soil.

Marine: Belonging to the sea.

Mass production: The making of large numbers of identical products in a factory, often using production line techniques.

Mercaptans: Organic compounds with the general formula R-SH, meaning that the thiol group (-SH) is attached to a radical.

Mesophilic microorganisms: Microorganisms whose optimum temperature for growth lies between 20-45°C.

Metabolism: All the chemical reactions that take place in living organism, comprising both anabolism and catabolism. Basal metabolism is the energy exchange of an animal at rest.

Metabolite: A substance that is involved in metabolism.

Methane: An odourless, colourless and asphyxiating gas that can explode under certain circumtances and that can be produced by solid wastes undergoing anaerobic decomposition.

Methane oxidizers: A group of Gram-negative bacteria capable of utilizing methane as their sole carbon and energy source.

Metropolis: The chief city, often the capital city, of a country or region.

Microaerophilic organisms: Organisms that requires low concentrations of oxygen for growth.

Microbicide: A chemical toxic to microorganisms.

Microbiocide: Misspelling of microbicide or else perhaps a tiny biocide.

Microinjection: The introduction of DNA into the nucleus of an oocyte, embryo or other cell by injection through a very fine needle.

Micronutrient: An element or compound that is required by living organisms, but very small amounts. Plants require a few grams to a few hundred grams per hectare of iron, manganese, zinc, born, copper, molybdenum and cobalt.

Microsatellite: A microsatellite is a simple sequence repeat (SSR). It might be a homopolymer (...TTTTTTT...), a dinucleotide repeat (....CACACACACACACA.....), trinucleotide repeat ('....AGTAGTAGTAGTAGT...') etc. Due to polymerase slip, during DNA replication there is a slight chance these repeat sequences may become altered; copies of the repeat unit can be created or removed. Consequently, the exact number of repeat units may differ between unrelated individuals. Considering all the known microsatellite markers, no two individuals are identical. This is the basis for forensic DNA identification and for testing of familial relationships e.g., paternity testing.

Migration: Movements particular animals carry out regularly, often between breeding places and winter feeding grounds.

Minamata: A bay and town in Japan that gave its name to a disease of the

Mineralization: The microbial breakdown of humus and other organic material in soil to inorganic substances.

Mineralize: To convert an element from an organic to an inorganic form.

Minimal tillage practices: Practices that allow farmers to reduce the tilling of the land to conserve topsoil and its nutrients.

Mitochondria: Organelles in plant and animal cells that contain the respiratory enzymes.

Mitosis: A process of chromosome duplication.

Molecular biology: A general term referring to study of the structure and function of proteins and nucleic acids in biological systems.

Molecular diffusion: The spontaneous intermixing of different substances by molecular movement, giving uniform concentrations.

Molecular weight: The relative weight of an atom or molecule based on a scale in which the H atom is assigned the weight of 1.0.

Molecule: The smallest part of a compound that retains all the properties of the compound.

Monitoring programme: The systematic measuring, quantitatively or qualitatively, of a phenomenon or the presence of a substance, over a period of time. Experiments and demonstrations are observed in this way. Monitoring programes are often use to provide information on the distribution in space or time of pollutants, so that effective measures may be developed to limit their harmful effects should the results of the programme indicate that remedial measures are necessary.

Monocline: A localized zone of steeply dipping beds in a region of horizontal to low.

Monoclonal Antibody: An antibody with very specific and often unique binding specificity which is secreted by a biologically cloned line of plasmacytoma cells in the absence of other related antibodies with different binding specificities. Differs from polyclonal antibodies, which are mixed populations of antibody molecules such as may be present in a serum specimen, within which many different individual antibodies have different binding specificities.

Monosaccharide: A sugar, a simple carbonhydrate generally having the formula $C_nH_{2n}O_n$ where n can vary from three to eight. The most common are five and six.

Mortality: The rate of removal of individuals from a population by death.

Motif: A recurring pattern of short sequence of DNA, RNA or protein that usually serves as a recognition site or active site. The same motif can be found in a variety of types of organisms.

mRNA: An RNA which contains sequences coding for a protein. The term mRNA is used only for a mature transcript with polyA tail and with all introns removed, rather than the primary transcript in the nucleus. As such, an mRNA will have a 5' untranslated region, a coding region, a 3' untranslated region and (almost always) a poly(A) tail. Typically about 2% of the total cellular RNA is mRNA.

Mulch: A material e.g., straw, paper, plastic sheeting, that is used to protect the surface of the soil from erosion where the mulch is composed of biodegradable material it becomes incorporated into the topsoil to become humus.

Multicopy Plasmids: Present in bacteria at amounts greater than one per chromosome. Vectors for cloning DNA are usually multicopy; there are sometimes advantages in using a single copy plasmid.

Multiple Cloning Site: An artificially constructed region within a vector molecule which contains a number of closely spaced recognition sequences for restriction endonucleases. This serves as a convenient site into which foreign DNA may be inserted.

Municipal waste: Substances discarded as unusable by private households, offices, shops, etc., but not the waste products of industrial processing or manufacturing. Municipal waste is composed typically of paper organic matter, plastics, metals and non-metallic minerals e.g., ash. Historically, the content of plastics has increased rapidly and the ash content has decreased. Such waste is generally collected for disposal by incineration, land-fill, composting or destructive distillation and in some areas it is used as fuel to generate heat or power.

Mutagen, mutagenic agent: Any agent that increases the frequency at which DNA is altered (mutated).

Mutagen: An agent *e.g.*, X-rays, gammarays, mustard gas that can induce mutation.

Mutagenicity: The capability of certain activating factors *e.g.*, chemicals, radiation to trigger off changes in the genetic matterial of a cell.

Mutation breeding: Commonly used practices in plant breeding and other areas in which chemicals or radiation are applied to whole organisms, for example plants or cells so changes in the organism's DNA will occur. Such changes are then evaluated for their beneficial effects such as disease resistance.

Mutation: A sudden change in the chromosomes of a cell, most mutations being due to changes in the DNA of individual genes, others to alterations in the structure or number of chromosomes.

Mutualism: An association in which both partners benefit.

Nanoplankton: The smallest of the phytoplankton.

Natality: The rate of addition of new individuals to a population by birth.

Natural resource ecosystem: A natural ecosystem in which one part is of use to humans.

Natural selection: The concept developed by Charles Darwin that genes which produce characteristics that are more favorable in a particular environment will be more abundant in the next generation.

Net productivity: The increase in energy content of an ecosystem after deducting the amount lost in respiration at all trophic levels.

Niche: The specific part of a habitat occupied by an organism. The role an organism plays in an ecosystem.

Nick translation: A method for incorporating radioactive isotopes (typically 32P) into a piece of DNA. The DNA is randomLy nicked by DNase I and then starting from those nicks DNA polymerase I digests and then replaces a stretch of DNA. Radio labeled precursor nucleotide triphosphates can thus be incorporated.

Nitrate: Salt of nitric acid.

Nitrification: The conversion by aerobic soil bacteria (nitrifying bacteria) of organic nitrogen compunds into nitrates (NO_3^-), which can be absorbed by green plants. Dead organic matter is broken down into substances such as ammonia, which reacts with calcium carbonate forming ammonium carbonate. Ammonium carbonate is oxidized to nitrite (NO_2^-) by nitrite bacteria (Nitrosomonas), and then nitrites are converted to nitrates by nitrate bacteria (Nitrobacter).

Non-coding strand: Anti-sense strand.

Non-systematical landfill area: A landfill area in which solid wastes are wasted randomLy without any precautions for human and environmental health and dumped without any covering material. Sometimes these solid wastes are burned; finally, dust, smoke and odor occur.

Nuclear reprogramming: Restoration of the correct embryonic pattern of gene expression in a nucleus derived from a somatic cell and introduced into an oocyte.

Pollen: Microspores of seed-producing plants. Each pollen grain contains a much reduced male gametophyte. Pollen grains are transferred by wind, water, birds or other animals to the ovules or stigmas where pollen tubes containing male nuclei grow out and penetrate the embryo sac.

Pollution: The direct or indirect alternation of the physical, thermal, biological or radioactive properties of any part of the environment in such a way as to create a hazard or potential hazard to health, safety or welfare of any living species. Pollution may occur naturally, but the term is more commonly applied to changes wrought by the emission of industrial pollutants or by the careless discharge or disposal of human domestic wastes r sewage.

Polyacrylamide Gel (Page): Used to separate proteins and smaller DNA fragments and oligonucleotides by electrophoresis. When run under conditions which denature proteins *i.e.* in the presence of 2-mercaptoethanol, SDS and possibly urea, molecules are separated primarily on the basis of size.

Polychlorinated biphenyl: An extremely toxic chemical contained in transformers and capacitors.

Polyethyleneterephytalate (PET): PET is one of these resins preferred for non-alcolic bevarage containers owing to its particularities of being a cheap, light but rigid material capable of retaining carbonation.

Polymer: A substance formed by the joining together (polymerization) of simple basic chemical units (monomers) in a regular pattern.

Polymerase Chain Reaction (PCR): A DNA amplification reaction involving multiple (30 or more) cycles of primer annealing, extension and denaturation, usually using a heat-stable DNA polymerase such as Taq polymerase. Paired primers are used, which are complementary to opposing strands of the DNA and which flank the area to be amplified. Under optimal conditions, single DNA sequence can be amplified a million-fold.

Polymerase: An enzyme which catalyzes the addition of a nucleotide to a nucleic acid molecule. There are a wide variety of RNA and DNA polymerases which have a wide range of specific activities and which operate optimally under different conditions. In general, all polymerases require templates upon which to build a new strand of DNA or RNA; however, DNA polymerases also require a primer to initiate the new strand, while RNA polymerases start synthesis at a specific promoter sequence.

Polymorphism: Variation within a DNA or RNA sequence.

Polynucleotide Kinase: Enzyme which catalyzes the transfer of the terminal phosphate of ATP to 5' hydroxyl termini of polynucleotides, either DNA or RNA. Usually derived from T4 bacteriophage.

Polypeptide: A chain of amino acids joined by peptide bonds. Another term for a protein.

Polysaccharide: Long chains of monosaccharide subunits.

Polyvinyl chloride (PVC) : One of the most common plastic, used in the manifacture of clothing, furniture, gramophone records and containers and produced by the polymerization of vinyl chloride.

Population: A group of individuals, sharing some feature in common and living in a particular defined area that is considered without regard to interrelationship among them.

Population density: The size of a population in relation to the area in which it occurs, expressed as the number of individuals per unit area.

Population dynamics: The study of changes in population densities with time.

Population ecology: The study of the factors that affect the number of individuals of a particular population present in a specified area over a period of time.

Porosity: The pencentage of pore space in a rock. Porosity in sedimentary rocks ranges from less than 1% to more than 50% and depends on the sorting, angularity and packing of the grains, as well as on the degree of cementation of the rock.

Post-translational modification: Modifications made to a polypeptide molecule after its initial synthesis, this includes proteolytic cleavages, phosphorylation, glycosylation, carboxylation, addition of fatty acid moieties, etc.

Post-translational processing: The reactions which alter a protein's covalent structure, such as phosphorylation, glycosylation or proteolytic cleavage.

Post-translational regulation: Any process which affects the amount of protein produced from a gene and which occurs after translation in the grand scheme of genetic expression. Actually, this is often just a buzz-word for regulation of the stability of the protein. The more stable a protein is, the more it will accumulate.

Potable: Water suitable for human consumption.

ppb: Abbreviation for parts per billion.

ppm: Abbreviation for parts per million.

PRE (Progesterone Response Element): A binding site in a promoter to which the activated progesterone receptor can bind. The progesterone receptor is essentially a transcription factor which is activated only in the presence of progesterone. The activated receptor will bind to a PRE and transcription of the adjacent gene will be altered.

Pre-adaptation: The possession of characteristics that provide an advantage for an organism when it is exposed to new conditions.

Precipitation: The settling out of water from cloud in the form of dew, rain, hail, snow etc. The formation of solid particles in a solution; the settling out of small particles.

Pre-mRNA: An RNA molecule which is transcribed from chromosomal DNA in the nucleus of eukaryotic cells and subsequently processed through splicing reactions to generate the mRNA which directs protein synthesis in the cytoplasm.

Primary economy: An economic system in which the principal activities and so the main sources of wealth and employment is connected with agriculture, mining and the obtaining of primary commodities.

Opportunist, opportunistic: An organism that causes disease only in hosts with impaired defense mechanisms, which might result from wounds, alcoholism and so on.

Optimum temperature: The temperature at which an organism grows most rapidly.

Order: A commonly used population classification category which in general usage is often employed to cluster together similar families.

Organ: A structure composed of different tissues coordinated to perform a special function.

Organelle: A specialized part of a cell analogous to an organ in higher forms of life.

Organic farming: Farming without the use of industrially made fertilizers and pesticides, according the principles laid down by Sir Albert Howard, Lady Eve Balfour and others and as modernized and interpreted in Britain by the Soil Association.

Organic matter: Amount of remainder after drying and incinerating of a sample into an oven at 625°C for 3 hours, which is taken from solid wastes or composts.

Organism: An individual plant, animal or microbe that can independently carry out all life functions.

Organotroph: An organism that uses an organic compound as the electron donor.

Origin of replication: Nucleotide sequences present in a plasmid which are necessary for that plasmid to replicate in the bacterial host.

Orthophosphate: The inorganic form of phosphate and the only form readily available for use by most plants and microorganisms.

Osmotic pressure: The pressure that develops when a pure solvent is separated from a solution by a membrane that allows only solvent molecules to pass through it.

Oxidation: The removal of an electron.

Oxidation pond: A shallow lagoon or basin in which waste water is purified by sedimentation accompanied by aerobic and anaerobic treatment.

Oxidizing agents: Any substance that oxidizes another substance and is itself reduced in the process.

Ozone: O_3 is formed by the influence of ultraviolet radiation in the earth's upper atmosphere. It is also formed by the simultaneous occurrence of nitrogen oxides and hydrocarbons in conjunction with solar radiation. O_3 is a powerful oxidation agent which can harm humans, plants and materials.

Ozone layer : A layer of the atmosphere, about 20-50 kilometers above the surface, in which the concentration of ozone is higher than elsewhere in the atmosphere due to the dissociation and reformation of oxygen molecules exposed to high frequency ultraviolet radiation.

Package treatment plant: A transportable unit for sewage treatment that is capable of achieving a desired quality of effluent.

Panel point: The connection point between members of a truss.

Nuclear transfer (NT): The generation of a new animal nearly identical to another one by injection of the nucleus from a cell of the donor animal into an enucleated oocyte of the recipient.

Nuclease: An enzyme which degrades nucleic acids. A nuclease can be DNA-specific (a DNase), RNA-specific (RNase) or non-specific. It may act only on single stranded nucleic acids or only on double stranded nucleic acids or it may be non-specific with respect to strandedness.

Nucleic acids: Ribonucleic acid (RNA) and deoxyribonucleic acid (DNA).

Nucleotide: A subunit of DNA or RNA consisting of a nitrogenous base (adenine, guanine, thymine or cytosine in DNA; adenine, guanine, uracil or cytosine in RNA), a phosphate molecule and a sugar molecule (deoxyribose in DNA and ribose in RNA). Thousands of nucleotides are linked to form a DNA or RNA molecule.

Nutrient budget: An estimate setting out for a particular living system the amounts of essential mineral nutrients which are taken up or lost.

Obligate aerobes: Those organisms that have an absolute requirement for oxygen gas.

Obligate anaerobes: Those organisms that cannot utilize oxygen gas. Some members of this group are killed by traces of oxygen.

Obligate intracellular parasites: Grow only inside living cells.

Oligotrophic: Applied to a mires and freshwater bodies that are poor in plant nutrients. Oligotrophic water bodies are unproductive and their waters are clear because planktonic organisms are sparse. Applied to any lake whose hypolimnion does not become depleted of oxygen during the summer. Even moderately productive lakes may be classified as oligotrophic if they are deep enough for the hypolimnion never to become deoxygenated.

Oligotrophic environment: An environment deficient in nutrients.

Oncogene: A gene in a tumor virus or in cancerous cells which, when transferred into other cells, can cause transformation. Functional oncogenes are not present in normal cells. A normal cell has many proto-oncogenes which serve normal functions and which under the right circumstances can be activated to become oncogenes. The prefix v — indicates that a gene is derived from a virus and is generally an oncogene.

Open community: A community that is readily colonized by other organisms because some niches remain unoccupied.

Open reading frame: Any region of DNA or RNA where a protein could be encoded. In other words, there must be a string of nucleotides in which one of the three reading frames has no stop codons.

Opencut mining: The working of coal or an ore by removing the overburden to expose the ore body, which is removed and may be partly processed on site.

Primary productivity: The rate at which energy is taken into an ecosystem through the activity of producers.

Primary Structure: Refers to the sequence of amino acid residues or nucleotides within protein or nucleic acid molecules, respectively.

Primary transcript: When a gene is transcribed in the nucleus, the initial product is the primary transcript, an RNA containing copies of all exons and introns. This primary transcript is then processed by the cell to remove the introns, to cleave off unwanted 3' sequence and to polyadenylate the 3' end. The mature message thus formed is then exported to the cytoplasm for translation.

Primary treatment: The removal of separable materials from wastewaters by sedimentation.

Primer extension: A reaction in which DNA is reverse transcribed from an RNA template to which a specific oligonucleotide primer has been annealed. The new cDNA product is an extension of the primer, which is synthesized at the 3' end of the primer in a direction extending toward the 5' end of the RNA. This reaction is useful for exploring the extreme 5' end of RNA molecules.

Primer: A small oligonucleotide (anywhere from 6 to 50 nt long) used to prime DNA synthesis. The DNA polymerases are only able to extend a pre-existing strand along a template; they are not able to take a naked single strand and produce a complimentary copy of it de-novo. A primer which sticks to the template is therefore used to initiate the replication. Primers are necessary for DNA sequencing and PCR.

Prion-related protein (PrP): A normal protein, expressed in the nervous system of animals, whose structure when altered by interaction with altered copies of itself is the cause of scrapie in sheep, BSE in cattle and Creutzfeldt-Jakob disease in humans.

Probe: Usually refers to a DNA or RNA molecule which has been labeled with 32P or with biotin, to facilitate its detection after it has specifically hybridized with a target DNA or RNA sequence. However, the term may also refer to antibody probes used in western blots.

Processing plant: A plant which is built up for recovery and reuse, composting, incineration, energy production, volume reduction, sanitary land filling to make wastes unharmful for environment.

Processing: With respect to proteins, generally used to refer to proteolytic post-translational modifications of a polypeptide. In the case of RNA, processing may involve the addition of a 5' cap and 3' poly-A tracks as well as splicing reactions in the nucleus.

Processivity: The extent to which an RNA or DNA polymerase adheres to a template before dissociating determines the average length (in kilobases) of the newly synthesized nucleic acid strands. Also applies to the action of exonucleases in digesting from the ends to the middle of a nucleic acid.

Producer: Autotrophic populations, usually of green plants, which procure energy from outside an ecosystem and direct it into the system.

Production ecology: The study of biomes in terms of the production and distribution of food and hence the flow of energy within them.

Production line: A manufacturing process that breaks fabrication into simple, discrete elements, each of which is performed by one person or group of people, in order to increase individual productivity.

Production rate: The number of organisms formed within an area during a given period of time.

Production residues: Wastes that result from production and distribution.

Production: Gross production rate; the rate of assimilation shown by organisms of a given trophic level. Gross primary production is the assimilation of organic matter or biocontent by a plant community during a specified period. Net primary production; the biomass or biocontent incorporated into a plant community during a specified period of time.

Productivity: Primary productivity; the amount of organic matter made in a given time by the atrophic organisms in an ecosystem. Net productivity; the amount of organic matter produced in excess of that used up by the producing organisms during respiration thus representing potential food for the consumers of the ecosystem.

Prokaryote: Organisms, namely, bacteria and cyanobacteria (formerly known as blue-green algae), characterized by the possession of a simple naked DNA chromosome, occasionally two such chromosomes, usually of circular structure, without a nuclear membrane and possessing a very small range of organelles, generally only a plasma membrane and ribosomes.

Prokaryotic: Applied to organism or cells whose genetic material is not enclosed by a nuclear membrane and that do not possess mitochondria or plastids. Bacteria and Cyanophyta are the only prokaryotic organisms.

Promoter: A specific sequence within a double-stranded DNA molecule that is recognized by an RNA polymerase, which binds to it and uses it to begin transcribing the DNA template into a new RNA. The location and orientation of the promoter within a DNA molecule determines the start site of the new RNA. Other proteins *e.g.*, transcriptional activators such as sigma factor are usually required for an RNA polymerase to recognize a promoter.

Promoter: The first few hundred nucleotides of DNA upstream (on the 5' side) of a gene, which control the transcription of that gene. The promoter is part of the 5' flanking DNA, *i.e.*, it is not transcribed into RNA, but without the promoter, the gene is not functional. Note that the definition is a bit hazy as far as the size of the region encompassed, but the promoter of a gene starts with the nucleotide immediately upstream from the cap site and includes binding sites for one or more transcription factors which cannot work if moved farther away from the gene.

Pronuclear injection: The use of a fine needle to inject DNA into the nucleus of an unfertilized egg.

Protein: A large molecule composed of one or more chains of amino acids in a specific order. The order is determined by the base sequence of nucleotides in the gene that codes for the protein. Proteins are required for the structure, function and regulation of the body's cells, tissues and organs; and each protein has unique functions. Examples are hormones, enzymes and antibodies.

Protista: The kingdom that comprises all the simple organisms.

Proto-Oncogene: A cellular oncogene like sequence which is thought to play a role in controlling normal cellular growth and differentiation.

Proto-oncogene: A gene present in a normal cell which carries out a normal cellular function, but which can become an oncogene under certain circumstances. The prefix c- indicates a cellular gene and is generally used for proto-oncogenes.

Prototroph, prototrophy: An organism that has on organic growth requirements other than a source of carbon and energy.

Protozoa: A group of organisms.

Pseudogene: Inactive but stable components of the genome which derived by duplication and mutation of an ancestral, active gene. Pseudo genes can serve as the donor sequence in gene conversion events.

Pseudoknot: A feature of RNA tertiary structure; best visualized as two overlapping stem-loops in which the loop of the first stem-loop participates as half of the stem in the second stem-loop.

Pseudomonas **sp.:** A common group of sulfur reducing bacteria causing accelerated corrosion of pipes.

Pseudorevertant: A mutant virus or organism which has recovered a wildtype phenotype due to a second-site mutation (potentially located in a different region of the genome or involving a different polypeptide) which has eliminated the effect of the initial mutation.

Psychrophiles: Organisms that grow best between - 5 and + 20^{0}C.

Pulsed field gel electrophoresis (PFGE): A gel technique which allows size-separation of very large fragments of DNA, in the range of hundreds of kb to thousands of kb. As in other gel electrophoresis techniques, populations of molecules migrate through the gel at a speed related to their size, producing discrete bands. In normal electrophoresis, DNA fragments greater than a certain size limit all migrate at the same rate through the gel. In PFGE, the electrophoretic voltage is applied alternately along two perpendicular axes, which forces even the larger DNA fragments to separate by size.

Pulverization: An intermediate step in refuse disposal in which refuse is broken into small particles, so reducing its volume.

Pumpimg station: An installation for raising sewage to a higher elevation or for pumping mains water supplies.

Pure culture: A culture that contains only a single strain of an organism.

Pyrolysis: A way of breaking down burnable waste by combustion in the absence of air. High heat is usually applied to the wastes in a closed chamber and all moiture evaporates and materials break down into various hydrocarbons in liquid and gas phase and carbon like residues.

Quota: The ratio of the quantity of recollected containers to the quantity of containers filled as of years, for the purpose of recycling and disposal of filled plastic or metal containers.

Radial drainage: River systems that form a radial pattern. Radial drainage is typical of high mountain areas or systems on volcanic cones.

Radical: A group of two or more atoms that acts as a single atom and goes through a reaction uncharged or is replaced by a single atom.

Radioactive waste: Waste that consists of or is contaminated with, radionuclide. According to their radioactive content, wastes are divided into three categories: Low-level, intermediate-level and high level.

Radioactivity: A property exhibited by unstable isotopes of elements that decay, emitting radiation, principally as α particles, β particles and X-rays.

Range management: The planning and management of the use of grazing land in order to sustain maximum livestock production consistent with the conservation of the range resource.

Raw sludge: Treatment sludge which is not dewatered dried and digested.

Reactor: A vessel in which a commercial fermentation process is carried out.

Receptor, receptor sites: Attachment sites on a cell surface.

Recombinant DNA molecules (rDNA): A combination of DNA molecules of different origin that are joined using recombinant DNA technologies.

Recombinant DNA technology: Procedure used to join together DNA segments in a cell-free system (an environment outside a cell or organism). Under appropriate conditions, a recombinant DNA molecule can enter a cell and replicate there, either autonomously or after it has become integrated into a cellular chromosome.

Recombination: The re-assortment of characters within linkage groups as a result of the crossing over which occurs during meiosis in reproductive tissue.

Recovery: Recovery is a general term used to describe the extraction of economically usable materials or energy from wastes. The concept may involve recycling or conversion into different and sometimes, unrelated uses.

Recycling: Procedure which is carried out without any chemical and biological treatment for some reusable materials such as paper, plastic, glass and can. These materials can be returned into economical processes.

Reducer: Heterotrophic individual which utilizes the chemical energy of organic matter while breaking it down to more simple substances.

Reduction: The removal of oxygen, the addition of hydrogen or the addition of electrons.

Regression: The dependence of one variable upon another independent variable.

Regressive: Applied to a body of water or to sediments associated with a lowering of sea level.

Relative humidity: The percentage of moisture in air compared to the maximum it might contain.

Renewable resource: A resource that can be exploited without depletion because it is constantly replenished. The includes agricultural crops and fish, provided stocks are not over fished and is extended to cover the energy of solar radiation, wind, waves and tides.

Repetitive DNA: A surprising portion of any genome consists not of genes or structural elements, but of frequently repeated simple sequences.

Replication: Synthesis of a copy. Cells replicate by increasing in size and dividing to produce two daughter cells identical with the original cell.

Reservoir: As used here, a substance in which the temperature remains constant.

Resistance management: Strategies that can delay the onset of resistance. For insect resistance management, this includes the use of a refuge in which the insect will not be challenged by the pesticide used in the rest of the field.

Resource: A means that is available for supplying an economic want. Minerals and fossil fuels are described as stock, resource or reserves.

Respiration: The process whereby oxygen is taken into an organism and carbon dioxide is given out.

Response element: By definition, a response element is a portion of a gene which must be present in order for that gene to respond to some hormone or other stimulus. Response elements are binding sites for transcription factors. Certain transcription factors are activated by stimuli such as hormones or heat shock. A gene may respond to the presence of that hormone because the gene has in its promoter region a binding site for hormone-activated transcription factor.

Restriction enzyme: A class of enzymes (restriction endonucleases) generally isolated from bacteria, which are able to recognize and cut specific sequences (restriction sites) in DNA. For example, the restriction enzyme BamHI locates and cuts any occurrence of-5'-GGATCC-3'| | | | | |3'-CCTAGG-5'.

Restriction fragment: The piece of DNA released after restriction digestion of plasmids or genomic DNA. One can digest a plasmid and isolate one particular restriction fragment. The term also describes the fragments detected on a genomic blot which carry the gene of interest.

Restriction map: A cartoon depiction of the locations within a stretch of known DNA where restriction enzymes will cut.

Restriction: To restrict DNA means to cut it with a restriction enzyme.

Retaining wall: A wall to hold a bank of soil in position.

Reverse osmosis: A process for the removal of dissolved ions from water is forced through a semi permeable membrane, retaining most ions while transmitting the water.

Reverse transcriptase: An enzyme which will make a DNA copy of an RNA template; a DNA-dependant RNA polymerase. RT is used to make cDNA; one begins by isolating polyadenylated mRNA, providing oligo-dT as a primer and adding nucleotide triphosphates and RT to copy the RNA into cDNA.

RFLP: Restriction fragment length polymorphism; the acronym is pronounced riflip. Although two individuals of the same species have almost identical genomes, they will always differ at a few nucleotides. Some of these differences will produce new restriction sites or remove them and thus the banding pattern seen on a genomic Southern will thus be affected.

Rhibonucleic acid: A chemical structure found in the cytoplasm that controls chemical reactions in a cell.

Rhizophere: The part of the soil immediately surrounding roots. Roots alter the nutrient status of the soil close to them by absorbing minerals and releasing other substances. This leads to an increase in the numbers of microorganisms and often alters the relative proportions of the different kinds of microorganisms present.

Riboprobe: A strand of RNA synthesized *in-vitro* usually radio labeled and used as a probe for hybridization reactions. An RNA probe can be synthesized at very high specific activity, is single stranded and can be used for very sensitive detection of DNA or RNA.

Ribose: A 5-carbon sugar found in nucleic acid.

Ribosome: A granule in the cytoplasm containing ribonucleic acid that controls the synthesis of protein.

Rigid: Capable of keeping a given shape under pressure.

Risk estimation: An actuarial technique, used in assessing the relative costs and benefits of a particular technology, that compares actual recorded incidence of death or injury to humans to the number of people using the technology, extended over many years.

RNAi (RNA interference): It is the mechanism by which small double stranded RNAs can interfere with expression of any mRNA having a similar sequence. Those small RNAs are known as siRNA, for short interfering RNAs. The mode of action for siRNA appears to be via dissociation of its strands, hybridization to the target RNA, extension of those fragments by an RNA-dependent RNA polymerase, then fragmentation of the target. Importantly, the remnants of the target molecule appears to then act as an siRNA itself; thus the effect of a small amount of starting siRNA is effectively amplified and can have long-lasting effects on the recipient cell.

RNase Protection Assay: This is a sensitive method to determine the amount of a specific mRNA present in a complex mixture of mRNA and/or the sizes of exons which comprise the mRNA of interest. A radioactive DNA or RNA probe is allowed to hybridize with a sample of mRNA, after which the mixture is digested with single strand specific nuclease. Only the probe which is hybridized to the specific mRNA will escape the nuclease treatment and can be detected on a gel. The amount of radioactivity which was protected from nuclease is proportional to the amount of mRNA to which it hybridized. If the probe included both intron and exons, only the exons will be protected from nuclease and their sizes can be ascertained on the gel.

RNase: Ribonuclease; an enzyme which degrades RNA. It is ubiquitous in living organisms and is exceptionally stable. The prevention of RNase activity is the primary problem in handling RNA.

Rotary pump: A pump in which the fluid is caused to flow by the rotary action of gears or similar moving parts.

Rotation: A turning around, as of a wheel on its axis.

rRNA: ribosomal RNA; any of several RNAs which become part of the ribosome and thus are involved in translating mRNA and synthesizing proteins. They are the most abundant RNA in the cell on a mass basis.

Run-off: Water from rain or snow that runs off the surface of the land and into streams and rivers.

S1 end mapping: A technique to determine where the end of an RNA transcript lies with respect to its template DNA (the gene).

S1 nuclease: An enzyme which digests only single-stranded nucleic acids.

Saline water or solution: Water or an aqueous solution containing an excessive amount of dissolved salts, usually over 10 000 mg/L.

Salinity: The degree of concentration of salt solutions, determined by measuring the density of the solution using a salinometer (a type of a hydrometer), by titration, by measuring the electrical conductivity of the solution, etc.

Sand clay: A mixture of sand and clay, used for road surface, clay becomes hard when it has baked in the sun.

Sanitary landfill area: A landfill area in which solid wastes are spread out as thin layers, compacted and covered with soil, daily. In this technique, sanitary precautions have been applied, accurately.

Saturation: A relative humidity of 100% measured by comparing the difference in readings between a dry bulb and wet bulb thermometer.

Screen: The portion of a well casing that is slotted or perforated to permit the flow of water into the well.

Screening 1: The operation of passing loose materials through a screen of known mesh so that constituent particles are separated into defined sizes.

Screening 2: To screen a library is to select and isolate individual clones out of the mixture of clones. For example, if you needed a cDNA clone of the pituitary glycoprotein hormone alpha subunit, you would need to make or buy a pituitary cDNA library, and then screen that library in order to detect and isolate those few bacteria carrying alpha subunit cDNA.

Secondary pollutant: A pollutant formed in the environment by the combination or reaction of other pollutants.

Secondary productivity: The procurement of energy by heterotrophs.

Secondary sorting: This operation will be made at places where solid wastes are dispatched for disposal or recycling.

Secondary thickening: In a woody perennial plant, the formation of secondary vascular tissue as a result of the activity of cambium in the stems and roots.

Secondary treatment: A process to remove the amount of dissolved organic matter in waste water and to reduce further the suspended solids.

Sedimentary cycle: The circulation of nutrients in an ecosystem which involves geological weathering and erosion with the eventual recovery of the elements by the uplift of marine sediments to form land masses.

Sedimentation: The separation of an insoluble solid from a liquid in which it is suspended by settling under the influence of gravity or centrifugation.

Selectable marker: A gene, usually encoding resistance to an antibiotic, added to a vector construct to allow easy selection of cells that contain the construct from the large majority of cells that do not.

Selection pressure: A measure of the effects of natural selection on the genetic composition of a population.

Selective breeding: Making deliberate crosses or mating of organisms so the offspring will have a desired characteristic derived from one of the parents.

Selective inhibitors: Substance added to growth media that inhibit one species of organism but not another.

Selective species: A species found most usually in a particular community, but also, rarely, in other communities.

Semipermeable: The passage of some materials but not others.

Seperate collection: Household and particularly industrial wastes will be collected in seperate containers or tins manually or with tools according to their types.

Septic tank: A watertight sedimentation tank for sewage in which solids settle and are decomposed anaerobically. A common facility for the treatment of household sewage in rural areas.

Sequence: As a noun, the sequence of a DNA is a buzz word for the structure of a DNA molecule, in terms of the sequence of bases it contains. As a verb, to sequence is to determine the structure of a piece of DNA; *i.e.*, the sequence of nucleotides it contains.

Settling tank: Clarifier, a tank or vat in which sedimentation or subsidence takes place.

Sewage: Domestic and industrial waste in a liquid or semi liquid state.

Shock loading: Any of several types of abrupt change in the environment in a biological treatment process.

Shotgun cloning: The practice of randomLy clipping a larger DNA fragment into various smaller pieces, cloning everything and then studying the resulting individual clones to figure out what happened. For example, if one was studying a 50 kb gene, it may be a bit difficult to figure out the restriction map. By randomLy breaking it into smaller fragments and mapping those, a master restriction map could be deduced. See also Shotgun sequencing.

Shotgun sequencing: A way of determining the sequence of a large DNA fragment which requires little brainpower but lots of late nights. The large fragment is shotgun cloned and then each of the resulting smaller clones (subclones) is sequenced. By finding out where the subclones overlap, the sequence of the larger piece becomes apparent. Note that some of the regions will get sequenced several times just by chance.

Single cell protein: Protein derived from unicellular organisms grown on a hydrocarbon substrate.

siRNA: Small Inhibitory RNA.

Slag: The non-metalic residue from the smelting of metalic ores that generally forms as a molten mass floating on the molten metal.

Slot blot: Similar to a dot blot, but the analyte is put onto the membrane using a slot-shaped template. The template produces a consistently shaped spot, thus decreasing errors and improving the accuracy of the analysis. See Dot blot.

Sludge disposal: Various processes for the terminal disposition of sludges created during the treatment of wastewaters.

Sludge: Thick mud often greasy.

Smog: Originally, a contraction of smoke and fog.

Smoke: An aerosol of minute solid or liquid particles formed by the incomplete combustion of a fuel.

SNP: Single Nucleotide Polymorphism is a position in a genomic DNA sequence that varies from one individual to another. It is thought that the primary source of genetic difference between any two humans is due to the presence of single nucleotide polymorphisms in their DNA. Furthermore, these SNPs can be extremely useful in genetic mapping to follow inheritance of specific segments of DNA in a lineage. SNP typing is the process of determining the exact nucleotide at positions known to be polymorphic.

snRNA: Small nuclear RNA; forms complexes with proteins to form snRNPs; involved in RNA splicing, polyadenylation reactions, other unknown functions (probably).

Softening: The process of removing the hardness-producing ions in exchange for less detrimental ions.

Soil drainage: The removal from the soil of water that is surplus to the requirements of the use to which the soil is to be put.

Soil map: A map that shows the distribution of soil types in relation to other features of the land surface.

Soil moisture: Water in the soil either held by capillary attraction or in the process of movement toward the water table.

Soil type: A subdivision of a soil series based on the texture.

Soil: Weathered, unconsolidated surface material in which plants anchor their roots and from which they derive nutrients and moisture.

Solid waste: They include materials which are wasted after using and treatment sludge. They must be regularly, continuously and accurately collected and disposed with respect to human and environmental health.

Solution hybridization: A method closely related to RNase protection. Solution hybridization is designed to measure the levels of a specific mRNA species in a complex population of RNA. An excess of radioactive probe is allowed to hybridize to the RNA, then single-strand specific nuclease is used to destroy the remaining unhybridized probe and RNA. The protected probe is separated from the degraded fragments and the amount of radioactivity in it is proportional to the amount of mRNA in the sample which was capable of hybridization. This can be a very sensitive detection method.

Solution: In soil, water entering the ground encounters organic matter containing carbon dioxide and acid ions which become dissolved in the water.

Somatic cells: Cells of body tissues other than the germ line.

Somatic: Pertaining to the soma or to the body wall of an animal.

Sorting: According to nature of transportation, wind or water can fractionate homogeneous rock debris into grains of similar sizes. The sorting of a sediment refers to the range of grain sizes within a particular sample.

Southern blot: A technique for analyzing mixtures of DNA, whereby the presence and rough size of one particular fragment of DNA can be ascertained, named for its inventor, Dr E. M. Southern.

Special waste (dangerous waste, hazardous waste, intractable waste): To qualify as special waste a substance must be sufficiently toxic to present a hazard to human health or risk of serious environmental contamination.

Species packing: Extensive diversification into species population within a comparatively narrow range of variation.

Species: A group of similar individuals having a common origin and continuous breeding system.

Spray: Liquid droplets greater than 10 micrometres in size, created by mechanical disintegration processes. Spray is a source of salt particles in the atmosphere.

SSR: Simple Sequence Repeat.

Stability: The ability of a structure to resist forces.

Stabilization: The increase of dominance that ends in a stable climax, produced by the invasion of species leading to the establishment of a population most completely fitted for the prevailing conditions.

Stabilize: Tend to hold steady, firm or balanced.

Stabilized: Treated to remain solidly packed-said of road soils.

Stable population: A population in which births and deaths are in balance so that discounting migrations, the size of the population remains constant.

Stable transfection: A form of transfection experiment designed to produce permanent lines of cultured cells with a new gene inserted into their genome. Usually this is done by linking the desired gene with a selectable gene *i.e.,* a gene which confers resistance to a toxin. Upon putting the toxin into the culture medium, only those cells which incorporate the resistance gene will survive and essentially all of those will also have incorporated the experimenter's gene.

Static stability: In the atmosphere, the condition in which small vertical displacements of a parcel of air cause gravitational restoring forces in the absence of horizontal wind. This is the case if the lapse rate is greater than the adiabatic lapse rate.

Sterilization: Rendering an object or substance free of all viable microorganisms or viruses.

Sticky ends: After digestion of a DNA with certain restriction enzymes, the ends left have one strand overhanging the other to form a short (typically 4 nt) single-stranded segment. This overhang will easily re-attach to other ends like it and are thus known as sticky ends. For example, the enzyme BamHI recognizes the sequence GGATCC and cut after first G in each strand.

Still: An apparatus for distilling used to prepare alcoholic drinks, distilled water and other purified liquids.

Stochastic: In statistics, applied to a random element.

Stratification: The arrangement of material in discrete layers. In the atmosphere, the forming of stable horizontal layers that do not intermingle, because the lapse rate is less than the adiabatic lapse rate.

Stratosphere: Upper layer of the atmosphere from 12 to 50 kilometres.

Stringency: A term used to describe the conditions of hybridization. By varying the conditions (especially salt concentration and temperature) a given probe sequence may be allowed to hybridize only with its exact complement (high stringency) or with any somewhat related sequences (relaxed or low stringency). Increasing the temperature or decreasing the salt concentration will tend to increase the selectivity of a hybridization reaction and thus will raise the stringency.

Structural proteins: Proteins that form part of the organism or virus.

Structure: The spatial and other arrangements of species within an ecosystem. The structure takes account of the composition of the biological community, including species, numbers, biomass, life cycle and spatial distribution; the quantity and distribution of the non-living materials. The range or gradient of conditions such as temperature, light etc.

Sub-cloning: If you have a cloned piece of DNA (say, inserted into a plasmid) and you need unlimited copies of only a part of it, you might sub-clone it. This involves starting with several million copies of the original plasmid, cutting with restriction enzymes and purifying the desired fragment out of the mixture. That fragment can then be inserted into a new plasmid for replication. It has now been subcloned.

Sublimation: The change in a substance between the solid and the gaseous phase without passing through the liquid phase.

Submersible pump: A pump designed to fit into a well and operate below the water level.

Substrate: The surface to which an organism is attached or upon which it moves. The material on which a microorganism grows. The particular substance or group of substances that an enzyme activates.

Succession: The replacement of one community by another as a result of changes in the environment.

Sulfate reducing bacteria: A group of bacteria capable of reducing sulfates in water to hydrogen sulfide gas. They have no sanitary significance and are classed as nuisance organisms.

Sulfur bacteria: Bacteria that oxidize hydrogen sulfide or sulfur to sulfuric or sulfurous acid.

Surface pressure: Normally, the atmospheric pressure inside a Stevenson Screen.

Surface runoff: Water flowing across the soil surface into a channel.

Suspension: As used here, the state of balance in which the body of a car is held on the springs and shock absorbers.

Sustainable capacity: Sustainable yield.

Sustainable development: Economic development that can continue indefinitely because it is based on the exploitation of renewable resources and causes insufficient environmental damage for this to pose an eventual limit.

Sustainable yield: The maximum extent to which a renewable resource may be exploited without depletion.

Symbiosis: A close and mutually beneficial association of organisms of different species. The occurrence of cellulose-digesting protozoans in the guts of wood-eating cockroaches and termites is a symbiotic relationship, as the insects cannot digest cellulose unaided and the protozoa cannot live independently.

Symbiotic relationship: Intimate relationship between members of different species.

Syndrome: A particular group of signs and symtoms that occur together.

Synecology: The study of the relationships between communities of species and their environment.

Synergism: A cooperative effort between two or more species of bacteria resulting in something the individual species could not have accomplished alone.

Synergistic action: The cooperative action of two distinct organisms such that the growth of one assists the growth or activity of the other.

Taq polymerase: A DNA polymerase isolated from the bacterium *Thermophilis aquaticus* and which is very stable to high temperatures. It is used in PCR procedures and high temperature sequencing.

TATA box: A sequence found in the promoter (part of the 5' flanking region) of many genes. Deletion of this site (the binding site of transcription factor TFIID) causes a marked reduction in transcription and gives rise to heterogeneous transcription initiation sites.

Taxonomy: The study of the methods of classifying organisms.

TDT, thermal death time: The amount of time needed to kill bacterial spores at a certain temperature.

Technosphere: That part of the physical environment built or modified by humans.

Tensiometer: An instrument used to measure the amount of water in the plant root area of a soil.

Teratogen: A substance that produces deformation of the fetus in the womb.

Terrestrial: Belonging to the Earth or to the mainland; existing on the mainland, in contrast to aquatic.

Tertiary treatment: A third stage in the treatment of waste water, usually involving the removal of soluble plant nutrients which might cause eutrophication were they released into still or slow-moving fresh water.

Texture: The size, shape and arrangement of the particles that make up a surface deposit, rock or soil.

Thallus: The body of an undifferentiated plant, such as a fungus.

Theodolite: An instrument used particularly in surveying for measuring horizontal and vertical angles.

Thermal pollution: The raising of the temperature of part of the environment by the discharge of substances whose temperature is higher than the ambient.

Thermocline: The layer of the water in a lake that lies between the epilimnion and the hypolimnion.

Thermograph: An instrument for recording changes in temperature as a line on a rotating drum.

Thermophilic microorganisms: Microorganisms that grow well at temperatures over 45^0C. Examples include bacteria in hot springs, manure heaps and fermenting hay ricks.

Thermosphere: That part of the upper atmosphere in which temperature increases with height.

Tissue culture: A process of growing a plant in the laboratory from cells rather than seeds. This technique is used in traditional plant breeding as well as when using techniques of agricultural biotechnology.

Tissue-specific expression: Gene function which is restricted to a particular tissue or cell type. For example, the glycoprotein hormone alpha subunit is produced only in certain cell types of the anterior pituitary and placenta, not in lungs or skin; thus expression of the glycoprotein hormone alpha-chain gene is said to be tissue-specific. Tissue specific expression is usually the result of an enhancer which is activated only in the proper cell type.

Tm: The melting point for a double-stranded nucleic acid. Technically, this is defined as the temperature at which 50% of the strands are in double-stranded form and 50% are single-stranded, *i.e.,* midway in the melting curve. A primer has a specific Tm because it is assumed that it will find an opposite strand of appropriate character.

Total solids: The weight of all solids, dissolved and suspended, organic and inorganic, per unit volume of water.

Toxicity: The degree to which a substaance is poisonous. Toxicity is divided into acute toxicity (aassimilaated once), subchronic toxicity (repeated assimilation over a short period of time) and into chronic toxicity (repeated assimilation over a long period of time)

Trace elements: Elements that is necessary in extremely small amounts for the proper functioning of metabolism in plants and animals. Most are probably constituents of enzymes. Higher plants need traces of copper, zinc, boron, molybdenum and manganese. Any element present in minute quantities in an organism, soil, water, etc.

Tracer: A substance used to determine the flow rate and direction of water movement in a stream or aquifer.

Traditional breeding: Modification of plants and animals through selective breeding. Practices used in traditional plant breeding may include aspects of biotechnology such as tissue culture and mutation breeding.

Transamination: A reaction in which an ammonium ion is transferred from one amino acid to an alfaketo acid, resulting in the synthesis of an acid.

Transcription factor: A protein which is involved in the transcription of genes. These usually bind to DNA as part of their function.

Transcription: The process of copying DNA to produce an RNA transcript. This is the first step in the expression of any gene. The resulting RNA, if it codes for a protein, will be spliced, polyadenylated, transported to the cytoplasm and by the process of translation will produce the desired protein molecule.

Transcriptional Start Site: The nucleotide of a gene or cistron at which transcription (RNA synthesis) starts; the most common triplet at which transcription begins in *E. coli* is CAT. Primer extension identifies the transcriptional start site.

Transfection: A method by which experimental DNA may be put into a cultured mammalian cell. Such experiments are usually performed using cloned DNA containing coding sequences and control regions (promoters, etc.) in order to test whether the DNA will be expressed. Since the cloned DNA may have been extensively modified (for example, protein binding sites on the promoter may have been altered or removed), this procedure is often used to test whether a particular modification affects the function of a gene.

Transfer station: A place or facility where wastes are transferred from smaller collection vehicles e.g., compactor trucks into larger transport hehicles *e.g.,* Over-the-road and off-road tractor trailers, railroad gondola cars or barges for movement to disposal area, usually landfills. In some transfer operations, compaction or seperation may be done at the station.

Transformation (with respect to bacteria): The process by which a bacterium acquires a plasmid and becomes antibiotic resistant. This term most commonly refers to a bench procedure performed by the investigator which introduces experimental plasmids into bacteria.

Transformation (with respect to cultured cells): A change in cell morphology and behaviour which is generally related to carcinogenesis. Transformed cells tend to exhibit characteristics known collectively as the transformed phenotype (rounded cell bodies, reduced attachment dependence, increased growth rate, loss of contact inhibition, etc.). There are different degrees of transformation and cells may exhibit only a subset of these characteristics. Not well understood, the process of transformation is the subject of intense research.

Transgene: A foreign gene which has been introduced into the germ line of an animal species.

Transgenic mouse: A mouse which carries experimentally introduced DNA. The procedure by which one makes a transgenic mouse involves the injection of DNA into a fertilized embryo at the pro-nuclear stage. The DNA is generally cloned and may be experimentally altered. It will become incorporated into the genome of the embryo. That embryo is implanted into a foster mother, who gives birth to an animal carrying the new gene. Various experiments are then carried out to test the functionality of the inserted DNA.

Transgenic: Containing genes altered by insertion of DNA from an unrelated organism. Taking genes from one species and inserting them into another species to get that trait expressed in the offspring.

Transient transfection: When DNA is transfected into cultured cells, it is able to stay in those cells for about 2-3 days, but then will be lost (unless steps are taken to ensure that it is retained). During those 2-3 days, the DNA is functional and any functional genes it contains will be expressed. Investigators take advantage of this transient expression period to test gene function.

Transition: A nucleotide substitution in which one pyrimidine is replaced by the other pyrimidine or one purine replaced by the other purine *e.g.*, A is changed to G or C is changed to T.

Translation: The process whereby mRNA directs the synthesis of a protein molecule; carried out by the ribosome in association with a host of translation initiation, elongation and termination factors. Eukaryotic genes may be regulated at the level of translation, as well as the level of transcription.

Translocation: The process by which a newly synthesized protein is directed toward a specific cellular compartment *i.e*, the nucleus, the endoplasmic reticulum.

Transpiration: The loss of water vapour from a plant, mainly through the stomata and to a small extent through the cuticle and lenticels.

Transposition: The movement of DNA from one location to another location on the same molecule or a different molecule within a cell.

Transposon: A transposable genetic element; certain sequence elements which are capable of moving from one site to another in a DNA molecule without any requirement for sequence relatedness at the donour and acceptor sites. Many transposons carry antibiotic resistance determinants and have insertion sequences at both ends and thus have two sets of inverted repeats.

Transversion: A nucleotide substitution in which a purine replaces a pyrimidine or vice versa *e.g.,* A is changed to T or T is changed to G.

Treatment sludge: Dewatered and dried materials which are produced after procedures such as physical, chemical and biological treatment of domestic and/or industrial waste waters.

tRNA: transfer RNA; one of a class of rather small RNAs used by cell to carry amino acids to the enzyme complex (the ribosome) which builds proteins, using an mRNA as a guide.

Trophic level: A particular step occupied by a population in the process of energy transfer within an ecosystem.

Tumor suppressor: A gene that inhibits progression towards neoplastic transformation. The best-known examples of tumor suppressors are the proteins p53 and Rb.

Turbulence: An irregular movement of a fluid in which, in general, no two particles of the fluid follow the same path. Most natural movement of fluids is turbulent rather than laminar and in air turbulence is a major cause of mixing.

Turn-over: The continuous, balanced process of generation and loss of cells or molecules in living systems. The turn-over time is the time needed for the replacement by turn-over of the cells or molecules equivalent to the total biomass of a population or the time taken for an individual organism to mature, die and undergo decomposition.

Ubiquitous: Occurring everywhere.

Upstream activator sequence: A binding site for transcription factors, generally part of a promoter region. A UAS may be found upstream of the TATA sequence and its function is to increase transcription. Unlike an enhancer, it cannot be positioned just anywhere or in any orientation.

Upstream/Downstream: In RNA, anything towards the 5' end of a reference point is upstream of that point. This orientation reflects the direction of both the synthesis of mRNA and its translation from the 5' end to the 3' end. In DNA, the situation is a bit more complicated. In the vicinity of a gene or in a cDNA, the DNA has two strands, but one strand is virtually a duplicate of the RNA, so its 5' and 3' ends determine upstream and downstream, respectively. In genomic DNA, two adjacent genes may be on different strands and thus oriented in opposite directions. Upstream or downstream is only used on conjunction with a given gene.

Urbanization: The migration of people in substantial numbers from rural to urban areas. Urbanization is characteristic of regions in the early stages of industrialization and is marked in third world countries.

Variety: Subdivision of a species for taxonomic classification. Used interchangeably with the term cultivar to denote a group of individuals that is distinct genetically from other groups of individuals in the species. An agricultural variety is a group of similar plants that by structural features and performance can be identified from other varieties within the same species.

Vector: A type of DNA, such as a plasmid or phage that is self-replicating and that can be used to transfer DNA segments among host cells. Also, an insect or other organism that provides a means of dispersal for a disease or parasite.

Vegetation: The plants of an area considered in general or as communities, but not taxonomically; the total plant cover in a particular area or on the Earth as a whole.

Vegetative cell: The growing or feeding form of a cell.

Velocity: Speed and direction. The wind velocity is the wind speed and the direction from which the wind blows. Velocity is sometimes used informally to mean speed alone.

Venturi effect: The acceleration of a fluid stream as it passes through a constriction in a channel. The acceleration is associated with a reduction in the pressure in the fluid.

Vertical transmission: Inheritance of a gene from parent to offspring.

Virulence: The relative capacity of a pathogen to overcome body defenses.

Virus: A non-cellular biological entity that can reproduce only within a host cell. Viruses consist of nucleic acid covered by protein; some animal viruses also are surrounded by a membrane. Inside the infected cell, the virus uses the synthetic capability of the host to produce progeny viruses.

Vitamins: Various substances that is essential in minute quantities to the nutrition of animals and plants.

Warm rain: Rain falling from water clouds as opposed to ice clouds.

Waste containing asbestos: Precautions for handling, disposal or reuse should be consistent with the hazard of asbestos dust at trace contaminant levels. Enclosure of such waste into a fixed substance should be done under conditions that prevent the release of asbestos fibers to the air. Waste contaminating asbestos may be disposed of under controlled conditions at landfill sites authorized to receive such waste.

Waste water: Polluted water from households and commercial and industrial sources which no longer corresponds to the condition of not having been influenced by man. A distinction is made between domestic waste water and commercial and industrial waste water.

Water table : The surface between the zone of saturation and the zone of aeration; that surface of a body of unconfined ground water at which the pressure is equal to that of the atmosphere.

Waterborne disease: A disease caused by a bacterium or organism able to live or be carried by water.

Western Blot: Proteins are separated by SDS-PAGE, then electrophoretically transferred to a solid-phase matrix such as nitrocellulose, then probed with a labeled antibody (or a series of antibodies).

Wet bulb: A thermometer bulb maintained wet with distilled water, usually by means of a muslin wick.

Wetland: An area covered permanently, occasionally or periodically by fresh or salt water up to a depth of 6 metres.

Wild dumping: Wastes of different kind and consistence are deposited without any plan and without permission.

Wildtype: The native or predominant genetic constitution before mutations, usually referring to the genetic constitution normally existing in nature.

Wind rose: A diagram summarizing the frequencies of winds of different strengths and directions as measured at a specified point over an extended period of time.

Wobble Position: The third base position within a codon, which can often (but not always) be altered to another nucleotide without changing the encoded amino acid.

Xanthophyll: A yellow chloroplast pigment.

X-chromosome: A chromosome associated with sex determination. In most animals, the female has two and the male has one X chromosome. The opposite occurs in birds, in which the equivalent is the Z chromosome.

Xenia: The immediate effect of pollen on some characters of the endosperm.

Xenobiotic: A chemical compound that is not produced by living organisms; a manufactured chemical compound.

Xenotransplantation: Transplantation of cells, tissues or organs from one species to another.

Xenotransplantation: The transplantation of tissue from one species to another species, typically from non-human mammals to humans. This technology has become very important because of a worldwide shortage of human organs for humans requiring a new organ. The most popular non-human species involved in this technology is the pig.

Xerophyte: A plant possessing xeromorphic characters.

Xerophytes: A plant very resistant to drought or that lives in very dry places.

X-linked disease: A genetic disease caused by an allele at a locus on X-chromosome. In X-linked recessive conditions, a normal female carrier passes on the allele on her X chromosome to an affected son.

X-linked: The presence of a gene on the X chromosome.

X-ray crystallography: The deduction of crystal structure from analysis of the diffraction pattern of X-rays passing through a pure crystal of a substance.

Xylem: A complex tissue specialized for efficient conduction of water and mineral nutrients in solution. Xylem may also function as a supporting tissue, particularly secondary xylem.

YAC: Yeast artificial chromosome. This is a method for cloning very large fragments of DNA. Genomic DNA in fragments of 200-500 kb is linked to sequences which allow them to propagate in yeast as a mini-chromosome including telomeres, a centromere and an ARS - an autonomous replication sequence. This technique is used to clone large genes and intergenic regions and for chromosome walking.

Yeast cloning vectors: The yeasts and especially *Saccaromyces cerevisiae* are favourite organisms in which to clone and express DNA. They are eukaryotes and so can splice out introns, the non-coding sequences in the middle of many eukaryotic genes.

Yeast: A unicellular ascomycete fungus, commonly found as a contaminant in plant tissue culture.

Z-DNA: A region of DNA that is flipped into a lefthanded helix, characterized by alternating purines and pyrimidines and which may be the target of a DNA-binding protein.

Zeolite: A group of hydrated sodium aluminosilicates, either natural or synthetic, with ion-exchange properties.

Zinc finger: A protein structural motif common in DNA binding proteins. Four Cys residues are found for each finger and one finger can bind a molecule of zinc.

Zone of elongation: The section of the young root or shoot just behind the apical meristem, in which the cells are enlarging and elongating rapidly.

Zoo blot: Hybridization of cloned DNA from one species to DNA from other organisms to determine the extent to which the cloned DNA is evolutionarily conserved.

Zoo FISH: Fluorescent *in situ* hybridization of DNA from one species on metaphase chromosomes of another species. Typically, the hybridization is done separately for DNA libraries representing each chromosome. The result is a fascinating picture of the regions of chromosomal homology between species.

Zoobiotic: Applied to an organism that lives parasitically on an animal.

Zoophyte: An animal which has a plant-like form.

Zooplankton: The floating and swimming small animals and protozoa found in marine environments, often in association with phytoplankton.

Zoospore: A spore that possesses flagella and is therefore motile.

Zygonema: Stage in meiosis during which synapsis occurs; coming after the leptotene stage and before the pachytene stage in the meiotic prophase.

Zygospore: A thick-walled resistant spore developing from a zygote resulting from the fusion of isogametes.

Zygote: A diploid cell formed by the fusion of two haploid gametes during fertilization in eukaryotic organisms with sexual reproduction. It is the first cell of the new individual.

Zymogen: Inactive enzyme precursor that after secretion is chemically altered to the active form of the enzyme.

Bibliography

Agarwal, M., Katiyar-Agarwal, S., Sahi. C., Gallie, D.R. and Grover, A. (2001). *Arabidopsis thaliana* Hsp100 protein:kith and kin. *Cell Stress Chap.*, 6: 219-224.

Agarwal, M., Sarkar, N. and Grover, A. (2003). Low molecular weight heat shock proteins in plants. *J. Plant Biol.*, 30: 141-149.

Alescio, T. (1960*a*). Osservazioni su culture organotipiche di polmone embrionale di topo. Arch. Ital. Anat. Rmbriol. 65: 323-363.

Alescio, T. (1960*b*). La culture du poumon embryonnaire de souris. Anat. Anz. 109: 144-149.

Anatomy & Physiology by Rod R. Seeley, Trent D. Stephens and Philip (Year) TaTa McGraw Hill, New Delhi.

Anonymous (1958). Nomenclature of cell strains. J. Nat. Cancer Inst. 20: 439.

Ansevin, K.D., and R. Buchsbaum. (1962). Capacity for histological reconstruction by mouse kidney cells in relation to age. *J. Gerontol.* 17: 130-137.

Ariizumi T., Kishitani S., Inatsugi R., Nishida I., Murata N., Toriyama K. (2002). An increase in unsaturation of fatty acids in phosphatidylglycerol from leaves improves the rates of photosynthesis and growth at low temperatures in transgenic rice seedlings. *Plant Cell Physiol.*, 43:751-758.

Asayama, S.I., and M. Furusawa. (1961). Sex differentiation of primordial gonads of the mouse embryo after cultivation *in vitro. Jap. J. Exp. Morphol.* 15: 34-47.

Ashok K. Rathoure and Meena Srivastava (2014). Royal Series of Zoological Sciences, Biotechnology, Immunology, Biological techniques and Biostatistics. Vol-1, 1st Edi. 2014. New Royal Book Company, Lucknow.

Auerbach, R. (1960). Morphogenetic interactions in the development of the mouse thymus glands. *Develop. Biol.* 2: 271-284.

Auerbach, R. (1961*a*). Genetic control of thymus lymphoid differentiation. *Proc. Natl. Acad. Sci.* 47: 1175-1181.

Auerbach, R. (1961*b*). Experimental analysis of the origin of cell types in the development of the mouse thymus. *Develop. Biol.* 3: 336-354.

Auerbach, R. (1963). Developmental studies of mouse thymus and spleen. *Nat. Cancer Inst. Monogr.* 11: 23-33.

Auerbach, R., and C. Grobstein. (1958). Inductive interaction of embryonic tissues after dissociation and reaggregation. *Exp. Cell Res.* 15: 384-397.

Barnett, T.M., Altohuler, C., McDaniel, N. and Mascarenhas, J.P. (1980). Heat shock induced proteins in plant cells. *Dev. Genet.*, 1: 331-340.

Barski, G. (1961). Clones cellulaires hybrids isolés à partir de cultures cellulaires mixtes. *Compt. Rend. Acad. Sci.* 253: 1186-1188.

Barski, G., and F. Cornefert. (1962). Characteristics of hybrid type cloned cell lines obtained from mixed cultures *in vitro. J. Nat. Cancer Inst.* 28: 801-821.

Barski, G., and J. Belehradek. (1963a). Transfert nucléaire intercellulaire en cultures mixtes. *Exp. Cell Res.* 29: 102-111.

Barski, G., and R. Cassigena. (1963b). Malignant transformation *in vitro* of cells from C57BL mouse normal pulmonary tissue. *J. Nat. Cancer Inst.* 30: 865-883.

Barski, G., J.L. Biedler, and F. Cornefert. (1961a). Modification of characteristics of an *in vitro* mouse cell line after an increase of its tumor-producing capacity. *J. Nat. Cancer Inst.* 26: 865-889.

Barski, G., S. Sorieul, and F. Cornefert. (1961b). Hybrid type cells in combined cultures of two different mammalian cell strains. *J. Nat. Cancer Inst.* 26: 1269-1291.

Batra, G., Chauhan, V.S., Singh, A., Sarkar, N.K. and Grover, A. (2007). Complexity of rice Hsp100 gene family: lessons from rice genome sequence data. *J. Biosci.*, 32:611-619.

Bennett, D. (1958). *In vitro* study of cartilage induction in *T/T* mice. Nature 181: 1286.

Bent, S.A., Schwaab, R.L., Collin, D.G., Jeffrey, R.D. (1987): Intellectual property rights in biotechnology worldwide. Stockton Press, New York.

Berman, I., and H.S. Kaplan. (1960). The functional capacity of mouse bone marrow cells growing in diffusion chambers. *Exp. Cell Res.* 20: 238-239.

Berwald, Y., and L. Sachs. (1963). *In vitro* cell transformation with chemical carcinogens. *Nature* 200: 1182-1184.

Biesele, J.J., J.L. Biedler, and D.J. Hutchison. (1959). Chromosomal status of drug resistant sublines of mouse leukemia L1210, *In: Genetics and Cancer. 13th Symp. Fundamental Cancer Res.* University of Texas Press, Austin. p. 295-307.

Bhojwani S S and M K Razdan, (2004). Plant Tissue Culture: Theory and Practice, *a revised edition*, Elsevier, New Delhi.

Biggers, J.D., L.M. Rinaldini, and M. Webb. (1957). The study of growth factors in tissue culture. *Symp. Soc. Exp. Biol.* 11: 264-297.

Biggers, J.D., P.J. Claringbold, and M.H. Hardy. (1956). The action of oestrogens on the vagina of the mouse in tissue culture. *J. Physiol.* 131: 497-515.

Biggers, J.D., R.B.L. Gwatkin, and R.L. Brinster. (1962). Development of mouse embryos in organ cultures of Fallopian tubes on a chemically defined medium. *Nature* 194: 747-749.

Biggers, J.D., R.B.L. Gwatkin, and S. Heyner. (1961). Growth of embryonic avian and mammalian tibiae on a relatively simple chemically defined medium. *Exp. Cell. Res.* 25: 41-58.

Billen, D., and G.A. Debrunner. (1960). Continuously propagating cells derived from normal mouse bone marrow. *J. Nat. Cancer Inst.* 25: 1127-1139.

Blumwald, E., Aharon, G.S. and Apse, M.P. (2000). Sodium transport in plant cells. *Biochemica et Biophysica Acta* 1465, 140-151.

Borghese, E. (1950a). The development *in vitro* of the submandibular and sublingual glands of *Mus musculus*. J. Anat. 84: 287-302.

Borghese, E. (1950b). Explantation experiments on the influence of the connective tissue capsule on the development of the epithelial part of the submandibular gland of *Mus musculus*. J. Anat. 84: 303-318.

Borghese, E. (1958). Organ differentiation in culture, In W.D. McElroy and B. Glass [ed.] *A Symposium on the Chemical Basis of Development*. Johns Hopkins Press, Baltimore. p. 704-773.

Borghese, E. (1961). The effect of ionizing radiations on mouse embryonic lungs developing *in vitro*. Ann. N.Y. Acad. Sci. 95: 866-872.

Borghese, E., and M.A. Venini. (1956). Culture *in vitro* di gonadi embrionale di *Mus musculus*. Symp. Genet. (Pavia) 5: 69-83.

Brand, K.G., and J. Syverton. (1962). Results of species-specific hemagglutination tests on transformed, nontransformed, and primary cell cultures. *J. Nat. Cancer Inst.* 28: 147-157.

Braun AC (1947). Thermal Studies on the factors responsible for tumour initiation in crown gall, *Am. J. Bot.*, Vol. 34 pp.234–240.

Bressan, R.A., Hasegawa, P.M. and Pardo, J.M. (1998). Plants use calcium to resolve salt stress. *Trends in Plant Sci.* 3:411-412.

Bruce W. B. Edmeades GO, Barker TC (2002). Molecular and physiological approaches to maize improvement for drought tolerance. *J. Exp. Bot.* 53: 13-25.

Butcher, D. N., and D. S. Ingram. (1976). Plant tissue culture. Arnold, London, pp 67.

Cameron, I.L. (1964). Is the duration of DNA synthesis in somatic cells of mammals and birds a constant? *J. Cell Biol.* 20:185-188.

Cann, H.M. and L.A. Herzenberg, (1963a). *In vitro* studies of mammalian somatic cell variations. II. Iso-immune cytotoxicity with a cultured mouse lymphoma and selection of resistant variants. *J. Exp. Med.* 117: 267-283.

Cann, H.M., and L.A. Herzenberg. (1963b). *In vitro* studies of mammalian somatic cell variation. I. Detection of H-2 phenotype in cultures mouse cell lines. *J. Exp. Med.* 117: 259-265.

Caplin S M and F C Steward, (1948). Effect of coconut milk on the growth of explants from carrot root, *Science*, 108:655–657.

Chen, J.M. (1952*a*). Studies on the morphogenesis of the mouse sternum. I. Normal embryonic development. *J. Anat.* 86: 373-387.

Chen, J.M. (1952*b*). Studies on the morphogenesis of the mouse sternum. II. Experiments on the origin of the sternum and its capacity for self-differentiation *in vitro. J. Anat.* 86: 387-401.

Chen, J.M. (1953). Studies on the morphogenesis of the mouse sternum. III. Experiments on the closure and segmentation of the sternal bands. *J. Anat.* 87: 130-149.

Chu, E.H.Y. (1962). Chromosomal stabilization of cell strains. *Nat. Cancer Inst. Monogr.* 7: 55-62.

Chu, E.H.Y., and V. Monesi. (1960). Analysis of X-ray induced chromosome aberrations in mouse somatic cells *in vitro. Genetics* 45: 981.

Chu, E.H.Y., K.K. Sanford, and W.R. Earle. (1958). Comparative chromosomal studies on mammalian cells in culture. II. Mouse sarcoma-producing cell strains and their derivatives. *J. Nat. Cancer Inst.* 21: 729-751.

Cleffmann, G. (1963). Agouti pigment cells *in situ* and *in vitro. Ann. N.Y. Acad. Sci.* 100: 749-761.

Conklin, J.L., M.M. Dewey, and R.H. Kahn. (1962). Cytochemical localization of certain oxidative enzymes. *Amer. J. Anat.* 110: 19-27.

Cocking E C. (1960). A method for the isolation of plant protoplast and vacuoles, *Nature*, Vol. 187:962–963.

Colmer T. D Flowers TJ, Munns R. (2006). Use of wild relatives to improve salt tolerance in wheat. *J. Exp. Bot.* 57: 1059-1078.

Connett, R.J.A., Barfoot, P.D. (1992): The development of gnetically modified varieties of agricultural crops by the seed industry. *In*: Plant genetic manipulation for crop protection (Eds. Gatehouse, A.M.R., Hilder, V.A. and Boulter, D.). pp. 45-72.

Coombs, R.R.A. (1962). Identification and characterization of cells by immunologic analysis with special reference to mixed agglutination. *Nat. Cancer Inst. Monogr.*7: 91-98.

Coombs, R.R.A., M.R. Daniel, B.W. Gurner, and A. Kelus. (1961). Species-characterizing antigens of L and ERK cells. *Nature* 189: 503-504.

Coriell, L.L., M.G. Tall, and H. Gaskill. (1958). Common antigens in tissue culture cell lines. *Science* 128: 198-199.

Davenport, H.W., V. Jensen, and L.A. Woodbury. (1948). The secretion of acid by the mouse stomach *in vitro. Gastroenterology* 11: 227-239.

D. Backs-Husemann and J. Reinert, (1970). Embryo formation by isolated single cells from tissue cultures of *Daucus carota*, *Protoplasma*, Vol. 70, pp. 49–60.

Dale, P.J., Marks, M.S., Brown, M.M., Woolston, C.J., Gunn, H.V., Mullineaux, P.M., Lewis, D.M., Friedt, W. (1998). Genetic modification of crop plants - recent achievements and future perspectives. *Proceedings of 2nd Balkan Symposium on field Crops.* (S. Stamenkovic, ed.), 1:9-11.

Davidson, P., and M.H. Hardy. (1952). The development of mouse vibrissae *in vivo* and *in vitro. J. Anat.* 86: 342-356.

Dawe, C.J., and L.W. Law. (1959). Morphologic changes in salivary-gland tissue of the newborn mouse exposed to parotid-tumor agent *in vitro. J. Nat. Cancer Inst.* 23: 1157-1177.

Day, M., and J.P. Green. (1962). The uptake of amino acids and the synthesis of amines by neoplastic mast cells in culture. *J. Physiol.* 164: 210-226.

De Bruyn, W.M., and E. Hansen-Melander. (1962). Chromosome studies in the MB mouse lymphosarcoma. *J. Nat. Cancer Inst.* 28: 1333-1354.

De Bruyn, W.M., R. Korteweg, and E. Kits van Waveren. (1949). Transplantable mouse lymphosarcoma T86157 (MB) studied *in vivo, in vitro* and at autopsy. *Cancer Res.* 9: 282-293.

de la Fuente, J. M., V. Ramirez-Rodriguez, J. L. Cabrera-Ponce, and L. Herrera-Estrella. (1997). Aluminum tolerance in transgenic plants by alteration of citrate synthesis. *Science* 276, no. 5318: 1566-68.

De la Pena A., Lorz, H., Chel, J. (1986): *Transgenic rice plants obtained by injecting DNA into young tillers. Nature,* 325, 274-276.

Defendi, V., and L.A. Manson. (1963). Analysis of the life-cycle in mammalian cells. *Nature* 198: 359-361.

Dodds, J. H., and L. W. Roberts. (1985). Experiments in plant tissue culture. Second edition.

Dulbecco, R., and M. Vogt. (1960). Significance of continued virus production in tissue cultures rendered neoplastic by polyoma virus. *Proc. Natl. Acad. Sci.* 46:1617-1623.

Dunn, T.B., and M. Potter. (1957). A transplantable mast-cell neoplasm in the mouse. *J. Nat. Cancer Inst.* 18: 587-596.

Eagle, H. (1955). Nutritional needs of mammalian cells in tissue culture. *Science* 122(3168):501–514.

Earle, W. R, J. C. Bryant, E. L. Schilling, and V. J. Evans. (1956). Growth of cell suspensions in tissue culture. *Ann. N. Y. Acad. Sci.* **63**:666–682.

Earle, W.R. (1928a). Studies upon the effect of light on blood and tissue cells. I. The action of light on white blood cells *in vitro. J. Exp. Med.* 48: 457-474.

Earle, W.R. (1928b). Studies upon the effect of light on blood and tissue cells. II. The action of light on erythrocytes *in vitro. J. Exp. Med.* 48: 667-681.

Earle, W.R. (1928c). Studies upon the effect of light on blood and tissue cells. III. The action of light on fibroblasts *in vitro. J. Exp. Med.* 48: 683-694.

Earle, W.R. (1943). Production of malignancy *in vitro*. IV. The mouse fibroblast cultures and changes seen in the living cells. *J. Nat. Cancer Inst.* 4: 165-212.

Earle, W.R., and A. Nettleship. (1943). Production of malignancy *in vitro*. V. Results of injections of cultures into mice. *J. Nat. Cancer Inst.* 4: 213-227.

Earle, W.R., E. Shelton, and E.L. Schilling. (1950). Production of malignancy *in vitro*. XI. Further results from reinjection of *in vitro* cell strains into strain C3H mice. *J. Nat. Cancer Inst.* 10: 1105-1113.

Edwards, R.G. (1961). Identification of the chromosome complements of new-born and adult living mice. *Nature* 192: 1316-1317.

Elias, J.J. (1957). Cultivation of adult mouse mammary gland in hormone-enriched synthetic medium. *Science* 126: 842-844.

Elias, J.J. (1962). Response of mouse mammary duct end-buds to insulin in organ culture. *Exp. Cell Res.* 27: 601-604.

Elias, J.J., and E. Rivera. (1959). Comparison of the responses of normal, precancerous and neoplastic mouse mammary tissues to hormones *in vitro*. *Cancer Res.*19: 505-511.

Ephrussi, B., and S. Sorieul. (1962). Mating of somatic cells *in vitro*, *In* D.J. Merchant and J.V. Neel [ed.] Approaches to the Genetic Analysis of Mammalian Cells. The University of *Michigan Press, Ann Arbor.* p. 81-97.

Evans D E, JOD Coleman and A Kearns, (2003). Plant Cell Culture, Bios Scientific Publishers, Taylor & Francis Group, London, p.1.

Evans, V.J., N.M. Hawkins, B.B. Westfall, and W.R. Earle. (1958). Studies on culture lines derived from mouse liver parenchymatous cells grown in long-term tissue culture. *Cancer Res.* 18: 261-266.

Evans, V.J., G.A. Parker, and T.B. Dunn. (1964). Neoplastic transformations in C3H mouse embryonic tissue *in vitro* determined by intraocular growth. I. Cells from chemically defined medium with or without serum supplement. *J. Nat. Cancer inst.* 32: 89-121.

F Constabel and J P Shyluk, (1994). Initiation Nutrition and Maintenance of Plant Cell and Tissue Cultures (Eds. I K Vasil and T A Thorpe), Kluwer Academic Publishers, Dordrecht, The Netherlands, pp. 6–7.

F Skoog and C O Miller, (1957). Chemical regulation of growth and organ formation in plant tissues cultured *in vitro*, *Symp. Soc. Exp. Bio.*, 11:118–130.

Fedoroff, S. (1962). Method for distinguishing between human and mouse cells in tissue culture. *Nature* 196: 394-395.

Fedoroff, S. (1966). Report on animal tissue culture nomenclature. *Tissue Culture Assoc. Comm. on Nomenclature.*

Fedoroff, S., and B. Cook. (1959). Effects of human blood serum on tissue culture. II. Development of resistance to toxic human serum in fibroblast-like cells (Earle's L strain) obtained from a C3H mouse. *J. Exp. Med.* 109: 615-632.

Fell, H.B. (1953). Recent advances in organ culture. *Sci. Progr.* 162: 212-231.

Fell, H.B. (1954). The effect of hormones and vitamin A on organ cultures. *Ann. N.Y. Acad. Sci.* 58: 1183-1187.

Fell, H.B. (1955). The effect of hormones on differentiated tissues in culture, *In* R.W. Smith, O.H. Gaebler, and C.N.H. Long [ed.] *The Hypophyseal Growth Hormone, Nature and Actions.* McGraw-Hill, New York. p. 138-148.

Fell, H.B. (1958). The physiology of skeletal tissue in culture. *Lect. Sci. Basis Med.* 6: 28-45.

Fell, H.B. (1964). The role of organ cultures in the study of vitamins and hormones. *Vit. Horm.* 22: 81-127.

Fell, H.B., and A.F.W. Hughes. (1949). Mitosis in the mouse: A study of living and fixed cells in tissue cultures. *Quart. J. Microscop. Sci.* 90: 355-380.

Fell, H.B. and E. Mellanby. (1950). Effects of hypervitaminosis A on foetal mouse bones cultivated *in vitro*; preliminary communication. *Brit. Med. J.* 2: 535-539.

Fell, H.B., (1956). Effect of excess vitamin A on organized tissues cultivated *in vitro*. *Brit. Med. Bull.* 12: 35-37.

Fell, H.B., and E. Mellanby. (1952). The effect of hypervitaminosis A on embryonic limb-bones cultivated *in vitro*. *J. Physiol.* 116: 320-349.

Fernandes, M.A.R., and I. Koprowska. (1963). Tissue culture studies on cells from mouse cervix subjected to carcinogenic treatment. *Acta Cytol.* 7: 215-223.

Fisher, G.A. (1959). Nutritional and amethopterin-resistant characteristics of leukemic clones. *Cancer Res.* 19: 372-376.

Francke, C. (1946). The effect of gonadotropins on explanted fragments of ovaries from immautre mice. *Endocrinology* 39: 430-431.

Franks, L.M. (1959). A factor in normal human serum that inhibits epithelial growth in organ cultures. *Exp. Cell Res.* 17: 579-581.

Franks, L.M. (1961). The growth of mouse prostate during culture *in vitro* in chemically defined and natural media, and after transplantation *in vivo*. *Exp. Cell Res.*22: 56-72.

Franks, L.M., and A.A. Barton. (1960). The effects of testosterone on the ultrastructure of mouse prostate *in vivo* and in organ cultures. *Exp. Cell Res.* 19: 35-50.

Frédéric, J. (1954). Effets de différentes longueurs d'onde du spectre visible sur des cellules vivantes cultivées *in vitro*. Compt. *Rend. Soc. Biol.* 148: 1678-1682.

G Morel and C Martin, (1952). Guerison de dahlias atteints d'une maladie a virus, *C R Acad. Sci.*, Paris, Vol. 235 pp.1324–1325.

Gaillard, P.J. (1942). *Hormones Regulating Growth and Differentiation in Embryonic Explants.* Masson, Paris. 82 p.

Gaillard, P.J. (1948). Growth, differentiation, and function of explants of some endocrine glands. *Symp. Soc. Exp. Biol.* 2: 139-144.

Gaillard, P.J. (1953). Growth and differentiation of explanted tissues. *Int. Rev. Cytol.* 2: 331-401.

Gaillard, P.J. (1961*a*). The influence of parathyroid extract on the explanted radius of albino mouse embryos. II. *Proc. Koninkl. Ned. Akad. Wetensch. Ser.* C64:119-128.

Gaillard, P.J. (1961*b*). Parathyroid and bone in tissue culture, p. 20-45. *In* R.O. Greep and R.V. Talmage [ed.] *The Parathyroids.* Charles C Thomas, Springfield, Ill.

Gaillard, P.J. (1962). A comparative study of the influence of thyroxine and of parathyroid extract on the histological structure of the explanted embryonic radius rudiment. *Acta Morphol. Neer.-Scand.* 5: 21-36.

Gaillard, P.J. (1963). Observations on the effect of thyroid and parathyroid secretions on explanted mouse radius rudiments. *Develop. Biol.* 7: 103-116.

Gelfant, S. (1960). A study of mitosis in mouse epidermis *in vitro*. III. Effects of glucolytic and Krebs' cycle intermediates. IV. Effects of metabolic inhibitors. *Exp. Cell Res.* 19: 65-82.

Geyer, R.P. (1958). Nutrition of mammalian cells in tissue culture. *Nutr.* Rev. 16: 321-323.

Gillette, R.W., A. Findley, and H. Conway. (1961). Effect of cortisone on skin maintained in organ culture. *J. Nat. Cancer Inst.* 27: 1285-1309.

Ginsburg, H.(1963). The *in vitro* differentiation and culture of normal mast cells from mouse thymus. *Ann. N.Y. Acad. Sci.* 103: 20-39.

Ginsburg, H., and L. Sachs. (1963). Formation of pure suspensions of mast cells in tissue culture by differentiation of lymphoid cells from the mouse thymus. *J. Nat. Cancer Inst.* 31: 1-39.

Gluecksohn-Waelsch, S., and T.R. Rota, (1963). Development in organ tissue culture of kidney rudiments from mouse embryos. *Develop. Biol.* 7: 432-444.

Goldhaber, P. (1960). Behavior of bone in tissue culture. *Pub. Amer. Ass. Adv. Sci.* 64: 349-372.

Gosal, S.S., Wani, S.H. (2009). Kang, M.S. Biotechnology and drought tolerance. *J. Crop Improv.,* 23:19-54.

Green, J.P., and M. Day. (1960). Heparin, 5-hydroxytryptamine and histamine in neoplastic mast cells. *Biochem. Pharmacol.* 3: 190-205.

Grobstein, C. (1950). Behavior of the mouse embryonic shield in plasma clot cutures. *J. Exp. Zool.* 115: 297-314.

Grobstein, C. (1953*a*). Epithelio-mesenchymal specificity in the morphogenesis of mouse submandibular rudiments *in vitro*. *J. Exp. Zool.* 124: 383-413.

Grobstein, C. (1953*b*). Analysis *in vitro* of the early organization of the rudiments of the mouse submandibular gland. *J. Morphol.* 93: 19-44.

Grobstein, C. (1953*c*). Inductive epithelio-mesenchymal interaction in cultured organ rudiments of the mouse. *Science* 118: 52-55.

Grobstein, C. (1955a). Inductive interaction in the development of the mouse metanephros. *J. Exp. Zool.* 130: 319-339.

Grobstein, C. (1955b). Tissue interaction in the morphogenesis of mouse embryonic rudiments *in vitro, In* D. Rudnick [ed.] *Aspects of Synthesis and Order in Growth.* Princeton University Press, Princeton, N.J. p. 233-256.

Grobstein, C. (1956). Trans-filter induction of tubules in mouse metanephrogenic mesenchyme. *Exp. Cell Res.* 10: 424-440.

Grobstein, C. (1957). Some transmission characteristics of the tubule-inducing influence of mouse metanephrogenic mesenchyme. *Exp. Cell Res.* 13: 575-587.

Grobstein, C. (1959). Autoradiography of the interzone between tissue in inductive interaction. *J. Exp. Zool.* 142: 203-213.

Grobstein, C. (1962). Interactive processes in cytodifferentiation. *J. Cell. Comp. Physiol.* 60 (Suppl. 1): 35-48.

Grobstein, C. and H. Holtzer. 1(955). *In vitro* studies of cartilage induction in mouse somite mesoderm. *J. Exp. Zool.* 128: 333-358.

Grobstein, C., and A.J. Dalton. (1957). Kidney tubule induction in mouse metanephrogenic mesenchyme without cytoplasmic contact. *J. Exp. Zool.* 135: 57-73.

Grobstein, C., and G. Parker. (1954). *In vitro* induction of cartilage in mouse somite mesoderm by embryonic spinal card. *Proc. Soc. Exp. Biol. Med.* 85: 477-481.

Grover, A. (2002). Molecular biology of stress responses. *Cell Stress Chap.*, 7: 1-5.

Grover, A., Aggarwal, P.K., Kapoor, A., Katiyar-Agarwal, S.,Agarwal, M., Chandramouli, A. (2003). Addressing abiotic stresses in agriculture through transgenic technology. *Curr Sci.*, 84: 355–367.

Guha S and Maheshwari S C. (1964). *In vitro* production of embryos from anthers of *Datura, Nature*, Vol. 204, p.497.

Guthrie, M.J. (1953). Enhancement of growth in the explanted ovary of the newborn mouse by inorganic phosphate and adenine. *Anat. Rec.* 115: 314-315.

Hanks, J.H. (1955). Nutrition of cells *in vitro, In An Introduction to Cell and Tissue Culture.* Burgess, Minneapolis. p. 74-82.

Hannah, M.A.; Heyer, A. G.; Hincha, D.K (2005). A global survey of gene regulation during cold acclimation in *Arabidopsis thaliana. PLoS Genet.*, 1, e26.

Hardy, M.H. (1949). The development of mouse hair *in vitro* with some observations on pigmentation. *J. Anat.* 83: 364-384.

Hardy, M.H. (1950). The development *in vitro* of the mammary glands of the mouse. *J. Anat.* 84: 388-393.

Hardy, M.H. (1951). The development of pelage hairs and vibrissae from skin in tissue culture. *Ann. N.Y. Acad. Sci.* 53: 546-561.

Hardy, M.H., J.D. Biggers, and P.J. Claringbold. (1953). Vaginal cornification of the mouse produced by oestrogens *in vitro. Nature* 172: 1196-1197.

Harris, M. (1964). *Cell Culture and Somatic Variation.* Holt, New York, 547 p.

Hasegawa, P.M., Bressan, R.A. and Pardo, J.M. (2000). The dawn of plant salt to tolerance genetics. *Trends in Plant Sci.* 5, 317-319.

Hasegawa, P.M., Bressan, R.A., Zhu, J.K. and Bohnert, H.J. (2000). Plant cellular and molecular responses to high salinity. *Annu. Rev. Plant Physiol. Plant Mol. Biol.* 51, 463-499.

Hauschka, T.S. (1957). Tissue genetics of neoplastic cell populations. *Can. Cancer Res. Conf.* 2 (1956): 305-345.

Hauschka, T.S. (1958). Correlation of chromosomal and physiologic changes in tumors. *J. Cell. Comp. Physiol.* 52: 197-267.

Hobbs, G.L., K.K. Sanford, V.J. Evans, and W.R. Earle. (1957). Establishment of a clone of mouse liver cells from a single isolated cell. *J. Nat. Cancer Inst.* 18:701-708.

Horsch, R.B., Fraley, R.T., Rogers, S.G., Sanders, P.R., Loyd, A., Hoffman, H. (1984). Inheritance of functional foreign genes in plants. *Science,* 223:496-498.

Hsieh, T.H.; Lee, J.T.; Yang, P.T.; Chiu, L.H.; Charng, Y.; Wang, Y.C.; Chan, M.T. (2002). Heterology expression of the *Arabidopsis crepeat/* dehydration response element binding factor 1 gene confers elevated tolerance to chilling and oxidative stresses in transgenic tomato. *Plant Physiol., 129:*1086-1094.

Hsu, T.C. (1959). Mammalian chromosomes *in vitro.* XI. Variability among progenies of a single cell, *In: Biol. Contrib. No. 5914, Univ. Texas, Austin.* p. 129-134.

Hsu, T.C. (1960). Mammalian chromosomes *in vitro.* XIII. Cyclic and directional changes of population strucutre. *J. Nat. Cancer Inst.* 25: 1339-1353.

Hsu, T.C. (1961). Chromosomal evolution in cell populations. Int. Rev. Cytol. 12: 69-161.

Hsu, T.C., D. Billen, and A. Levan. (1961a). Mammalian chromosomes *in vitro.* XV. Patterns of transformation. *J. Nat Cancer Inst.* 27: 515-541.

Hsu, T.C., and D.J. Merchant. (1961b). Mammalian chromosomes *in vitro.* XIV. Genotypic replacement in cell populations. *J. Nat. Cancer Inst.* 26: 1075-1083.

Hsu, T.C., and D.S. Kellogg (1959). Genetics of *in vitro* cells, *In Genetics and Cancer. 13th Symp. Fundamental Cancer Res.* University of Texas Press, Austin. p. 183-204.

Hsu, T.C., and D.S. Kellogg (1960). Mammalian chromosomes *in vitro.* XII. Experimental evolution of cell populations. *J. Nat. Cancer Inst.* 24: 1067-1093.

Hsu, T.C., and O. Klatt (1958). Mammalian chromosomes *in vitro.* IX. On genetic polymorphism in cell populations. *J. Nat. Cancer Inst.* 21: 437-473.

Hungerford, D.A. (1955). Chromosome numbers of ten day fetal mouse cells. *J. Morphol.* 97: 497-510.

I. Takebe, G. Labib and G. Melchers, (1971). Regeneration of whole plants from isolated mesophyll protoplasts of tobacco, *Naturwissenschaften,* 58:318–320.

I. Zaenen, H. van Larebeke, H. Teuchy, M van Montagu and J Schell (1974). Supercoiled circular DNA in crown gall inducing *Agrobacterium* strains, *J. Mol. Biol.*, 86:109–127.

Ingalls, T.H., E.F. Ingenito, and F. J. Curley. (1963). Acquired chromosomal anomalies induced in mice by injection of a teratogen in pregnancy. Science 141: 810-812.

Ingram, R.L. (1962). Maintenance of organized adult liver tissue *in vitro*. *Exp. Cell Res.* 28: 370-380.

Jacobs, B.B. (1963). *In vivo* assay of function of mouse ovaries following culture in hormone enriched medium. *Exp. Cell Res.* 32: 431-441.

Ishizaki-Nishizawa, O.; Fuji, T.; Azume, M.; Sekiguchi, K.; Murata, N.; Ohtani, T.; Toguri, T. (1996). Low-temperature resistance of higher plants is significantly enhanced by a nonspecific cyanobacterial desaturase. *Nat. Biotechnol.*, 14:1003-1006.

J. H. Harrison, (1982). *Foreword*, (Eds. J. H. Dodds and L. W. Roberts), *Experiment in Plant Tissue Culture*, Cambridge University Press, p.vii.

Kahn, R. H. (1958). Organ culture in experimental biology. *Univ. Michigan Med. Bull.* 24: 242-252.

Kite, J.H., and D.J. Merchant. (1961). Studies of some antigens of the L-strain mouse fibroblast. *J. Nat. Cancer Inst.* 26: 419-434.

Katiyar-Agarwal, S., Agarwal, M., Gallie, D. and Grover, A. (2001). Search for the cellular functions of plant Hsp100/ Clp family proteins. *Crit. Rev. lant Sci.*, 20: 277-295.

Kemp, J.M., Kemp, J.M., Chen, D.F., Gilmour, D.M., Flavell, R.B. (1989). Agroinfection of wheat: inoculation of in vitro grown seedling and embryos. *Plant Science*, 63, 237-245.

Kidd, G.H. (1985). The new plant genetics: restructing the global seed industry. *In:* The world Biotech Report 1, Online, London, pp. 311-321.

Klein, E. (1960). On substrate-induced enzyme formation in animal cells cultured *in vitro*. *Exp. Cell Res.* 21: 421-429.

Klein, E. (1961). Studies on the substrate-induced arginase synthesis in animals cell strains cultured *in vitro*. *Exp. Cell Res.* 22: 226-232.

Knezevic, D., Zecevic, V., Marinkovic, I., Konstatinov, K., Mladenovic-Drinic, S., Andjelkovic, M., Micanovic, D. (1998). Prospect and problems of genetically modified cultivars, development and impact on conventional plant breeding. Proceedings of International Symposium Breeding of Small Grains, pp. 103-110.

Kodama, H., Hamada, T., Horiguchi, G., Nishimura, M., Iba, K. (1994). Genetic enhancement of cold tolerance by expression of a gene for chloroplast *w*-3 fatty acid desaturase in transgenic tobacco. *Plant Physiol.*, 105:601-605.

Konstatinov, Lj. K., Mladenovic-Drinic, S.D. (1998). Biotechnology in intellectual property protection in breeding. Proceedings of 2nd Balkan Symposium on field Crops. (S. Stamenkovic, ed.), 1, 157-160.

Kotak, S., Larkindale, J., Lee, U., von Koskull-Doring, P., Vierling, E., and Scharf, K.D. (2007). Complexity of the heat stress response in plants. *Curr. Opin. Plant Biol.*, 10, 310-316.

Koziorowska, J. (1962). The influence of ovarian hormones and insulin on the mouse mammary glands cultivated *in vitro*. Acta Med. Pol. 3: 237-245.

Krishna, P. and Gloor, G. (2001). The Hsp90 family of proteins in *Arabidopsis thaliana*. *Cell Stress Chap.*, 6:238–246.

Kuff, E.L., and V.J. Evans. (1961). α-Glucuronidase activities of cultured cells derived from C3H mouse liver. *J. Nat. Cancer Inst.* 27: 667-678.

Kumar Ashok (2011). Molecular Biology and Recombinant DNA Technology: A Practical Book; 1st Ed. Narendra Publishing House (P) Ltd. New Delhi. ISBN: 978-93-80428-32-1.

Kumar Ashok (2012). Role of PGPR in the Management of Chromium Contaminated Soil, *In*: Toxicity of Heavy Metals to Legumes and Bioremediation, Editors: Almas Zaidi, Pervaze Ahmad Wani, Mohammad Saghir Khan, Springer-Vienna. pp. 163-178 DOI: 10.1007/978-3-7091-0730-0_10.

Kumar Ashok (2013). GCMS Screening for Phytocontents in the Essential Oil of *Coleus forskohlii*, *In*: Medicinal Plants: Phytochemistry, Pharmacology and Therapeutics. Vol. 3, Editor Dr. Vijay Gupta, Daya Publication House, New Delhi, pp. 79-124.

Kumar Ashok (2013). Transgenesis via Genetic Engineering: A crop Improvemental Approach *In*: Crop Improvement in the Era of Climate Change, Editor Dr. Rajib Roychowdhury, I.K. International Publication House Pvt. Ltd. pp. 285-319

Kumar Ashok (2013). Wound healing and *Ficus arnottiana* Miq.—A Review, *In*: Natural products: Research Reviews, Vol. 2, Editor Dr. Vijay Gupta, Daya Publication House, New Delhi pp. 293-302.

Kumar Ashok (2014). Microbial Biomass Production, *In*: Microbial Biotechnology: Progress and Trends, Editors Dr. Hongzhang Chen, Dr. Farshad Darvishi, CRC Press / Taylor & Francis Group 6000 Broken Sound Parkway NW, Suite 300, Boca Raton, FL 33487. ISBN 9781782245202 K23526.

Kumar Ashok and Srivastava Meena (2012). Molecular Cytogenetics; 1st Edi. Narendra Publishing House (P) Ltd. New Delhi; ISBN: 938-04-287-9-1.

Kumar, M.S., Kumar, G., Srikanthbabu, V. and Udayakumar, M. (2007). Assessment of variability in acquired thermotolerance: potential option to study genotypic response and the relevance of stress genes. *J Plant Physiol.*, 164: 111-125.

Kumar, P.A. (2006). Bt crops. *In*: Extended summaries, National Seminar Transgenic Crops Indian Agricul.: Status, Risks and Acceptance. Hisar, India. pp. 1-3.

Lasfargues, E.Y. (1957*a*). Cultivation and behaviour *in vitro* of the normal mammary epithelium of the adult mouse. *Anat. Rec.* 127: 117-129.

Lasfargues, E.Y. (1957*b*). Cultivation and behavior *in vitro* of the normal mammary epithelium of the adult mouse. II. Observations on the secretory activity. *Exp. Cell Res.* 13: 553-562.

Lasfargues, E.Y. (1957*c*). Comparative behaviour *in vitro* of the normal and neoplastic mammary epithelium of the mouse. *Proc. Amer. Ass. Cancer Res.* 2: 224.

Lasfargues, E.Y. (1960). Action de l'oestradiol et de la progestérone sure des cultures de glandes mammaires de jeunes souris. *Compt. Rend. Soc. Biol.* 154: 1720-1722.

Lasfargues, E.Y. (1962). Concerning the role of insulin in the differentiation and functional activity of mouse mammary tissues. *Exp. Cell Res.* 28: 531-542.

Lasfargues, E.Y., and D.G. Feldman. (1963). Hormonal and physiological background in the production of B particles by the mouse mammary epithelium in organ culture. *Cancer Res.* 23: 191-196.

Lasfargues, E.Y., and M.R. Murray. (1959). Hormonal influences on the differentiation and growth of embryonic mouse mammary gland in organ culture. *Develop. Biol.* 1: 413-435.

Lasfargues, E.Y., D.H. Moore, and M.R. Murray. (1958). Maintenance of the milk factor in cultures of mouse mammary epithelium. *Cancer Res.* 18: 1281-1285.

Lasnitzki, I. (1954). The effect of oestrone alone and combined with 20-methylcholanthrene on mouse prostate glands grown *in vitro. Cancer Res.* 14: 632-639.

Lasnitzki, I. (1955*a*). The effect of testosterone propionate on organ cultures of the mouse prostate. *J. Endocrinol.* 12: 236-240.

Lasnitzki, I. (1955*b*). The influence of A hypervitaminosis on the effect of 20-methylcholanthrene on mouse prostate glands grown *in vitro. Brit. J. Cancer* 9: 434-441.

Lasnitzki, I. (1961*a*). The effect of radiation on the normal and oestrone-treated mouse vagina grown *in vitro. Brit J. Radiol.* 34: 356-361.

Lasnitzki, I. (1961*b*). Effect of excess vitamin A on the normal and oestrone-treated mouse vagina grown in chemically defined media. *Exp. Cell Res.* 24: 37-45.

Lasnitzki, I. (1961*c*). Action and interaction of radiation, oestrogen and vitamin A on the mouse vagina grown *in vitro. Colloq. Int. Centre Nat. Res. Sci.* 101: 73-84.

Lasnitzki, I. (1961*d*). The effect of X rays on cellular differentiation in organ culture. *Ann. N.Y. Acad. Sci.* 95: 873-881.

Lasnitzki, I. (1962). Hypovitaminosis-A in the mouse prostate gland cultured in chemically defined medium. *Exp. Cell Res.* 28: 40-51.

Lasnitzki, I. (1965). The action of hormones on cell and organ cultures, p. 591-658. *In* E.N. Willmer [ed.] *Cells and Tissue in Culture.* Vol 1. Academic Press, New York.

Lasnitzki, I. (1958). The effect of carcinogens, hormones and vitamins on organ cutlures. *Int. Rev. Cytol.* 7: 79-121.

Lasnitzki, I., and J.A. Lucy. (1961). Amino acid metabolism and arginase activity in mouse prostate glands grown *in vitro* with and without 20-methylcholanthrene. *Exp Cell Res.* 24: 379-392.

Levan, A., and J.J. Biesele. (1958). Role of chromosomes in cancerogenesis, as studied in serial tissue culture of mammalian cells. *Ann. N.Y. Acad. Sci.* 71: 1022-1053.

Levan, A., and T.C. Hsu. (1960). The chromosomes of two mouse strains from mammary carcinomas of the mouse. *Hereditas* 46: 231-240.

Leskien, D., Flitner, M. (1997). Intellectual Property Rights and Plant Genetic Resources: Options for a Sui Generis System. *Issues in Genetic Resources,* 6.

Levintow, L., and H. Eagle. (1961). Biochemistry of cultured mammalian cells. *Annu. Rev. Biochem.* 30: 605-640.

Levitt, J. (1980). Responses of plants to environmental stress. In: *Chilling, Freezing and High Temperature Stress.* New York Academic Press, 1.

Lieberman, M. (1958). Cultivation of mouse thymus in diffusion chambers *in vivo*. *Proc. Amer. Ass. Cancer Res.* 2: 321.

Lostroh, A.J. (1959). The response of ovarian explants from post-natal mice to gonadotropins. *Endocrinology* 65: 124-132.

Lostroh, A.J. (1960). *In vitro* response of mouse testis to human chorionic gonadotropin. *Proc. Soc. Exp. Biol. Med.* 103: 25-27.

Lostroh, A.J. (1963). Effects of insulin and of DL-aldosterone on protein synthesis by mouse uteri in organ culture. *Exp. Cell Res.* 32: 327-332.

Lucas, D.R. (1958). Inherited retinal dystrophy in the mouse: its appearance in eyes and retinae cultured *in vitro*. *J. Embryol. Exp. Morphol.* 6: 589-592.

Lucas, D.R., and O.A. Trowell. (1958). *In vitro* culture of the eye and the retina of the mouse and rat. *J. Embryol. Exp. Morphol.* 6: 178-182.

Ludovici, P.P., C. Ashford, and N.F. Miller. (1962*a*). Studies on chemically induced and "spontaneous" alterations of morphology and growth potential in human cell culture. *Cancer Res.* 22: 788-796.

Ludovici, P.P., C. Ashford, and N.F. Miller. (1962*b*). Studies on the chemicals required to induce alterations of morphology and growth potential in human cell culture. *Cancer Res.* 22: 797-803.

M E Curtin, (1983). Harvesting profitable product from plant tissue culture, *Biotechnology,* Vol.83 pp.649–657.

Magee, W.E., M.R. Sheek, and B.P. Sagik. (1958). Methods of harvesting mammalian cells grown in tissue culture. *Proc. Soc. Exp. Biol. Med.* 99: 390-392.

Maio, J.J., and H.V. Rickenberg. (1960). The α-galactosidase of mouse strain L-cells and mouse organs. *Biochem. Biophys. Acta* 37: 101-106.

Manson, L.A., G.V. Foschi, and J. Palm. (1962*a*). *In vivo* and *in vitro* studies of histocompatibility antigens isolated from a cultured mouse cell line. *Proc. Nat. Acad. Sci.* 48: 1816-1821.

Manson, L.A., G.V. Foschi, J.F. Duplan, and O.B. Zaalberg. (1962*b*). Isolation of transplantation antigens from a leukemic cell grown i*n vitro*. Ann. N.Y. Acad. Sci. 101: 121-130.

Marks, M.S., Kemp, J.M., Woolston, C.J., Dale, P.J. (1989). *Agroinfection of wheat: a comparison of Agrobacterium strains. Plant Science,* 63, 247-256.

Martin, L. (1959). Growth of the vaginal epithelium of the mouse in tissue culture. *J. Endocrinol.* 18: 334-342.

Martinovitch, P.N. (1938). The development *in vitro* of the mammalian gonad. Ovary and ovogenesis. *Proc. Roy. Soc. B* 125: 232-249.

Martinovitch, P.N. (1939). The effect of subnormal temperature on the differentiation and survival of cultivated *in vitro* embryonic and infantile rat and mouse ovaries. *Proc. Roy. Soc. B* 128: 138-143.

McCarthy, B.J., and B.H. Hoyer. (1964). Identity of DNA and diversity of messenger RNA molecules in normal mouse tissues. *Proc. Nat. Acad. Sci.* 52: 915-922.

McCulloch, E.A., and J.E. Till. (1962). The sensitivity of cells from normal mouse bone marrow to gamma radiation *in vitro* and *in vivo*. *Radiat. Res.* 16: 822-832.

McKenna, J.M., and W.S. Blakemore. (1962). Serological comparisons among tissue culture cell lines. *Nature* 195: 1009-1010.

McLaren, A., and J. D. Biggers. (1958). Successful development and birth of mice cultivated *in vitro* as early embryos. *Nature* 182: 877-878.

Melchers G, Sacristan M D, and Holder A A. (1978). Somatic hybrid plants of potato and tomato regenerated from fused protoplasts, *Carlsberg Res Commun* 43:203–218.

Merchant, D.J., and J.V. Neel [ed.] (1962). *Approaches to the Genetic Analysis of Mammalian Cells.* The University of Michigan Press, Ann Arbor. 97 p.

Merchant, D.J., R.H. Kahn, and W.H. Murphy. (1964). Handbook of Cell and Organ Culture, 2nd ed. Burgess, Minneapolis. 263 p.

Miller, C. O. F Skoog, M. Saltza and F. M. Strong, (1955). Kinetin, a cell division factor from deoxyribonucleic acid, *J. Am. Chem. Soc.,* 77:1329.

Mintz, B. (1962*a*). Experimental study of the developing mammalian egg: removal of the zona pellucida. *Science* 138: 594-595.

Mintz, B. (1962*b*). Incorporation of nucleic acid and protein precursors by developing mouse eggs. *Amer. Zool.* 2: 432.

Mintz, B. (1962*c*). Formation of genotypically mosaic mouse embryos. *Amer. Zool.* 2: 432.

Mintz, B. (1963). Growth *in vitro* of t^{12}/t^{12} lethal mutant mouse eggs. *Amer. Zool.* 2: 432.

Mitsutani, M., Y. Ohnuki, Y.H. Nakanishi, and C.M. Pomerat. (1960). The development of a near-diploid *in vitro* strain from a smoke-condensate induced mouse tumor. *Texas Rep. Biol. Med*. 18: 455-469.

Moretti, R.L., and K.B. DeOme. (1962). Effect of insulin on glucose uptake by normal and neoplastic mouse mammary tissues in organ culture. *J. Nat. Cancer Inst*.29: 321-329.

Morgan, J.F. (1958). Tissue culture nutrition. *Bacteriol. Rev*. 22: 20-45.

Morgan, J.F., L.F. Guerin, and H.J. Morton. (1956). The effect of low temperature and storage on the viability and mouse strain specificity of ascitic tumor cells. *Cancer Res*. 16: 907-912.

Murray, M.R. (1959). Uses of tissue culture in the study of malignancy, p. 469-516. *In* F. Homburger [ed.] The Pathophysiology of Cancer, *2nd ed*. Hoeber-Harper, New York.

Murray, M.R., and G. Kopech. (1953). A Bibliography of the Research in Tissue Culture, *1884-1950*. Academic Press, New York. 2 vol.

Murray, M.R., and G. Kopech. (1965). Current Tissue Culture Literature. *Vol. 5*. October House, New York.

Murray, M.R., and G. Kopech. (1966). Current Tissue Culture Literature. [1961-64]. Vols. *1-4*. October House, New York.

New, D.A.T. (1962). Action of vitamin A on rodent skin and buccal epithelium in organ culture, *Annu. Rep. Strangeways Res. Lab., Cambridge, England*. p. 20.

New, D.A.T., and K.F. Stein. (1963). Cultivation of mouse embryos *in vitro*. *Nature* 199: 297-299.

Parker, R.C. (1961). Methods of Tissue Culture, *3rd ed*. Hoeber-Harper, New York. 358 p.

Ohta, Y. (1986): High efficiency genetic transformation of mize by mixture of pollen and exogenous DNA. P.A.N.Sci. USA, 83, 715-719.

Oxtoby, E. Hughes, M.A. (1990). Engineering herbicide tolerance into crops. Tibtech, 8, 61-65.

Carlson P S, H H Smith and R D Dearing, (1972). Parasexual interspecific plant hybridization, *P. Soc. Natl. Acad. Sci.*, USA, 69:.2292–2294.

Paul, J. (1958). A note on nomenclature of cell strains. *Virology* 5: 175.

Paul, J. (1960). Environmental influences on the metabolism and composition of cultured cells. *J. Exp. Zool.* 142: 475-505.

Paul, J. (1961). Cell and Tissue Culture, 2nd ed. Livingstone, Edinburgh and London. 312 p.

Paul, J., and M.G. Struthers. (1963). Actinomycin D-resistant RNA synthesis in animal cells. Biochem. Biophys. *Res. Commun.* 11: 135-139.

Pearce, G.W. (1963). Tissue culture in the study of muscular dstrophy, p. 178-191. *In* G.H. Bourne and M.N. Golarz [ed.] *Muscular Dystrophy in Man and Animals*. Hafner, New York.

Pearson, H.E. (1962). Reaction of certain mouse and hamster tumor tissue cultures to polyoma virus. *Proc. Soc. Exp. Biol. Med.* 111: 332-334.

Peppers, E.V., B.B. Westfall, H.A. Kerr, and W.R. Earle. (1960). Note on the catalase activity of several mammalian cell strains after long cultivation *in vitoro. J. Nat. Cancer Inst.* 25: 1065-1068.

Phillips, H.J., and J.E. Terryberry. (1957). Counting actively metabolizing tissue cultured cells. *Exp. Cell Res.* 13: 341-347.

Pinkel, D. (1963). Successful cultivation of spleen fragments in organ culture. *Proc. Soc. Exp. Biol. Med.* 112: 242-245.

Pinto, Y. M., R. A. Kok, and D. C. Baulcombe. (1999). Resistance to rice yellow mottle virus (RYMV) in cultivated African rice varieties containing RYMV transgenes. *Nature Biotechnology* 17(7): 702-707.

Prop, F.J.A. (1959). Organ culture of total mammary gland of the mouse. *Nature* 184: 379-380.

Prop, F.J.A. (1960). Development of alveoli in organ cultures of total mammary glands of six weeks old virgin mice. *Exp. Cell Res.* 20: 256-258.

Prop, F.J.A. (1961). Sensitivity to prolactin of mouse mammary glands *in vitro. Exp. Cell Res.* 24: 629-631.

Reid, T.R., and M.P. Gifford. (1952). A quantitative study of the effects of X-radiation on cells *in vitro.* J. Nat. Cancer Inst. 13: 431-439.

Rainer, D.H., Bottino, P., Gordon, M.P, Nester, E.W. (1990). Agrobacterium mediated transformation of rice (*Oryza sativa* L.). *Bio/Technology*, 8:33-38.

Rathoure Ashok K. (2014). Basics of Biotechnology, Vol-1, Vol-2 and Vol-3; Narendra Publishing House (P) Ltd. New Delhi-110006., 1st Edn. 2014

Rathoure Ashok K. and Srivastava Meena (2014). Cell Biology and Genetics; 1st Edi. Astral International Publisher (P) Ltd. New Delhi. ISBN 9789351243199

Rathoure Ashok K. (2013). Fundamentals of Biochemical Engineering, 1st Edn. 2013. Global Vision Publishing House, Daryaganj, Delhi ISBN: 9788182205819

Ribaut J-M., Poland D. (2004). http://www.cimmyt.org/english/docs/proceedings/molecApproaches/pdfs/MolecularApproaches.p

Ritossa, F.M. (1962). A new puffing pattern induced by temperature shock and DNP in *Drosophila. Experientia*, 18: 571–573.

Rivera, E.M. (1963). Hormonal requirements for survival and growth of mouse primary mammary ducts in organ culture. *Proc. Soc. Exp. Biol. Med.* 114: 735-738.

Rivera, E.M., and H.A. Bern. (1961). Influence of insulin on maintenance and secretory stimulation of mouse mammary tissues by hormones in organ culture. *Endocrinology* 69: 340-353.

Rivera, E.M., J.J. Elias, H.A. Bern, N.P. Napalkov, and D. Pitelka. (1963). Toxic effects of steroid hormones on organ cultures of mouse mammary tumors, with a comment on the occurrence of viral inclusion bodies. *J. Nat. Cancer Inst.* 31: 671-687.

Roosa, R.A., and L.A. Herzenberg. (1959). The selection of variants resistant to folic acid antagonists and 5-fluorouridine in cell cultures of a lymphocytic neoplasm. *Proc. Amer. Ass. Cancer Res.* 3: 58.

Rothfels, K.H., and R.C. Parker. (1959). The karyotypes of cell lines recently established from normal mouse tissues. *J. Exp. Zool.* 142: 507-520.

Sachs, L., and D. Medina. (1961). *In vitro* transformation of normal cells by polyoma virus. *Nature* 189: 457-460.

Salzburger, B. (1962). Étude du développement de l'ovarie de souris greffé dans l'embryon depoulet après culture *in vitro. Arch. Anat. Microscop. Morphol. Exp.*51: 1-10.

Sahi C. Singh, A., Kumar, K., Bumwald, E. and Grover, A. (2006). Salt stress response in rice: genetics, molecular biology, and comparative genomics. *Functional & Integrative Genomic,* DOI 10.1007/s10142-006-0032-5.

Sakamoto A., Sulpice R., Hou C.X., Kinoshita, M., Higashi S.I., Kanaseki T., Nonaka H., Moon B.Y., Murata N. (2004). Genetic modification of the fatty acid unsaturation of phosphatidylglycerol in chloroplasts alters the sensitivity of tobacco plants to cold stress. *Plant Cell & Environment,* 27: 99-105.

Sanchez, Y. and Lindquist, S. (1990). HSP104 required for induced thermotolerance. *Science* 248: 1112-1114.

Sanders, D. (2000). Plant biology: The salty tale of Arabidopsis. *Curr. Biol.* 10, 486-488.

Sanford, K.K, H.B. Andervont, G.L. Hobbs, and W.R. Earle. (1961a). Maintenance of the mammary tumor agent in long term cultures of mouse mammary carcinoma. *J. Nat. Cancer Inst.* 26: 1185-1191.

Sanford, K.K., A.B. Covalesky, L.T. Dupree, and W.R. Earle. (1961b). Cloning of mammalian cells by a simplified capillary technique. *Exp. Cell Res.* 23: 361-372.

Sanford, K.K. (1958). Clonal studies on normal cells and their neoplastic transformation *in vitro. Cancer Res.* 18: 747-752.

Sanford, K.K. (1962). Transformations in relation to malignancy. Acta Cytol. 6: 400-401.

Sanford, K.K., B.B. Westfall, E.H.. Chu, E.L. Kuff, A.B. Covalesky, L.T. Dupree, G.L. Hobbs, and W.R. Earle. (1961). Alterations in morphology, arginase and â-glucuronidase within a clone of mouse tumor cells *in vitro. J. Nat. Cancer Inst.* 26: 1193-1219.

Sanford, K.K., G.D. Likely, and W. R. Earle, (1954). The development of variations in transplantability and morphology within a clone of mouse fibrobalsts transformed to sarcoma-producing cells *in vitro. J. Nat. Cancer Inst.* 15: 215-237.

Sanford, K.K., G.D. Likely, V.J. Evans, C.J. Mackey, and W.R. Earle. (1952). The production of sarcomas from cultured tissues of hepatoma, melanoma and thyroid tumors. *J. Nat. Cancer Inst.* 12: 1057-1077.

Sanford, K.K., G.L. Hobbs, and W.R. Earle. (1956). The tumor-producing capacity of strain L mouse cells after 10 years *in vitro. Cancer Res.* 15: 162-166.

Sanford, K.K., R.M. Merwin, G.L. Hobbs, J.M. Young, and W.R. Earle. (1959). Clonal analysis of variant cell lines transformed to malignant cells in tissue culture. *J. Nat. Cancer Inst.* 23: 1035-1059.

Sanford, K.K., R.M. Merwin, G.L. Hobbs, M.C. Fioramonti, and W.R. Earle. (1958). Studies on the difference in sarcoma-producing capacity of two lines of mouse cells derived *in vitro* from one cell. *J. Nat. Cancer Inst.* 20: 121-145.

Sanford, K.K., T.B. Dunn, A.B. Covalesky, L.T. Dupree, and W.R. Earle. (1961). Polyoma virus and the production of malignancy *in vitro*. *J. Nat. Cancer Inst.*26: 331-357.

Sanford, K.K., W.R. Earle, and G.D. Likely. (1948). The growth *in vitro* of single isolated tissue cells. *J. Nat. Cancer Inst.* 9: 229-246.

Sanford, K.K., W.R. Earle, E. Shelton, E.I. Shilling, E.M. Duchesne, G.D. Likely, and M.M. Becker. (1950). Production of malignancy *in vitro*. XII. Further transformations of mouse fibroblasts to sarcomatous cells. *J. Nat. Cancer Inst.* 11: 351-375.

Sato, G., and V. Buonassisi. (1961). The culture of differentiated tumors. *Abstr. 1st meeting Amer. Soc. Cell Biol.* p. 189.

Scharf, K.D., Siddique, M., and Vierling, E. (2001). The expanding family of *Arabidopsis thaliana* small heat stress proteins and a new family of proteins containing alpha-crystallin domains (Acd proteins). *Cell Stress Chap.*, 6: 225-237.

Schindler, R., M. Day, and G.A. Fisher. (1959). Culture of neoplastic mast cells and their synthesis of 5-hydroxytryptamin and histamine *in vitro*. *Cancer Res.* 19:47-51.

Scott, D.B.M., A.M. Pakoskey, and K.K. Sanford. (1960). Analysis of enzymatic activities of clones derived from variant cell lines transformed to malignant cells in tissue culture. *J. Nat. Cancer Inst.* 25: 1365-1379.

Seaman, A.R. (1956). The *in vitro* cultivation of the prostate gland of the adult mouse in alkaline fluid medium. *Exp. Cell Res.* 11: 283-288.

Seaman, A.R., and S. Stahl. (1956). The uptake of I^{131} by the thyroid gland of the adult mouse after *in vitro* cultivation. *Exp. Cell Res.* 11: 220-221.

Serrano, R., Culiañz-Maciá, A. and Moreno, V. (1999). Genetic engineering of salt and drought tolerance with yeast regulatory genes. *Sci Hortic* 78, 261-269.

Shelton, E. and W.R. Earle. (1951). Production of malignancy *in vitro*. XIII. Behaviour of recovery cultures. *J. Nat. Cancer Inst.* 11: 817-837.

Shelton, E., V.J. Evans, and G.A. Parker. (1963). Malignant transoformation of mouse connective tissue grown in diffusion chambers. *J. Nat. Cancer Inst.* 30: 377-392.

Shinozaki K. and Yamaguchi-Shinozaki K. (2007). Gene networks involved in drought stress response and tolerance. *J. Exp. Bot.* 58: 221-227.

Shinozaki, K., Yamaguchi-Shinozaki, K., Seki, M. (2003). Regulatory network of gene expression in the drought and cold stress responses. *Curr. Opin. Plant Biol.*, 6:410-417.

Shinozaki, K.; Yamaguchi-Shinozaki, K. (1996). Molecular response to drought and cold stress. *Curr. Opin. Plant Biol.*, 7, 161-167.

Sidman, R.L. (1956a). Histogenesis of brown adipose tissue *in vivo* and in organ culture. *Anat. Rec.* 124: 581-595.

Sidman, R.L. (1956b). The direct effect of insulin on organ culture of brown fat. *Anat. Rec.* 124: 723-734.

Sidman, R.L. (1961). Tissue culture studies of inherited retinal dystrophy. Dis. Nerv. Syst. (Monogr. Suppl.) 22(4): 14-20.

Sidman, R.L. (1963). Organ culture analysis of inherited retinal dystrophy in rodents. *Nat. Cancer Inst. Monogr.* 11: 227-246.

Sidman, R.L., and P. Mottla. (1961). Cell division and migration in organ cultures of mouse retina. *Excerpta Med.* (Sect. I) 15: 558.

Singla, S.L., Pareek, A. and Grover, A. (1997). High temperature stress. In: *Physiological Ecology of Plants.* (Ed M.N.V. Prasad), John Wiley and Sons, pp. 101-127.

Smith E F and Townsend C O. (1907). A plant tumour of bacteriological origin, *Science*, Vol. 25, pp.671–673.

Sorieul, S. and B. Ephrussi. (1961). Karyological demonstration of hybridization of mammalian cells *in vitro*. *Nature* 190: 653-654.

Souza, M. T., Jr. (1999). Analysis of the resistance in genetically engineered papaya against papaya ringspot potyvirus, partial characterization of the PRSV. Brazil. Bahia isolate, and development of transgenic papaya for Brazil. Cornell University.

Stevenson, R.E. (1962). Analytic Cell Culture. *Nat. Cancer Inst. Monogr.* 7:290.

Steward F C and S M Caplin, (1951). A tissue culture from potato tubers, The synergistic action of 2,4-D and coconut milk, *Science*, 113:518–520.

Stewart, D.C., and P.L. Kirk. (1954). The liquid medium in tissue culture. *Biol. Rev.* 29: 119-153.

Street, H. E. (1973). Plant tissue and cell culture. Blackwell Scientific Publications, Oxford, 320

Sui, N.; Li, M.; Zhao, S.J.; Li, F.; Liang, H.; Meng, Q.W. (2007). Over expression of glycerol-3-phosphate acyl transferase gene improves chilling tolerance in tomato. *Planta*, *226*, 1097-1108.

Sunderland, N., and M. Roberts. (1977). New approach to pollen culture. *Nature*, 270:236-238.

Swim, H.E. (1959). Microbiological aspects of tissue culture. *Annu. Rev. Microbiol.* 13: 141-176.

Szabó, G. (1954). Studies on the cultivation of teeth *in vitro*. *J. Anat.* 88: 31-44.

T. Yamada, T Shoji and Y Sinoto, (1963). Formation of calli and free cells in the tissue culture of *Tradescantia reflexa*, *Bot. Mag. Tokyo*,76:332–339.

Taiz, L. and Zeiger, E. (1998). Plant Physiology. Sunderland, Massachusetts: Sinauer Associates, Inc.

Tarkowski, A.K. (1959a). Experiments on the development of isolated blastomeres of mouse eggs. Nature 184: 1286-1287.

Tarkowski, A.K. (1959b). Experimental studies on regulation in the development of isolated blastomeres of mouse eggs. Acta Theriol. 3: 191-267.

Tarkowski, A.K. (1961). Mouse chimaeras developed from fused eggs. Nature 190: 857-860.

Tarkowski, A.K. (1963). Studies on mouse chimaeras developed from eggs fused in vitro. Nat. Cancer Inst. Monogr. 11: 51-71.

Thomashow, M.F. (1998). Role of cold-responsive genes in plant freezing tolerance. Plant Physiol., 118, 1-8.

Till, J.E. (1961a). Radiation effects on the division cycle of mammalian cells in vitro. Ann. N.Y. Acad. Sci. 95: 911-919.

Till, J.E. (1961b). Radiosensitivity and chromosome number in strain L mouse cells in tissue culture. Radiat. Res. 15: 400-409.

Ting, I. P. (1982). Plant physiology. Addison-Wesley, Reading, Massachusetts, 642 pages.

Tissieres, A., Mitchell, H. K. and Tracey, U. M. (1974). Protein synthesis in salivary glands of Drosophila melanogaster: relation to chromosome puffs J. Mol. Biol., 84: 389–398.

Todaro, G.J., and H. Green. (1963). Quantitative studies of the growth of mouse embryo cells in culture and their development into established cell lines. J. Cell Biol.17: 299-313.

Trowell, O.A. (1959). The culture of mature organs in a synthetic medium. Exp. Cell Res. 16: 118-147.

Trowell, O.A. (1961a). Cytocidal effects of radiation on organ cultures. Ann. N.Y. Acad. Sci. 95: 849-865.

Trowell, O.A. (1961b). Problems in the maintenance of mature organs in vitro. Colloq. Int. Centre Nat. Res. Sci. 101: 237-254.

Torres, A. C., A. T. Ferreira, P. E. Melo, E. Romano, M. A. Campos, J. A. Peters, J. A. Buso, and D. de Castro Monte. (1999). Transgenic plants of Achat potato resistant to the mosaic virus (PVY) . BIOTECNOLOGIA Ciência & Desenvolvimento, no. 7.

Umezawa, T., Nakashima, K., Miyakawa, T., Kuromori, T., Tanokura, M., Shinozaki, (2006). Engineering drought tolerance in plants: discovering and tailoring genes to unlock the future. Current Opinion in Biotechnology, 17:113-122.

Van de Kerckhove, D. (1958). L'ovaire périnatal de la souris blanche en culture organotypique. Compt. Rend. Ass. Anat. 104: 754-759.

Vierling, E. (1991). The roles of heat shock proteins in plants. Annu. Rev. Plant Physiol. Plant Mol. Biol., 42: 579–620.

Vogt, M., and R. Dulbecco. (1960). Virus-cell interaction with a tumor-producing virus. *Proc. Nat. Acad. Sci.* 46: 365-370.

W. H. Muir, (1952). Culture conditions favouring the isolation and growth of single cells from higher plants *in vitro*, PhD Thesis, University of Wisconsin, Madison.

Wahid, A., Gelani, S., Ashraf, M. and Foolad, M.R. (2007). Heat tolerance in plants: an overview. *Environ. Expt. Bot.*, 61: 199-223.

Wang WX, Vinocur B, Shoseyov O, Altman A (2001). Biotechnology of plant osmotic stress tolerance: physiological and molecular considerations. *Acta Hortic* 560:285–292.

Wang, W., Vincour, B., Shoseyov, O. and Altman, A. (2004). Role of plant heat shock proteins and molecular chaperones in the abiotic stress response. *Trends Plant Sci.*, 9: 244–252.

Wang, W., Vinocur, B. and Altman, A. (2003). Plant responses to drought, salinity and extreme temperatures: towards genetic engineering for stress tolerance. *Planta,* 218:1-14.

Wani Shabir H. and Gosal Satbir S. (2011). Introduction of OsglyII gene into Indica rice through particle bombardment for increased salinity tolerance. *Biologia Plantarum* 55 (3): 536-540 (NAAS 8.6/10)

Wani, S.H.; Sandhu, J.S.; Gosal, S.S. (2008). Genetic engineering of crop plants for abiotic stress tolerance. *In*: Advanced Topics in Plant Biotechnology and Plant Biology. Malik, C.P.; Kaur, B.; Wadhwani, C.; Eds. MD Publications New Delhi, pp. 149-183.

Watson, J. D., M. Gilman, J. Witkowski, and M. Zoller (1983). Recombinant DNA. Scientific American Books. W. H. Freeman and Company, New York, NY.

Waymouth, C. (1954). The nutrition of animal cells. *Int. Rev. Cytol.* 3: 1-68.

Waymouth, C. (1960). Growth in tissue culture *In* W.W. Nowinski [ed.] *Fundamental Aspects of Normal and Malignant Growth.* Elsevier, Amsterdam., p. 546-587.

Waymouth, C. (1965). Construction and use of synthetic media *In:* E.N. Willmer [ed.] *Cells and Tissues in Culture, Vol. 1* Academic Press, New York., p. 99-142.

Wells, L.J., and E. Borghese (1961). Sviluppo embrionale *in vitro* del pancreas di topo. *Boll. Zool.* 28: 235-239.

Wells, L.J., and E. Borghese (1963). Development of the pancreas of the mouse embryo *in vitro*: acini and islets. *Gen Comp. Endocrinol.* 3: 265-273.

Westfall, B.B. (1962). Characterization of cells in tissue culture. Nat. Cancer Inst. Monogr. 7: 147-157.

Westfall, B.B., E.V. Peppers, V.J. Evans, K.K. Sanford, N.M. Hawkins, M.C. Fioramonti, H.A. Kerr, G.L. Hobbs, and W.R. Earle. (1958). The arginase and rhodanese activities of certain cell strains after long cultivation *in vitro. J. Biophys. Biochem. Cytol.* 4: 567-570.

Wetherell, D. F. (1982). Introduction to in vitro propagation. Avery Publishing Group Inc.

White, P.R. (1957). Proceedings of the decennial review conference on tissue culture. *J. Nat. Cancer Inst.* 19: 467-843.

White, P.R. (1963). The Cultivation of Animal and Plant Cells, *2nd ed.* Ronald, New York. 228 p.

Whitfield, J.F., and R.H. Rixon. (1959). Effects of X radiation on multiplication and nucleic acid synthesis in cultures of L strain mouse cells. *Exp. Cell Res.* 18: 126-137.

Whitfield, J.F., R.H. Rixon, and T. Youdale. (1961). Effects of ultraviolet light on multiplication and deoxyribonucleic acid synthessis in cultrues of L strain mouse cells. Exp. Cell Res. 22: 450-454.

Whitfield, J.F., R.H. Rixon, and T. Youdale. (1962). Prevention of mitotic decay in irradiated suspension cultures of L mouse cells by agmatine. *Exp. Cell Res.* 27:143-147.

Whitmore, G.F., J.E. Till, R.B.L. Gwatkin, L. Siminovitch, and A.F. Graham. (1958). Increase of cellular constituents in X-irradiated mammalian cells. *Biochem. Biophys. Acta* 30: 583-590.

Whitten, W.K. (1956). Culture of tubal mouse ova. *Nature* 177: 96.

Whitten, W.K. (1957). The effect of progesterone on the development of mouse eggs *in vitro. J. Endocrinol.* 16: 80-85.

Wiegand, R. (1998). Plant genomics: new approach to crop improvement and food quality enhancement. XVII International Congress of Genetics, Beijing, China, Aug. 10-15.

Willmer, E.N. (1960a). Tissues in culture and in the body. *Symp. Soc. Exp. Biol.* 14: 28-40.

Willmer, E.N. (1960b). Cytology and Evolution. Academic Press, New York. pp. 430.

Wolff, E. (1952). Sur la différenciation sexuelle des gonades de souris explantées *in vitro. Compt. Rend. Acad. Sci.* 234: 1712-1714.

Wolff, E. and J.P. Weniger. (1954). Recherches préliminaires sur les chimères d'organs embryonnaires d'oiseaux et de mammifères en culture *in vitro. J. Embryol. Exp. Morphol.* 2: 161-171.

Woods, M.W., K.K. Sanford, D. Burk, and W.R. Earle. (1959). Glycolytic properties of high and low sarcoma-producing lines and clones of mouse tissue culture cells. *J. Nat. Cancer Inst.* 23: 1079-1088.

Yoshioka, W. (1960). Studies on the isologous transplantation of tooth germs in mice. II. Effects of hormones on the isologous transplantations of tooth germs previously cultured *in vitro. Arch. Histol. Jap.* 20: 19-34.

Xin, Z.; Browse, J. (2001). Cold comfort farm: the acclimation of plants to freezing temperatures. *Plant Cell Environ.,* 23, 893-902.

Zhai, W., X. Li, W. Tian, Y. Zhou, X. Pan, S. Cao, X. Zhao, B. Zhao, Q. Zhang, and L. Zhu. (2000). Introduction of a blight resistance gene, Xa21, into five Chinese rice varieties through an Agrobacterium mediated system. *Science in China (Series C)* 43, No. 3:361-368.

Zhang J. Z. Creelman RA, Zhu JK., (2004). From laboratory to field. Using information from Arabidopsis to engineer salt, cold, and drought tolerance in crops, *Plant Physiol.* 135: 615-621.

Zhang Z, Tian HQ, Russell SD. (1999). Immunogold scanning electron microscopic localization of myosin on isolated sperm cells of tobacco (*Nicotiana tabacum* L.). *Protoplasma* 208:123–28.

Zheng Z-L, Yang Z. (2000). The Rop GTPase switch turns on polar growth in pollen.*Trends Plant Sci.* 5:298–303.

Zhu, J.-K. (2001). Plant salt tolerance. *Trends in Plant Sci.* 6, 66-71.

Zinkl G.M., Zweibel BI, Grier DG, Preuss D. (1999). Pollen-stigma adhesion in *Arabidopsis*: a species-specific interaction mediated by hydrophobic molecules in the pollen exine. *Development* 126:5431–40.

Appendices

Appendix-1

Calculation of Logarithm and Logarithm Table

Logarithm Definition

When b is raised to the power of y is equal x:

$b^y = x$

Then the base b logarithm of x is equal to y:

$\log_b(x) = y$

For example when:

$2^4 = 16$

Then $\log_2(16) = 4$

Logarithm as Inverse function of Exponential function

The logarithmic function,

$y = \log_b(x)$

is the inverse function of the exponential function,

$x = b^y$

So if we calculate the exponential function of the logarithm of x (x>0),

$f(f^{-1}(x)) = b^{\log_b(x)} = x$

Or if we calculate the logarithm of the exponential function of x,

$f^{-1}(f(x)) = \log_b(b^x) = x$

Natural logarithm (ln)

Natural logarithm is a logarithm to the base e:

$\ln(x) = \log_e(x)$

When e constant is the number:

$$e = \lim_{x \to \infty} \left(1 + \frac{1}{n}\right)^n = \lim_{x \to 0}(1 + n)^{\frac{1}{n}} = 2.71828183...$$

Inverse Logarithm calculation

The inverse logarithm (or anti logarithm) is calculated by raising the base b to the logarithm y:

$x = \log^{-1}(y) = b^y$

Logarithmic function

The logarithmic function has the basic form of:

$f(x) = \log_b(x)$

Common logarithm (with base 10)

We know that

$1 = 10^0 \Rightarrow \log_{10}1 = 0$

$10 = 10^1 \Rightarrow \log_{10}10 = 1$

$100 = 10^2 \Rightarrow \log_{10}100 = 2$

$100 = 10^3 \Rightarrow \log_{10}1000 = 3$

And

$0.1 = 10^{-1} \Rightarrow \log_{10}0.1 = {}^\wedge 1$

$0.01 = 10^{-2} \Rightarrow \log_{10}0.01 = {}^\wedge 2$

$0.001 = 10^{-3} \Rightarrow \log_{10}0.001 = {}^\wedge 3$

$0.0001 = 10^{-4} \Rightarrow \log_{10}0.001 = {}^\wedge 4$

Where ^1, ^2, ^3 and ^4 represent -1, -2, -3 and -4.

Basic Laws

For Positive numbers m and n,

$\log(m \times n) = \log m + \log n$

$\log(m / n) = \log m - \log n$

$\log m^n = n \log m$

Remember just one more fact:

If 1<x<10, then 0<log x<1

Let us do some problems on multiplication.

1. Multiply 256 and 768

Solution: $256 = 2.56 \times 10^2$ and $768 = 7.68 \times 10^2$

Now, $\log(256 \times 768) = \log 256 + \log 768$

$= \log(2.56 \times 10^2) + \log(7.68 \times 10^2)$

$= 2.4082 + 2.8854$

$= 5.2936$

$256 \times 768 = $ antilog 5.2936

$\qquad = 1.966 \times 10^5$

$\qquad = 196600$

Express each number in the standard form. That is put a decimal after the first digit and multiply by the appropriate power of 10. The logarithm of a number has two parts the first of which is the exponent of 10, called the characteristic, and the second part is a decimal called the mantissa, which is read from the log tables. The characteristic can be positive or negative. The negative characteristic is written with a bar above the number. The mantissa is always a positive decimal less than 1. To multiply two numbers, find the logarithm of each number and add them. Then find the antilogarithm of the mantissa (fraction part) from anti-log table (which will be a decimal between 1 and 10) and multiply by 10 raised to the characteristic to get the product.

2. Multiply 67846 and 0.0839

Solution: $67846 = 6.7846 \times 10^4$ and $0.0839 = 8.39 \times 10^{-2}$

Now, $\log (67846 \times 0.0839) = \log 67846 + \log 0.0839$

$\qquad = \log (6.7846 \times 10^4) + \log (8.39 \times 10^{-2})$

$\qquad = 4.8315 + \bar{2}.9238$

$\qquad = 3.7553$

$67846 \times 0.0839 = $ antilog 3.7553

$\qquad = 5.6925 \times 10^3$

$\qquad = 5692.5$

The bar above the characteristic is written to show that only the characteristic part is negative and the mantissa part is positive.

3. Multiply 0.04532 and 0.03487

Solution: $0.04532 = 4.532 \times 10^{-2}$ and $0.03487 = 3.487 \times 10^{-2}$

Now, $\log (0.04532 \times 0.03487) = \log 0.04532 + \log 0.03487$

$\qquad = \log (4.532 \times 10^{-2}) + \log (3.487 \times 10^{-2})$

$\qquad = \bar{2}.6563 + \bar{2}.5425$

$\qquad = \bar{3}.1988$

$0.04532 \times 0.03487 = $ antilog 3.1988

$\qquad\qquad = 1.581 \times 10^{-3}$

$\qquad\qquad = 0.00581$

Now let us do some problems on division.

4. Divide 826 by 347

Solution: $826 = 8.26 \times 10^2$

$347 = 3.47 \times 10^2$

Now, $\log (826 \div 347) = \log 826 - \log 347$

$\quad = \log (8.26 \times 10^2) + \log (3.47 \times 10^2)$

$\quad = 2.9170 - 2.5403$

$\quad = 0.3767$

$826 \times 347 = $ antilog 0.3767

$\quad = 2.381 \times 10^0$

$\quad = 2.381$

To divide a number by another number, find their logarithm and subtract the logarithm of the divisor from the logarithm of the dividend. Then find the antilogarithm of the mantissa from anti-log table and multiply by 10 raised to the characteristic to get the result.

5. Divide 273 by 9876

Solution: $273 = 2.73 \times 10^2$

$9876 = 9.876 \times 10^3$

Now, $\log (273 \div 9876) = \log 273 - \log 9876$

$\quad = \log (2.73 \times 10^2) + \log (9.876 \times 10^3)$

$\quad = 2.8315 - 3.9946$

$\quad = {}^\wedge 2.4416$

$273 \times 9876 = $ antilog 2.4416

$\quad = 2.764 \times 10^{-2}$

$\quad = 0.02764$

We can find square root of a number using log tables.

6. Find the square root of 5468

Solution: Square root of 5468

$$\sqrt{5468} = 5468^{\frac{1}{2}}$$

$$\log \sqrt{5468} = \log 5468^{\frac{1}{2}}$$

$$\log \sqrt{5468} = \frac{1}{2}\log 5468$$

$$= \frac{1}{2}\log(5.468 \times 10^3)$$

$$= \frac{1}{2} \times 3.7378$$

$$\sqrt{5468} = anti\log 1.8689$$

$$= 7.394 \times 10^1$$

$$= 73.94$$

To find the square root of a number, find its logarithm and divide it by 2 and then find its antilogarithm.

7. Find the square root of 0.8745

Solution: Square root of $0.8745 = 0.8745^{\frac{1}{2}}$

$$\log \sqrt{0.8745} = \log 0.8745^{\frac{1}{2}}$$

$$= \frac{1}{2}\log(8.745 \times 10^{\overline{1}})$$

$$= \frac{1}{2} \times (\overline{1}.9418)$$

$$= \frac{1}{2}\overline{2} + 1.9418$$

$$= \overline{1} + 9709$$

$$\sqrt{0.8745} = \text{antilog } \overline{1}.9709$$

$$= 9.352 \times 10^{-1}$$

$$= 0.9352$$

Finally let us do the following calculation.

Calculate $\sqrt[3]{\dfrac{375 \times 123^{\frac{3}{2}}}{476^{11}}}$

$$\log \sqrt[3]{\frac{375 \times 123^{\frac{3}{2}}}{476^{11}}} = \log 375^{\frac{1}{3}} + \log 123^{\frac{3}{2}} - \log 476^{11}$$

$$= \frac{1}{3}\log 375 + \frac{3}{2}\log 123 - 11\log 476$$

$$= \frac{1}{3}\log(3.75 \times 10^2) + \frac{3}{2}\log(1.23 \times 10^2) - 11\log(4.76 \times 10^2)$$

$$= \frac{1}{3}(2.5740) + \frac{3}{2}(2.0899) - 11(2.6776)$$

$$= 0.8580 + 3.1349 - 29.4536$$

$$= \overline{26}.5393$$

$$\therefore \sqrt[3]{\frac{375 \times 123^{\frac{3}{2}}}{476^{11}}} = \text{antilog } \overline{26}.5393$$

$$= 3.492 \times 10^{-26}$$

Log Table

Table of base 10, base 2 and base e (ln) logarithms

x	$\log_{10} x$	$\log_2 x$	$\log_e x$
0	undefined	undefined	undefined
0+	undefined	undefined	undefined
0.0001	-4.000000	-13.287712	-9.210340
0.001	-3.000000	-9.965784	-6.907755
0.01	-2.000000	-6.643856	-4.605170
0.1	-1.000000	-3.321928	-2.302585
1	0.000000	0.000000	0.000000
2	0.301030	1.000000	0.693147
3	0.477121	1.584963	1.098612
4	0.602060	2.000000	1.386294
5	0.698970	2.321928	1.609438
6	0.778151	2.584963	1.791759
7	0.845098	2.807355	1.945910
8	0.903090	3.000000	2.079442
9	0.954243	3.169925	2.197225
10	1.000000	3.321928	2.302585
20	1.301030	4.321928	2.995732
30	1.477121	4.906891	3.401197
40	1.602060	5.321928	3.688879

Contd.....

Table Contd.....

x	$\log_{10} x$	$\log_2 x$	$\log_e x$
50	1.698970	5.643856	3.912023
60	1.778151	5.906991	4.094345
70	1.845098	6.129283	4.248495
80	1.903090	6.321928	4.382027
90	1.954243	6.491853	4.499810
100	2.000000	6.643856	4.605170
200	2.301030	7.643856	5.298317
300	2.477121	8.228819	5.703782
400	2.602060	8.643856	5.991465
500	2.698970	8.965784	6.214608
600	2.778151	9.228819	6.396930
700	2.845098	9.451211	6.551080
800	2.903090	9.643856	6.684612
900	2.954243	9.813781	6.802395
1000	3.000000	9.965784	6.907755
10000	4.000000	13.287712	9.210340

Appendix- 2

Microbiological Equipment

Water bath

A laboratory water bath is a tool used to maintain a very stable temperature much like an incubator. Water baths can hold often temperatures within a tenth of a degree Celsius; the water is often circulated. Sometimes beads are used as a waterless option. Scientific water baths are also used in commercial kitchens to cook sous-vide.

Principle: In a lab or a kitchen it is often essential to keep a liquid mixture at an exact temperature without a gradient of heat (bottom being hotter than top) to make it cook properly. To do this scientists and cooks often submerge the vessel needing this controlled environment into a bath of water at a controlled tempezrature. The advantage is that the water in the wath presents the heated material with a constant temperature that will not exceed 100°C (the boiling point of water) so that over heating or scorching is avoided. The laboratory water bath is slightly more complex than the kitchen version (the double boiler) as the temperature can be controlled through sensors to within a degree of the desired temperature.

Operating Procedure:

1. Ensure that sufficient amount of water is available in the water bath.
2. Ensure that the instrument is properly connected to power supply.
3. Fill the bath to the level little above the falls bottom
4. Switch on the supply. Put the toggle switch ON.
5. Set the thermostat knob to the required temperature and rising in the temperature is indicated by glowing the Red Indicator Lamp.
6. When required temperature is reached, the Red Indicator Lamp will go OFF.
7. The bath is then allowed to work.

8. After completion of heating process, reduce the temperature to zero, by rotating the temperature setting knob to zero position. Switch off the power supply and allow the bath to cool to the desired temperature before the control knob is turned backwards. This is to eliminate unnecessary strain on the thermostat.

9. Report any discrepancy observed during operation of the instrument to Department head and notify the defect to Utility department to rectify the defect. Affix BREAK DOWN label on the instrument till it get rectified.

Autoclave

An autoclave is a device used to sterilize equipment and supplies by subjecting them to high pressure saturated steam at 121°C or more, typically for 15–20 minutes depending on the size of the load and the contents. It was invented by Charles Chamberland in 1879, although a precursor known as the steam digester was created by Denis Papin in 1679. The name comes from Greek auto, ultimately meaning self and Latin clavis meaning key- a self-locking device.

Relationship between the Pressure and Temperature of Steam at Sea Level

Pressure (psi)	Temperature (°C)
0	100
5	110
10	116
15	121
20	126
25	130
30	135
40	141

Principle: A basic principle of chemistry is that when the pressure of a gas increases, the temperature of the gas increase proportionally. For example, when free flowing steam at a temperature of 100°C is placed under a pressure of 1 atmosphere above sea level pressure – that is, about 15 pounds of pressure per square inch (Psi) the temperature rises to 121°C. Increasing the pressure to 20 psi raises the temperature to 126°C. The relationship between temperature and pressure is shown in table 3.1. In this way steam is a gas, increasing its pressure in a closed system increases its temperature. As the water molecules in steam become more energized, their penetration increases substantially. This principle is used to reduce cooking time in the home pressure cooker and to reduce sterilizing time in the autoclave. It is important to note that the sterilizing agent is the moist heat, not the pressure.

Uses: Autoclaving is used to sterilize culture media, instruments, dressings, intravenous equipment, applicators, solutions, syringes, transfusion equipment, and numerous other items that can withstand high temperatures and pressures. The laboratory technician uses it to sterilize bacteriological media and destroy pathogenic cultures. The autoclave is equally valuable for glassware and metal ware, and is among the first instruments ordered when a microbiology laboratory is established.

Principle of autoclave

Autoclaves are also used on large industrial scale. Large industrial autoclaves are called retorts, but the same principle applies for common household pressure cooker used in the home canning of foods.

Limitations and Disadvantages: The autoclave also has certain limitations. For example, some plastic ware melts in the high heat, and sharp instruments often become dull. Moreover, many chemicals breakdown during the sterilization process and oily substances cannot be treated because they do not mix with water. Heat requires extra time to reach the center of solid materials, such as canned meats, because such materials do not develop the efficient heat-distributing convection currents that occur in liquids. Heating large containers also requires extra time. Table 3 shows the different time requirements for sterilizing liquids in various container sizes. Unlike sterilizing aqueous solutions, sterilizing the surface of a solid requires that steam actually contact it.

Rules implied for Autoclaving: Articles should be placed in the autoclave so that steam can easily penetrate them. Air should be evacuated so that the chamber fills with steam.

Laminar flow

Laminar flow, sometimes known as streamLine flow, occurs when a fluid flows in parallel layers, with no disruption between the layers. At low velocities the fluid tends to flow without lateral mixing, and adjacent layers slide past one another like playing cards. There are no cross currents perpendicular to the direction of flow, nor eddies or swirls of fluids. In laminar flow the motion of the particles of fluid is very orderly with all particles moving in straight lines parallel to the pipe walls. In fluid dynamics, laminar flow is a flow regime characterized by high momentum diffusion and low momentum convection. When a fluid is flowing through a closed channel such as a pipe or between two flat plates, either two types of flow may occur depending on the velocity of the fluid: laminar flow or turbulent flow. Laminar flow is the opposite of turbulent flow which occurs at higher velocities where eddies or small packets of fluid particles form leading to lateral mixing. In nonscientific terms laminar flow is smooth, while turbulent flow is rough. The type of flow occurring in a fluid in a channel is important in fluid dynamics problems. The dimensionless Reynolds number is an important parameter in the equations that describe whether flow conditions lead to laminar or turbulent flow. In the case of flow through a straight pipe with a circular cross-section, Reynolds numbers of less than 2100 are generally considered to be of a laminar type; however, the Reynolds number upon which laminar flows become turbulent is dependent upon the flow geometry. When the Reynolds number is much less than 1, Creeping motion or Stokes flow occurs. This is an extreme case of laminar flow where viscous (friction) effects are much greater than inertial forces. The common application of laminar flow would be in the smooth flow of a viscous liquid through a tube or pipe. In that case, the velocity of flow varies from zero at the walls to a maximum along the centerline of the vessel. The flow profile of laminar flow in a tube can be calculated by dividing the flow into thin cylindrical elements and applying the viscous force to them.

For example, consider the flow of air over an aircraft wing. The boundary layer is a very thin sheet of air lying over the surface of the wing (and all other surfaces of the aircraft). Because air has viscosity, this layer of air tends to adhere to the wing. As the wing moves forward through the air, the boundary layer at first flows smoothly over the streamLined shape of the airfoil. Here the flow is called laminar and the boundary layer is a laminar layer. Prandtl applied the concept of the laminar boundary layer to airfoils in 1904.

Principle of laminar air flow: When fresh air is passed in the laminar air flow it replaces the contaminated air inside and keeps it contamination free. Laminar Air Flow is based on the flow of air current to create uniform velocity, along parallel lines, which helps in transforming microbial culture in aseptic conditions.

Applications

1. **Life Science Research:** The clean work area provides an excellent work space for small laboratory appliances, microscopes, pipetting, or similar applications.

2. **Pharmacy:** For use in compounding sterile drug preparations.

3. **Animal or Plant:** For procedures requiring work-in-progress protection from outside potentially harmful contaminants.

Types of Laminar Air Flow

Vertical Laminar Air Flow Cabinet: These are designed to meet the filtration, illumination, Noise and vibration requirement and US federal standard 209 B BS 5290, providing air to meet class 100 (class1) conditions. to the extent applicable. This vertical laminar down flow configuration find extensive application in Scientific, Medical and Industrial application where localized high quality, clean working environment is essential. These are designed to provides an atmosphere free from airborne particles with laminar airflow flowing downward the worktable. It provides effective and satisfactory long term sterile working conditions for microbiological investigation, tissue culture studies. Toxic preparation etc. On vertical laminar flow is used, and the experiment held do not require eye hand co-ordination. In semi-mechanized procedures this equipment is frequently' used.

Construction

1. **Cabinet**: Laminar airflow cabinet is constructed out of 18 mm Duro Board Teak Wood, which is terminate and insect proof fire and weather resistant, Front, Back, Top and exterior surfaces are covered with white DECOLAM or FORMICA interior surfaces are epoxy painted.

2. **Upper Chamber**: Its top is fitted with pre-filters for filtration. it is made of re-useable synthetic fiberglass, and is washable also. It retains all major impurities of air sucked inside the laminar flow.

3. **Main Chamber**: It consists of main work surface, which is made of MICA TOP or stainless steel.

4. **Side Panels**: Made of 6-mm thick transparent Plexiglass framed in anodized aluminum angle frame.

5. **Front Panels**: Made of folding transparent glass. It can be folded upwards while working inside the main chamber.

6. **Protective Screen**: Non-Shedding, non-corrosive protects filters, white stove painted protective screen in the main chamber.

7. **Exhaust Fan**: Exhaust is fitted below the main chamber it sucks the used air from the main chamber and throws out of the laminar flow. An exhaust do not is also provided here, which takes this air out of the room. Exhaust can be provided at an extra cost. (Optional)

8. **Airflow and Filtration**: Laminar flow principle involves double filtration of air. Atmospheric air is drawn through prefilter and is made to pass through high efficiency particulate air filter (HEPA). Filter having efficiency rating as high as 99.99% with cold DOP and 99.97% hot DOP. Thus retaining all airborne particles of size 0.3 micron and larger. Double filtered air blows in laminar flow through the work table at designed velocity of 90ft.min +20%.

9. **Blower Motor Assembly**: Duly balanced, direct drive motor blower units sized to provide adequate airflow volume over the entire surface of HEPA filter.

10. **Lighting**: Work are properly illuminated by diffused glare free fluorescent light.

11. **UV Germicidical Light**: Are fitted inside the cabinet / work-area.

12. **Easy Mobility**: The whole body is provided with four Nos. castor wheels at the bottom for easy mobility to any place.

Ceiling Suspended Laminar Air Flow (CLAF)

Ceiling suspended laminar air flow (CLAF) is used for OT applications, pharma filling and packing line etc. CLAF provides ultra clean sterile HEPA filtered CLASS 100 air in an isolated area where the highly sensitive process activities are carried-out. Clean air CLAF available in complete stainless steel construction or GI construction with PU coated finish. Equipped with MINIPLEAT HEPA with dynamically balanced ultra-low noise blowers for optimum airflow. Differential pressure monitoring done through MAGNEHELIC gauges. Various sizes can be manufactured and supplied to suit the specific site conditions.

Precaution of Laminar Air Flow

1. Put off the shoes before entering to operate the apparatus.
2. Wash the hands with detergent or soap.
3. One should not tank inside the chamber while performing microbial culture transfer, failing which chances of contamination may be more which may come either through mounth, sneezing or air.

Incubator

An incubator is an instrument that consists of cooper/steel chamber, around which warm water or air is circulated by electric currents or by means of small gas flame.

Colony Counter

A colony counter is an instrument used to count colonies of bacteria or other microorganisms growing on an agar plate. Early counters were merely lighted surfaces on which the plate was placed, with the colonies marked off with a felt-tipped pen on the outer surface of the plate while the operator kept the count manually. More recent counters attempt to count the colonies electronically, by identifying individual areas of dark and light according to automatic or user-set thresholds, and counting the resulting contrasting spots.

Microorganism enumeration: Such counters are used to estimate the density of microorganisms within a liquid culture. An appropriate dilution, or several dilutions within the estimated appropriate range, is spread using sterile technique on the agar plate, which is then incubated under the appropriate conditions for growth until individual colonies appear. Each colony marks the spot where a single organism was originally placed, thus the number of colonies on the plate equals the number of organisms within the volume of liquid spread on the plate. That concentration is then extrapolated by the known dilution from the original culture, to estimate the concentration of organisms within that original culture. The maximum number of colonies which may be effectively counted on a single plate is somewhere between 100 and 1,000, depending on the size of the colony and the type of organism.

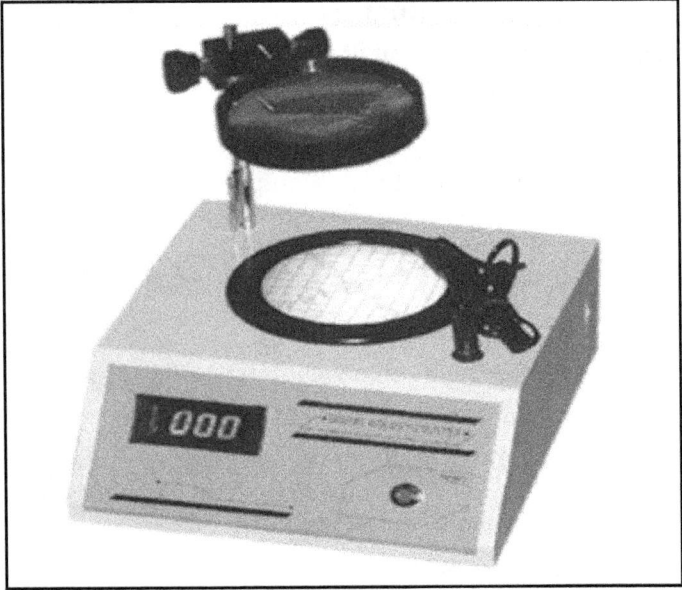

Colony counter

Appendix -3

KARL FISCHER TITRATION

Introduction: Karl Fischer Titration is a widely used method for determining the micro amount of water in a variety of products. Karl Fischer titration is a classic titration method in analytical chemistry that uses coulometric or volumetric titration to determine trace amounts of water in a sample. It was invented in 1935 by the German chemist Karl Fischer., the iodometric titration method that bears his name has become an increasingly popular analytical technique for quantifying water in a variety of industries. During this time, Karl Fischer titration has evolved from an esoteric novelty to a widely used instrumental method employed in Research and Development, Production and Quality Control.

Principle

1. Fundamental Reaction

The fundamental principle behind the Karl Fischer Titration is based on the Bunsen Reaction between iodine and sulfur dioxide in an aqueous medium shown below:

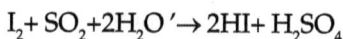

$$I_2 + SO_2 + 2H_2O' \rightarrow 2HI + H_2SO_4$$

Karl Fischer discovered that this reaction could be modified to be used for the determination of water in a non-aqueous system containing an excess of sulfer dioxide. He used a primary alcohol (methanol) as the solvent, and a base (pyridine) as the buffering agent. So the reagent changed into:

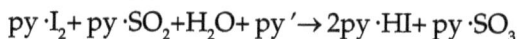

$$py \cdot I_2 + py \cdot SO_2 + H_2O + py' \rightarrow 2py \cdot HI + py \cdot SO_3$$

2. Function of Pyridine

In classical Karl Fischer Reaction pyridine is used as a basic reagent. And as a ligand it can complex the I_2 and SO_2, which can lower the vapor pressure of both I_2 and SO_2, shifting the equilibrium further to the right of the reaction equation.

3. Function of Anhydrous Methanol

During the titration py·SO_3 can reacts with H_2O, which varies the stoichiometry of H_2O and I_2 from 1:1 to 2:1:

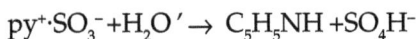

$$py^+·SO_3^- + H_2O' \rightarrow C_5H_5NH + SO_4H^-$$

To prevent such side reaction, excessive anhydrous methanol is added as it can react with **py$^+$·SO$_3^-$**, which lower the concentration of **py$^+$·SO$_3^-$**

$$CH_3OH + py^+·SO_3^-' \rightarrow C_5H_5N(H)SO_4CH_3$$

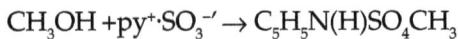

4. Advancement of Karl Fischer Reaction

Classical Karl Fischer reagent contained pyridine, a noxious carcinogen, as the base. The reagents most frequently used today are pyridine-free and contain imidazole or primary amines instead. And the reactive alcohol methanol can be replaced by 2-(2-Ethoxyethoxy)ethanol or another suitable alcohol. The reaction can be summarized by this equation:

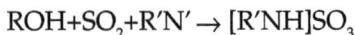

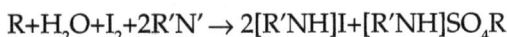

$$ROH + SO_2 + R'N' \rightarrow [R'NH]SO_3$$

$$R + H_2O + I_2 + 2R'N' \rightarrow 2[R'NH]I + [R'NH]SO_4R$$

In this reaction, the alcohol reacts with sulfur dioxide (SO_2) and base to form an intermediate alkyl sulfite salt, which is then oxidized by iodine to an alkyl sulfate salt. This oxidization reaction consumes water.

Procedure

1 Preparation for Titration

Before the titration being carried out, some preparing work should be done. Mostly the pH of the sample solution, the standardization of KF reagent and the pre-treatment of sample is concerned.

1.1 Select a Proper pH Range

Karl Fischer Titration is sensitive to the pH and the rate of the reaction depends on the pH value of the solvent, or working medium. When pH is between 5 and 8, the titration proceeds normally. However, when the pH is lower than 5, the titration speed is very slow, On the other hand, when pH is higher than 8, titration rate is fast, but only due to an interfering etherification side reaction which produce water, resulting in an vanishing endpoint. Thus, the optimal pH range for the Karl Fischer Reaction is from 5 to 8, and highly acidic or basic samples need to be buffered to bring the overall pH into that range.

1.2 Standardization of KF Reagent

Karl Fischer reagent decomposes on standing. Because decomposition is particularly rapid immediately after preparation, it is common practice to prepare the reagent a day or two before it is to be used. Ordinarily, its strength must be standardized against a standard solution of water in methanol or the solid sample of $(CHOH)_2(COONa)_2·2H_2O$.

It is obvious that great care must be exercised to keep atmospheric moisture from contaminating the Karl Fischer reagent and the sample. All glassware must be carefully dried before use, and the standard solution must be stored out of contact with air. It is also necessary to minimize contact between the atmosphere and the solution during the titration.

1.3 Pre-treatment of the Titrand

As the property of titrand differs from one to another, Karl Fischer Titration can be directly applied to only part of the materials to be titrated. For the rest there must be some treatment brought into the method to eliminate the interfering factors. For example, the hydrosulfide in the sample, causing a higher result of the titration by a red-ox reaction with I_2, must be removed in a addition reaction by adding alkene.

Under most circumstances, the interfering factors include:

(a) The sample itself, not water only, reacts with Karl Fischer reagent.

(b) Incomplete reaction, usually caused by incomplete extract of the water in sample.

(c) Uncertain reaction.

2. Volumetric Karl Fischer Titration Method

In volumetric Karl Fischer, iodine is added mechanically to a solvent containing the sample by the titrator's burette during the titration. Water is quantified on the basis of the volume of Karl Fischer reagent consumed.

Volumetric is best suited for determination of water content in the range of 100 ppm to 100%.

There are two main types of Karl Fischer Titration reagent system.

(a) In one-component volumetric KF, the titrating reagent (also known as a CombiTitrant, or a Composite) contains all of the chemicals needed for the Karl Fischer Reaction, namely iodine, sulfur dioxide, and the base, dissolved in a suitable alcohol. Methanol is typically used as the working medium in the titration cell. One-component volumetric reagents are easier to handle, and are usually less expensive than two-component reagent.

(b) In two-component volumetric KF, the titrating agent (usually known as Titrant) contains only iodine and methanol, while the Solvent containing the other Karl Fischer Reaction component is used as the working medium in the titration cell. Two-component reagents have better long-term stability and faster titration time than one-component reagents, but are usually more costly and have lower solvent capacity.

A volumetric titrator is usually applied in practical work and it performs the following three key functions:

1. It dispenses KF titrating reagent containing iodine into the cell using the burette

2. It detects the endpoint of the titration using the double platinum pin indicator electrode

3. It calculates the end result based on the volume of KF reagent dispensed using the on-board microprocessor.

3. Coulometric Karl Fischer Titration Method

In coulometric Karl Fischer, iodine is generated electrochemically *in situ* during the titration. Water is quantified on the basis of the total charge passed (Q), as measured by current (amperes) and time (seconds), according to the following relationship:

$$Q = 1 \text{ C (Coulomb)} = 1 \text{ A} \times 1 \text{ s where } 1 \text{ mg } H_2O = 10.72 \text{ C}$$

Coulometry is best suited for determination of water content in the range of 1 ppm to 5%.

There are two main types of coulometric KFT reagent systems:

(a) In conventional, or fritted-cell, coulometric KF, a diaphragm or frit separates the anode from the cathode that form the electrolytic cell known as the generator electrode. The purpose of the frit is to prevent the iodine generated at the anode from being reduced back to iodide at the cathode instead of reacting with water.

(b) In fritless-cell coulometric KF, an innovative cell design is used that through a combination of factors, but without a frit, makes it nearly impossible for iodine to reach the cathode and get reduced to iodide instead of reacting with water.

The advantages of the fritless cell include:

- Uses only one reagent

  Lower reagent cost

- Titration cell much easier to clean

  Reduced downtime

  Lower maintenance cost

- Long-term drift (background) value more stable

  Can use reagent longer without refilling

- Refilling of electrolyte suitable for automation

  Reduced downtime

  Increased lab safety

Also there exists a coulometric titrator which performs the following three key functions:

1. It generates iodine at the anode of the titration cell, instead of dispensing KF reagent as in volumetric titration

2. It detects the endpoint of the titration using the double platinum pin indicator electrode

3. It calculates the end result based on the total charge passed (Q), in Coulombs, using the on-board microprocessor.

Karl Fischer's Original Reagents

In 1935 the German chemist Karl Fischer needed a method for moisture determination in sulphur dioxide. He mixed a reagent containing pyridine, sulphur dioxide and iodine according to the Bunsen equation without the excess of water.

He formulated:

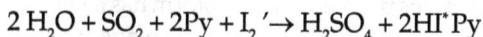

$$2\,H_2O + SO_2 + 2Py + I_2' \rightarrow H_2SO_4 + 2HI^\bullet Py$$

Py = pyridine

He validated the reagent by adding known amounts of water but never attempted to modify his formulation. In the next 40 years the Karl Fischer titration was slightly modified, but there was no significant progress. The KF titration was disliked by the laboratory technicians since it was difficult to determine the end-point, the reagent contained pyridine and was malodorous.

First Generation of Pyridine-free Karl Fischer Reagents

In the beginning of the 80s Eugen Scholz at Riedel-de Haën in Germany started investigations on KF reagents. The objective was to develop a reagent without the pyridine odour. After a few months he formulated the following reaction equation:

1. **Step**

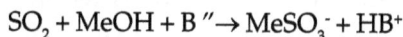

$$SO_2 + MeOH + B'' \rightarrow MeSO_3^- + HB^+$$

2. **Step**

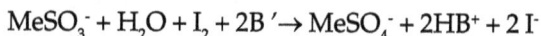

$$MeSO_3^- + H_2O + I_2 + 2B' \rightarrow MeSO_4^- + 2HB^+ + 2I^-$$

B = Base

He discovered that the methanol takes part in the reaction forming the methyl sulphite, one active species in the KF titration. As Anders Cedergren noticed some years before the pyridine was just a buffering agent and not a reactive part. According to the results it was possible to replace the unpleasant pyridine with the odourless imidazole. The second advantage of the imidazole is its higher basicity which leads to a faster reaction speed and more stable endpoints. Within a short period of time, various reagents for general use in one-component titration, two-component titration and coulometric titration had been formulated.

Second Generation of Pyridine-free Karl Fischer Reagents: Specialities

Water determination in a variety of different products had been possible at that point. But there were still a large group of samples which underwent side reactions with the ingredients of the KF reagents. Acids and bases change the pH which supports side reactions and fats and oils do not dissolve. A very typical side reaction is the generation of ketals from ketones and methanol. During this reaction water is formed and causes false results and fading end-points.

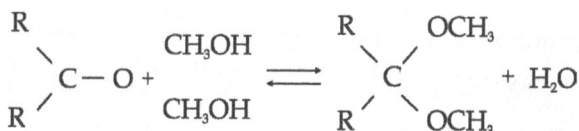

Therefore, it was necessary to develop reagents which did not undergo side reactions while keeping their reactivity. Systematic investigations of various organic solvents showed that halogenated alcohols react according to equation (2a) and do not form by-products with carbonyl compounds. Chloroform also has a positive effect on the KF titration and in addition it dissolves a variety of compounds which are insoluble in methanol. In coulometric determination, the conductivity of such compounds generates problems. Chloroform has a very low dielectric constant, thereby making it impossible to form a coulometric reagent based on pure chloroform. On the other hand, a suitable alcohol is necessary to keep the exact stochiometry of the Karl Fischer reaction. A conductivity of at least 10 mS/cm is also required in the reagent. Trifluoroethanol is the solution: it improves the conductivity and does not undergo side reactions.

Third Generation of Karl Fischer Reagents: Environmentally friendly

In the late 80s health and environment became important points in public discussion. Carbontetrachloride, which was part of all commercial coulometric catholytes for KF titration, was forbidden in the USA because of its cancerogenity. Halogenated hydrocarbons became more expensive to dispose. Therefore attempts were made to remove these solvents from KF reagents. Unfortunately, we found that they were needed as reaction partners, not only as solvents. Carbon tetrachloride and chloroform were reduced in the cathodic KF reaction.

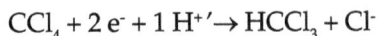

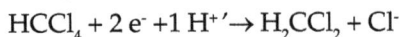

$$CCl_4 + 2 e^- + 1 H^{+\prime} \rightarrow HCCl_3 + Cl^-$$
$$HCCl_4 + 2 e^- + 1 H^{+\prime} \rightarrow H_2CCl_2 + Cl^-$$

These reductions form electrochemical inert products (chloride, chloroform and methylene chloride) which could not be oxidised at the anode. In a catholyte without halogenated hydrocarbons, methyl sulphite is reduced. The reduction products diffuse into the anode compartment of the coulometric cell where they act as water. We found that ammonium salts can be used as a reactive agent in KF catholytes. In this case, hydrogen ions are reduced to hydrogen which evaporates out of the cell and does not disturb the anodic reaction. For analysis of ketones the halogenated alcohols can be replaced by glycol ethers and long chain alcohols.

Forth Generation of Karl Fischer Reagents: non-hazardous

Environmentally friendly is not automatically also friendly for mankind. A lot of KF reagents have still been based on methanol. Methanol is considered toxic and displays the skull and crossbone on the label. Our next goal was to make a reagent line which protects the people in the lab as good as possible from the danger of hazardous chemicals.

Advantage: The popularity of the Karl Fischer titration is due in large part to several critical advantages that it holds over other methods of quantifying water, including:

1. High accuracy and precision,
2. Selectivity for water,

3. Small sample quantities required,

4. Easy sample preparation,

5. Short analysis duration,

6. Nearly unlimited measuring range (1ppm to 100%),

7. Suitability for analyzing solids, liquids, and gases,

8. Independence of presence of other volatiles

9. Suitability for automation.

Disadvantage: The water has to be accessible and easily brought into methanol solution. Many common substances, especially foods such as chocolate, release water slowly and with difficulty, and require additional efforts to reliably bring the total water content into contact with the Karl Fischer reagents.

Appendix -4

HIGH-PERFORMANCE LIQUID CHROMATOGRAPHY (HPLC)

The technique of high performance liquid chromatography is so called because of its improved performance when compared to classical column chromatography. It is also called as high pressure liquid chromatography since high pressure is used when compared to classical column chromatography. Liquid chromatography was defined in the early 1900's by the work of the Russian botanist, Mikhail S. Tswett. His pioneering studies focused on separating compounds (leaf pigments), extracted from plants using a solvent, in a column packed with particles. Tswett filled an open glass column with particles. Two specific materials that he found useful were powdered chalk (calcium carbonate) and alumina. He poured his sample (solvent extract of homogenized plant leaves) into the column and allowed it to pass into the particle bed. This was followed by pure solvent. As the sample passed down through the column by gravity, different coloured bands could be seen separating because some components were moving faster than others. He related these separated, different-coloured bands to the different compounds that were originally contained in the sample. He had created an analytical separation of these compounds based on the differing strength of each compound's chemical attraction to the particles. The compounds that were more strongly attracted to the particles slowed down, while other compounds more strongly attracted to the solvent moved faster. This process can be described as follows: the compounds contained in the sample distribute or partition differently between the moving solvent, called the mobile phase and the particles, called the stationary phase. This causes each compound to move at a different speed, thus creating a separation of the compounds.

The acronym HPLC, coined by the late Prof. Csaba Horváth for his 1970 Pittcon paper originally indicated the fact that high pressure was used to generate the flow required for liquid chromatography in packed columns. In the beginning, pumps only had a pressure capability of 500 psi (35 bar). This was called high pressure liquid chromatography (HPLC). The early 1970s saw a tremendous leap in technology. These new HPLC instruments could develop up to 6,000 psi (400 bar) of pressure and incorporated improved injectors, detectors and columns. HPLC really began to take hold in the mid-to late-1970s. With continued advances in performance during this time (smaller particles, even higher pressure), the acronym remained the same, but the name was changed to high-performance liquid chromatography (HPLC). High-performance liquid chromatography (HPLC) is now one of the most powerful tools in analytical chemistry. It has the ability to separate, identify and quantitate the compounds that are present in any sample that can be dissolved in a liquid. Today, compounds in trace concentrations as low as parts per trillion (ppt) may easily be identified. HPLC can be and has been, applied to just about any sample, such as pharmaceuticals, food, nutraceuticals, cosmetics, environmental matrices, forensic samples and industrial chemicals. High-performance liquid chromatography (or high-pressure liquid chromatography, HPLC) is a chromatographic technique that can separate a mixture of compounds and is used in biochemistry and analytical chemistry to identify, quantify and purify the individual components of the mixture.

HPLC typically utilizes different types of stationary phases, a pump that moves the mobile phase(s) and analyte through the column and a detector that provides a characteristic retention time for the analyte. The detector may also provide other characteristic information (*i.e.,* UV/Vis spectroscopic data for analyte if so equipped). Analyte retention time varies depending on the strength of its interactions with the stationary phase, the ratio/composition of solvent(s) used and the flow rate of the mobile phase. With HPLC, a pump (rather than gravity) provides the higher pressure required to propel the mobile phase and analyte through the densely packed column. The increased density arises from smaller particle sizes. This allows for a better separation on columns of shorter length when compared to ordinary column chromatography.

Principle

The principle of separation in normal phase mode and reverse phase mode is adsorption. When a mixture of components is introduced in to a HPLC column, they travel according to their relative affinities towards the stationary phase. The component which has more affinity towards the adsorbent travels slower. The component which has less affinity towards the stationary phase travels faster. Since no two components have the same affinity towards the stationary phase, the components are separated.

Instrumentation

A liquid chromatograph consists of a reservoir containing the mobile phase, a pump to force the mobile phase through the system at high pressure, an injector to introduce the sample into the mobile phase, a chromatographic column, a detector and a data collection device such as a computer, integrator or recorder.

Modern HPLC essentially comprises of the following main components namely:

1. Solvent reservoir and degassing system
2. Pressure, flow and temperature
3. Pumps
4. Sample injection system

5. Column
6. Detectors
7. Recorders and Integrations
8. Microprocessor control.

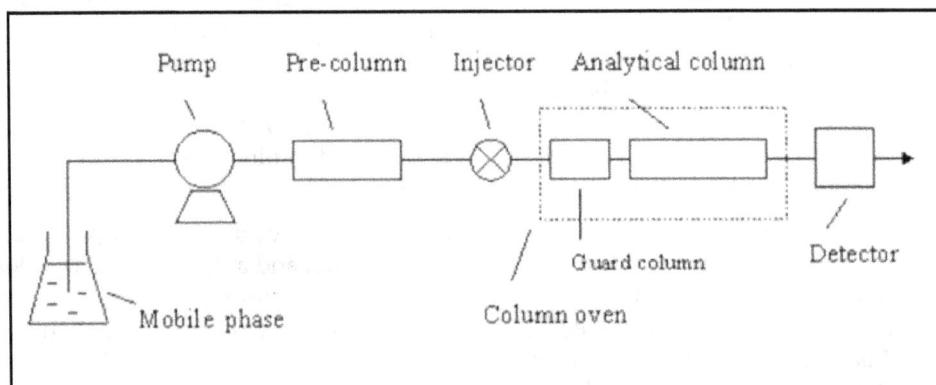

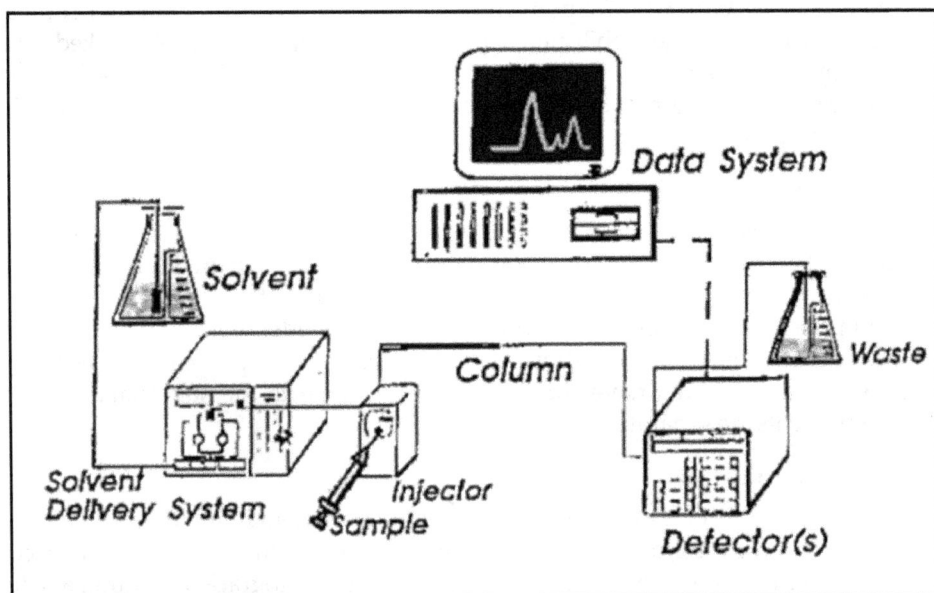

High-Performance Liquid Chromatography (HPLC) System

1. Solvent Reservoir and Degassing System

Mobile phase consisting of a mixture of organic solvents or an aqueous-organic mixture or a buffer solution may be employed depending upon the chromatography method vis-à-vis the detector to be used. Solvents-reservoir comprises of a 1 dm³ glass bottle having a lid and a 1/8 inch diameter ptfe-tube to convey the mobile phase from the reservoir to the degasses and then to the pump. The solvents used must be of high purity, preferably HPLC grade and filtered through 0.45µ filter.

Degassing: Several gases are soluble in organic solvents. When solvents are pumped under high pressure, gas bubbles are formed which will interfere with the separation process, steady baseline and the shape of the peak. Hence degassing of solvents is important. This can be done by using any one of the following technique:

a. **Vacuum filtration:** which can remove the air bubbles. But it is not always reliable and complete.

b. **Helium purging:** *i.e.* by passing helium through the solvent. This is very effective but Helium is expensive.

c. **Ultrasonication:** by using ulrtasonicator, which converts ultra-high frequency to mechanical vibrations. This causes the removal of air bubbles.

2. Pressure, Flow and Temperature

Pressure: HPLC columns are packed usually up to 700 times atmospheric pressure and, therefore, the operating inlet-column-pressure in HPLC may be to a maximum of 200 times atmospheric pressure.

Hence, 1 N atmospheric pressure=10^5 Pa (Pascal)

or $\qquad$ 1 Pa= 1 Nm^{-2}

or $\qquad$ 1 Bar= 10^5 Pa

Pressures may also be expressed as psi *i.e.* pounds per square inch or in kg cm^{-2}

$$1 \text{ kg cm}^{-2}=0.981 \text{ bar}=14.2 \text{ psi}$$

However, it is pertinent to mention here that most of the analytical HPLC is performed using pressures between 25 to 100 bar only.

Flow: The flow can be measured periodically at the column outlet by collecting the liquid for a known period and thereafter, either measuring the volume or weighing it physically.

Temperature: In reality, the maintenance of strict 'temperature control' plays a vital role in measuring retention-data correctly and precisely. It makes use of the refractometer detectors specifically.

3. Pumps: The two major functions of the pump in a modern HPLC are, namely:

(i) To pass the mobile-phase through the column at a high pressure and

(ii) At a constants a controlled flow rate.

HPLC makes use of two types of pumps. They are:

(a) **Constant Pressure pump:** A constant-pressure pump acts by applying a constant pressure to the mobile-phase. The flow rate through the column is determined by the flow resistance of the column.

(b) **Constant Flow Pump:** A constant flow pump affords and maintains a given flow of liquid. The pressure developed entirely depends upon the flow resistance.

In a constant-pressure pump the flow rate will change if the flow resistance changes. Whereas in the constant flow pumps the changes in flow resistance are compensated duty by a change of pressure. Therefore, it is always advisable to use constant flow pump in HPLC determination.

Salient feature of HPLC pump are as follow:

(i)   Interior of the pump must not be corroded by any solvent to be used in the system,

(ii) Variable-flow-rate device must be available to monitor flow rate,

(iii) Solvent flow must be non-pulsing,

(iv) Changing from one mobile-phase to another must be convenient an

(v)   It should be easy to dismantle and repair.

4. Sample Injection System: There are in all three different modes of sample injection system that are used in HPLC:

(a) **Septum Injectors:** This is injecting the sample through a rubber septum. This is not common, since the septum has to withstand high pressure.

(b) **Stop-flow SeptumLess Injection:** In which the flow of mobile phase is stopped for a while and the sample is injected through a valve device.

(c) **Rheodyne Injector (loop valve type):** It is the most popular injector. This has a fixed volume loop like 2µl to over 100 µl. Injector has two modes *i.e.* load position when the sample is loaded in the loop and inject mode, when the sample is injected.

5. Column: The column is made up of stainless steel, glass, polyethylene and PEEK (Poly ether ether ketone). Most widely used are stainless steel which can withstand high pressure.

Following are the various dimensions of HPLC columns:

Material	Stainless-steel (highly polished surface)
External Diameter	6.35 mm (or 0.25 inch)
Internal Diameter	4-5 mm (usual:4.6 mm)
Length	5-30 cm
Particle Size	1µ to 20µ
Particle Nature	Spherical, uniform sized, porous material

(i) **Fittings:** Each end of the column is adequately fitted with a stainless-steel or frit with a mesh of 2 µm or less so as to retain the packing material (usually having a particle diameter 10, 5 and 3 µm).

(ii) **Performance:** Inside the column the concentration of a band of solute decreases as it moves through the system. The column performance or the efficiency of a column entirely depends on the amount of spreading that taken place.

The efficiency or performance of a column may be measured by the following expression:

$$N=16(V_R/W_B)^2 \quad .... (1)$$

$$H=L/N \quad ...... (2)$$

Where, V_R = Retention volume of a solute

W_R =Volume occupied by a solute (or Peak-Width). Evidently, for a more efficient column, W_B will be smaller at a given value of V_R.

N = Plate number of the column (dimensionless)

H= Plate height of the column (mm×µm)

L= Length of the column (cm)

Based on equation (2) one may clearly observe that for a more efficient column 'N' gets larger and correspondingly 'H' gets smaller.

(iii) Types of Packing: Broadly speaking three types of packing are invariably used in HPLC column:

(a) Styrene-divinylbenzene copolymers

(b) Porous-layer beads

(c) Porous-silica particles

6. Detectors

An appropriate detector has the ability to sense the presence of a compound and send its corresponding electrical signal to a computer data station. A choice is made among many different types of detectors, depending upon the characteristics and concentrations of the compounds that need to be separated and analyzed, as discussed below:

(i) Bulk-property detector

(a) Refractive-index detector: Differential refractometer detectors measure the difference between the refractive index of the mobile phase alone and that of the mobile phase containing chromatographed compounds as it emerges from the column. Refractive index detectors are used to detect non UV absorbing compounds, but they are less sensitive than UV detectors.

(b) Conductivity detector: Based upon electrical conductivity, the response is recorded. This detector is used when the sample has conducting ions like anions and cations.

(ii) Solute-property detector

(a) UV-detector: A beam of UV radiation passed through the flow cell and into the detector. As compounds elute from the column, they pass through the cell and absorb the radiation resulting in measurable energy level changes.

(b) Fluorometric detectors: These are sensitive to compounds that are inherently fluorescent or that can be converted to fluorescent derivative either by chemical transformation of the compound or by coupling with fluorescent reagents at specific functional groups.

(iii.) Multipurpose detector: A multipurpose detector essentially comprises of three detector combined and housed together in a single unit. A typical example of such a detector is the one developed by Perkin-Elmer known as Perkin-Elmer '3D' System.

The functions of the three different detectors:

(a) Fluorescence function: It can monitor emission above 280 nm, based on excitation at 254 nm.

(b) UV-function: It is fixed wavelength 254 nm detector.

(c) Conductance function: The mental inlets and outlets tubes serve as electrodes to measure the conductance of the ions.

iv.) Electrochemical detector: Electrochemical detectors with carbon paste electrodes may be used to measure nanogram quantities of easily oxidised compounds. Potentiometric, voltametric or polarographic electrochemical detectors are useful for quantification of species that can be oxidised or reduced at working electrodes.

(a) Amperometric detector: This detector is based on the reduction or oxidation of the compounds when a potential is applied. The diffusion current recorded is proportional to the concentration of the compound eluted. This is applicable when compounds have functional groups which can be either oxidised or reduced. This is highly sensitive detector.

7. Recorders and Integrations

Recorders: Recorders are used to record the responses obtained from detectors after amplification, if necessary. They record the baseline and all the peaks obtained, with respect to time. Retention time for all the peaks can be founds out from such recordings, but the area of individual peaks cannot be known.

Integrators: Integrators are improved version of recorders with some data processing capability. They can record the individual peaks with retention time, height and width of peaks, peak area, percentage of area, etc. Integrators provide more information on peaks than recorders. Now a day's computers and printers are used for recording and processing the obtained data and for controlling several operations.

8. Microprocessor Control

Microprocessor based analytical equipment is no longer an uncommon phenomenon towards the modernization, automation and handling of sophisticated devices, for instance: a microprocessor scans the array of diodes many times a second in a diode array detector; a microprocessor does the temperature programming of a constants temperature chamber of HPLC unit.

Working of HPLC

A reservoir holds the solvent (called the mobile phase, because it moves). A high-pressure pump (solvent delivery system or solvent manager) is used to generate and meter a specified flow rate of mobile phase, typically milliliters per minute. An injector (sample manager or autosampler) is able to introduce (inject) the sample into the

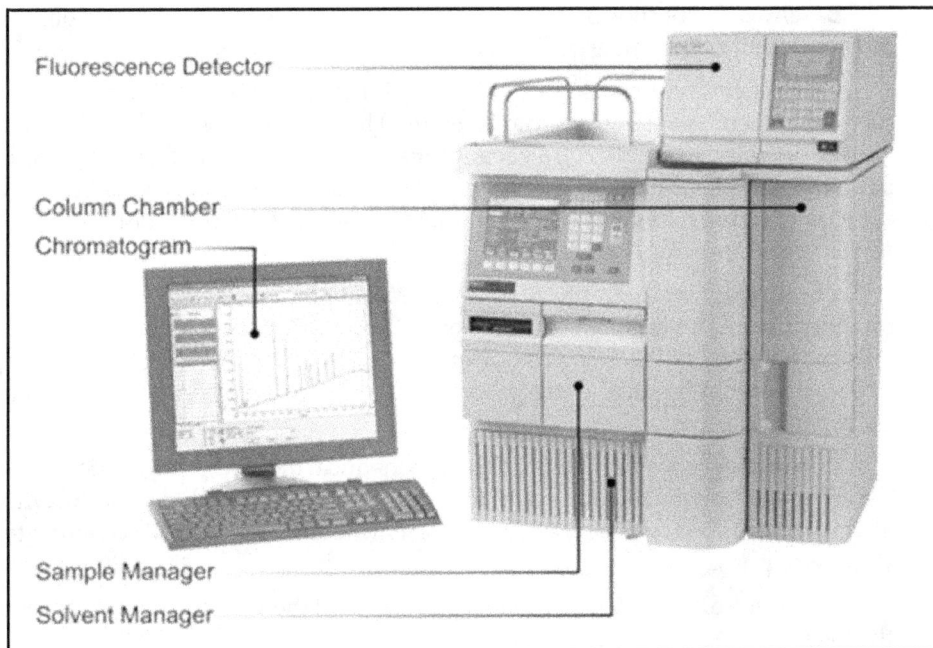

Typical HPLC (Waters Alliance) System

continuously flowing mobile phase stream that carries the sample into the HPLC column. The column contains the chromatographic packing material needed to effect the separation. This packing material is called the stationary phase because it is held in place by the column hardware. A detector is needed to see the separated compound bands as they elute from the HPLC column (most compounds have no colour, so we cannot see them with our eyes). The mobile phase exits the detector and can be sent to waste or collected, as desired. When the mobile phase contains a separated compound band, HPLC provides the ability to collect this fraction of the eluate containing that purified compound for further study. This is called preparative chromatography. The high-pressure tubing and fittings are used to interconnect the pump, injector, column and detector components to form the conduit for the mobile phase, sample and separated compound bands. The detector is wired to the computer data station, the HPLC system component that records the electrical signal needed to generate the chromatogram on its display and to identify and quantitate the concentration of the sample constituents.

HPLC Nomenclature

Alumina: A porous, particulate form of aluminum oxide (Al_2O_3) used as a stationary phase in normal-phase adsorption chromatography. Alumina has a highly active basic surface; the pH of 10% aqueous slurry is about 10. It is successively washed with strong acid to make neutral and acidic grades (slurry pH 7.5 and 4, resp.). Alumina is more hygroscopic than silica. Its activity is measured according to the Brockmann scale for water content; *e.g.*, Activity Grade I contains 1% H_2O.

Baseline: The portion of the chromatogram recording the detector response when only the mobile phase emerges from the column.

Cartridge: A type of column, without endfittings, that consists simply of an open tube wherein the packing material is retained by a frit at either end. SPE cartridges may be operated in parallel on a vacuum-manifold. HPLC cartridges are placed into a cartridge holder that has fluid connections built into each end. Cartridge columns are easy to change, less expensive and more convenient than conventional columns with integral endfittings.

Chromatogram: A graphical or other presentation of detector response or other quantity used as a measure of the concentration of the analyte in the effluent versus effluent volume or time. In planar chromatography *e.g.*, thin-layer chromatography or paper chromatography, chromatogram may refer to the paper or layer containing the separated zones.

Chromatography: A dynamic physicochemical method of separation in which the components to be separated are distributed between two phases, one of which is stationary (stationary phase) while the other (mobile phase) moves relative to the stationary phase.

Column Volume (Vc): The geometric volume of the part of the tube that contains the packing (internal cross-sectional area of the tube multiplied by the packed bed length, L). The interparticle volume of the column, also called the interstitial volume, is the volume occupied by the mobile phase between the particles in the packed bed. The void volume (V_0) is the total volume occupied by the mobile phase *i.e.*, the sum of the interstitial volume and the intraparticle volume also called pore volume.

Detector: A device that indicates a change in the composition of the eluent by measuring physical or chemical properties *e.g.*, UV/visible light absorbance, differential refractive index, fluorescence or conductivity. If the detector's response is linear with respect to sample concentration, then, by suitable calibration with standards, the amount of a component may be quantitated. Often, it may be beneficial to use two different types of detectors in series. In this way, more corroboratory or specific information may be obtained about the sample analytes. Some detectors *e.g.*, electrochemical, mass spectrometric are destructive *i.e.*, they effect a chemical change in the sample components. If a detector of this type is paired with a non-destructive detector, it is usually placed second in the flow path.

Display: A device that records the electrical response of a detector on a computer screen in the form of a chromatogram. Advanced data recording systems also perform calculations using sophisticated algorithms *e.g.*, to integrate peak areas, subtract baselines, match spectra, quantitate components and identify unknowns by comparison to standard libraries.

Efficiency: A measure of a column's ability to resist the dispersion of a sample band as it passes through the packed bed. An efficient column minimizes band dispersion or band spreading. Higher efficiency is important for effective separation, greater sensitivity and/or identification of similar components in a complex sample mixture. Nobelists Martin and Synge, by analogy to distillation, introduced the concept of plate height (H or H.E.T.P., height equivalent to a theoretical plate) as a measure of chromatographic efficiency and as a means to compare column performance. Presaging HPLC and UPLC technology, they recognized that a homogeneous bed packed with the smallest possible particle size (requiring higher pressure) was key to maximum efficiency.

Chromatographers often refer to a quantity that they can calculate easily and directly from measurements made on a chromatogram, namely plate number (N), as efficiency. Plate height is then determined from the ratio of the length of the column bed to N (H = L/N). It is important to note that calculation of N or H using these methods is correct only for isocratic conditions and cannot be used for gradient separations.

Eluate: The portion of the eluent that emerges from the column outlet containing analytes in solution. In analytical HPLC, the eluate is examined by the detector for the concentration or mass of analytes therein. In preparative HPLC, the eluate is collected continuously in aliquots at uniform time or volume intervals or discontinuously only when a detector indicates the presence of a peak of interest. These fractions are subsequently processed to obtain purified compounds.

Eluotropic Series: A list of solvents ordered by elution strength with reference to specified analytes on a standard sorbent. Such a series is useful when developing both isocratic and gradient elution methods. Trappe coined this term after showing that a sequence of solvents of increasing polarity could separate lipid fractions on alumina. Later, Snyder measured and tabulated solvent strength parameters for a large list of solvents on several normal-phase LC sorbents. Neher created a very useful nomogram by which equi-eluotropic (constant elution strength) mixtures of normal-phase solvents could be chosen to optimize the selectivity of TLC separations. A typical normal-phase eluotropic series would start at the weak end with non-polar aliphatic hydrocarbons, *e.g.*, pentane or hexane, then progress successively to benzene (an aromatic hydrocarbon), dichloromethane (a chlorinated hydrocarbon), diethyl ether, ethyl acetate (ester), acetone (ketone) and, finally, methanol (an alcohol) at the strong end.

Elute: To chromatograph by elution chromatography. The process of elution may be stopped while all the sample components are still on the chromatographic bed (planar thin-layer or paper chromatography) or continued until the components have left the chromatographic bed.

Note: The term elute is preferred to develop (a term used in planar chromatography), to avoid confusion with the practice of method development, whereby a separation system (combination of mobile and stationary phases) is optimized for a particular separation.

Elution Chromatography

A procedure for chromatographic separation in which the mobile phase is continuously passed through the chromatographic bed. In HPLC, once the detector baseline has stabilized and the separation system has reached equilibrium, a finite slug of sample is introduced into the flowing mobile phase stream. Elution continues until all analytes of interest have passed through the detector.

Elution Strength: A measure of the affinity of a solvent relative to that of the analyte for the stationary phase. A weak solvent cannot displace the analyte, causing it to be strongly retained on the stationary phase. A strong solvent may totally displace all the analyte molecules and carry them through the column unretained. To achieve a proper balance of effective separation and reasonable elution volume, solvents are often blended to set up an appropriate competition between the phases, thereby optimizing both selectivity and separation time for a given set of analytes. Dipole moment, dielectric constant, hydrogen bonding, molecular size and shape and surface tension may give some indication of elution strength. Elution strength is also determined by the separation mode. An eluotropic series of solvents may be ordered by increasing strength in one direction under adsorption or normal-phase conditions; that order may be nearly opposite under reversed-phase partition conditions.

Fluorescence Detector: Fluorescence detectors excite a sample with a specified wavelength of light. This causes certain compounds to fluoresce and emit light at a higher wavelength. A sensor, set to a specific emission wavelength and masked so as not to be blinded by the excitation source, collects only the emitted light. Often analytes that do not natively fluoresce may be derivatized to take advantage of the high sensitivity and selectivity of this form of detection.

Flow Rate: The volume of mobile phase passing through the column in unit time. In HPLC systems, the flow rate is set by the controller for the solvent delivery system (pump). Flow rate accuracy can be checked by timed collection and measurement of the effluent at the column outlet. Since a solvent's density varies with temperature, any calibration or flow rate measurement must take this variable into account. Most accurate determinations are made, when possible, by weight, not volume. Uniformity and reproducibility of flow rate is important to many LC techniques, especially in separations where retention times are key to analyte identification or in gel-permeation chromatography where calibration and correlation of retention times are critical to accurate molecular-weight-distribution measurements of polymers. Often, separation conditions are compared by means of linear velocity, not flow rate. The linear velocity is calculated by dividing the flow rate by the cross-sectional area of the column. While flow rate is expressed in volume/time (*e.g.*, mL/min), linear velocity is measured in length/time *e.g.*, mm/sec.

Gel-Permeation Chromatography

Separation based mainly upon exclusion effects due to differences in molecular size and/or shape. Gelpermeation chromatography and gel filtration chromatography describe the process when the stationary phase is a swollen gel. Both are forms of size-exclusion chromatography. Porath and Flodin first described gel-filtration using dextran gels and aqueous mobile phases for the size-based separation of biomolecules. Moore applied similar principles to the separation of organic polymers by size in solution using organic-solvent mobile phases on porous polystyrene-divinylbenzene polymer gels.

Gradient: The change over time in the relative concentrations of two (or more) miscible solvent components that form a mobile phase of increasing elution strength. A step gradient is typically used in solid-phase extraction; in each step, the eluent composition is changed abruptly from a weaker mobile phase to a stronger mobile phase. It is even possible, by drying the SPE sorbent bed in between steps, to change from one solvent to another immiscible solvent. A continuous gradient is typically generated by a low or high-pressure mixing system according to a pre-determined curve representing the concentration of the stronger solvent B in the initial solvent A over a fixed time period. A hold at a fixed isocratic solvent composition can be programmed at any time point within a continuous gradient. At the end of a separation, the gradient program can also be set to return to the initial mobile phase composition to re-equilibrate the column in preparation for the injection of the next sample. Sophisticated HPLC systems can blend as many as four or more solvents or solvent mixtures into a continuous gradient.

Injector: A mechanism for accurately and precisely introducing (injecting) a discrete, predetermined volume of a sample solution into the flowing mobile phase stream. The injector can be a simple manual device or a sophisticated autosampler that can be programmed for unattended injections of many samples from an array of individual vials or wells in a predetermined sequence. Sample compartments in these systems may even be temperature controlled to maintain sample integrity over many hours of operation. Most modern injectors incorporate some form of syringe-filled sample loop that can be switched on- or offline by means of a multi-port valve. A well-designed, minimal-internal-volume injection system is situated as close to the column inlet as possible and minimizes the spreading of the sample band. Between sample injections, it is also capable of being flushed to waste by mobile phase or a wash solvent, to prevent carryover.

Samples are best prepared for injection, if possible, by dissolving them in the mobile phase into which they will be injected; this may prevent issues with separation and/or detection. If another solvent must be used, it is desirable that its elution strength be equal to or less than that of the mobile phase. It is often wise to mix a bit of a sample solution with the mobile phase offline to test for precipitation or miscibility issues that might compromise a successful separation.

Inlet: The end of the column bed where the mobile phase stream and sample enter. A porous, inert frit retains the packing material and protects the sorbent bed inlet from particulate contamination. Good HPLC practice dictates that samples and mobile phases should be particulate-free; this becomes imperative for small-particle columns whose inlets are much more easily plugged. If the column bed inlet becomes clogged and exhibits higher-than-normal backpressure, sometimes, reversing the flow direction while directing the effluent to waste may dislodge and flush out sample debris that sits atop the frit. If the debris has penetrated the frit and is lodged in the inlet end of the bed itself, then the column has most likely reached the end of its useful life.

Ion-Exchange Chromatography: This separation mode is based mainly on differences in the ion-exchange affinities of the sample components. Separation of primarily inorganic ionic species in water or buffered aqueous mobile phases on small particle, superficially porous, high-efficiency, ion-exchange columns followed by conductometric or electrochemical detection is referred to as ion chromatography (IC).

Isocratic Elution: A procedure in which the composition of the mobile phase remains constant during the elution process.

Liquid Chromatography: A separation technique in which the mobile phase is a liquid. Liquid chromatography can be carried out either in a column or on a plane (TLC or paper chromatography). Modern liquid chromatography utilizing smaller particles and higher inlet pressure was termed high-performance or high-pressure liquid chromatography (HPLC) in 1970. In 2004, ultra-performance liquid chromatography dramatically raised the performance of LC to a new plateau.

Mobile Phase: A fluid that percolates, in a definite direction, through the length of the stationary-phase sorbent bed. The mobile phase may be a liquid or a gas (gas chromatography) or a supercritical fluid. In gas chromatography the expression carrier gas may be used for the mobile phase. In elution chromatography, the mobile phase may also be called the eluent, while the word eluate is defined as the portion of the mobile phase that has passed through the sorbent bed and contains the compounds of interest in solution.

Normal-Phase Chromatography: An elution procedure in which the stationary phase is more polar than the mobile phase. This term is used in liquid chromatography to emphasize the contrast to reversed-phase chromatography.

Peak: The portion of a differential chromatogram recording the detector response while a single component is eluted from the column. If separation is incomplete, two or more components may be eluted as one unresolved peak. Peaks eluted under optimal conditions from a well-packed, efficient column, operated in a system that minimizes bandspreading, approach the shape of a Gaussian distribution. Quantitation is usually done by measuring the peak area less often, peak height (the distance measured from the peak apex to the baseline) may be used for quantitation. This procedure requires that both the peak width and the peak shape remain constant.

Plate Number: A number indicative of column performance (mechanical separation power or efficiency, also called plate count, number of theoretical plates or theoretical plate number. It relates the magnitude of a peak's retention to its width. In order to calculate a plate count, it is assumed that a peak can be represented by a Gaussian distribution (a statistical bell curve). At the inflection points (60.7% of peak height), the width of a Gaussian curve is twice the standard deviation (ó) about its mean (located at the peak apex). As shown in Figure U, a Gaussian curve's peak width measured at other fractions of peak height can be expressed in precisely defined multiples of ó. Peak retention (retention volume, VR or retention time, tR) and peak width must be expressed in the same units, because method of calculating N is aN is a dimensionless number.

Preparative Chromatography: The process of using liquid chromatography to isolate a compound in a quantity and at a purity level sufficient for further experiments or uses. For pharmaceutical or biotechnological purification processes, columns several feet in diameter can be used for multiple kilograms of material. For isolating just a few micrograms of a valuable natural product, an analytical HPLC column is sufficient. Both are preparative chromatographic approaches, differing only in scale.

Resolution: The separation of two peaks, expressed as the difference in their corresponding retention times, divided by their average peak width at the baseline. Rs = 1.25 indicates that two peaks of equal width are just separated at the baseline. When Rs = 0.6, the only visual indication of the presence of two peaks on a chromatogram is a small notch near the peak apex. Higher efficiency columns produce narrower peaks and improve resolution for difficult separations; however, resolution increases by only the square root of N. The most powerful method of increasing resolution is to increase selectivity by altering the mobile/stationary phase combination used for the chromatographic separation.

Retention Factor (k): A measure of the time the sample component resides in the stationary phase relative to the time it resides in the mobile phase; it expresses how much longer a sample component is retarded by the stationary phase than it would take to travel through the column with the velocity of the mobile phase. Mathematically, it is the ratio of the adjusted retention time and the hold-up time $k = tR'/tM$.

Retention Time (tR): The time taken for a particular compound to travel through the column to the detector is known as its retention time.

The time between the start of elution (typically, in HPLC, the moment of injection or sample introduction) and the emergence of the peak maximum. The adjusted retention time, tR', is calculated by subtracting from tR the hold-up time (tM, the time from injection to the elution of the peak maximum of a totally unretained analyte).

Reversed-Phase Chromatography: An elution procedure used in liquid chromatography in which the mobile phase is significantly more polar than the stationary phase, *e.g.*, a microporous silica-based material with alkyl chains chemically bonded to its accessible surface.

Note: Avoid the incorrect term reverse phase.

Selectivity (Separation Factor, ó): A term used to describe the magnitude of the difference between the relative thermodynamic affinities of a pair of analytes for the specified mobile and stationary phases that comprise the separation system. The proper term is separation factor (ó). It equals the ratio of retention factors, $k2/k1 = 1$, then both is always e" 1. If ó by definition, ó peaks co-elute and no separation is obtained. It is important in preparative chromatography to maximize á for highest sample loadability and throughput.

Sensitivity (S): The signal output per unit concentration or unit mass of a substance in the mobile phase entering the detector *e.g.,* the slope of a linear calibration curve. For concentration-sensitive detectors *e.g.*, UV/VIS absorbance, sensitivity is the ratio of peak height to analyte concentration in the peak. For mass-flow-sensitive detectors, it is the ratio of peak height to unit mass. If sensitivity is to be a unique performance characteristic, it must depend only on the chemical measurement process, not upon scale factors.

The ability to detect or measure an analyte is governed by many instrumental and chemical factors. Well-resolved peaks eluting from high efficiency columns (narrow peak width with good symmetry for maximum peak height) as well as good detector sensitivity and specificity are ideal. Both the separation system interference and electronic component noise should also be minimized to achieve maximum sensitivity.

Solid-Phase Extraction (SPE): A sample preparation technique that uses LC principles to isolate, enrich and/or purify analytes from a complex matrix applied to a miniature chromatographic bed. Offline SPE is done (manually or via automation) with larger particles in individual plastic cartridges or in micro-elution plate wells, using low positive pressure or vacuum to assist flow. Online SPE is done with smaller particles in miniature HPLC columns using higher pressures and a valve to switch the SPE column online with the primary HPLC column or offline to waste, as appropriate. SPE methods use step gradients to accomplish bed conditioning, sample loading, washing and elution steps. Samples are loaded typically under conditions where the k of important analytes is as high as possible, so that they are fully retained during loading and washing steps. Elution is then done by switching to a much stronger solvent mixture. The goal is to remove matrix interferences and to isolate the analyte in a solution and at a concentration, suitable for subsequent analysis.

Speed: A benefit of operating LC separations at higher linear velocities using smaller-volume, smaller-particle analytical columns or larger-volume, larger-particle preparative columns. Order-of-magnitude advances in LC speed came in 1972 with the use of 10 µm particles and pumps capable of delivering accurate mobile-phase flow at 6000 psi, in 1976 with 75-µm preparative columns operated at a flow rate of 500 mL/min and in 2004 with the introduction of UPLC technology 1.7 µm-particle columns operated at 15,000 psi. High-speed analytical LC systems must not only accommodate higher pressures throughout the fluidics; injector cycle time must be short; gradient mixers must be capable of rapid turnaround between samples; detector sensors must rapidly respond to tiny changes in eluate composition; and data systems must collect the dozens of points each second required to plot and to quantitate narrow peaks accurately. Together, higher resolution, higher speed and higher efficiency typically deliver higher throughput. More samples can be analyzed in a workday. Larger quantities of compound can be purified per run or per process period.

Stationary Phase: One of the two phases forming a chromatographic system. It may be a solid, a gel or a liquid. If a liquid, it may be distributed on a solid. This solid may or may not contribute to the separation process. The liquid may also be chemically bonded to the solid (bonded phase) or immobilized onto it (immobilized phase). The expression chromatographic bed or sorbent may be used as a general term to denote any of the different forms in which the stationary phase is used. The use of the term liquid phase to denote the mobile phase in LC is discouraged. This avoids confusion with gas chromatography where the stationary phase is called a liquid phase (most often a liquid coated on a solid support). Open-column liquid-liquid partition chromatography (LLC) did not translate well to HPLC. It was supplanted by the use of bonded-phase packings. LLC proved incompatible with modern detectors because of problems with bleed of the stationary-phase-liquid coating off its solid support, thereby contaminating the immiscible liquid mobile phase.

Appendix -5

Management of Heavy Metal Pollution

Waste

Waste is an unavoidable by product of most human activity. Waste can be, in the form of solid or liquid, posed the harmful nuisance. Most solid waste is either sent to landfills or to incinerators. Ocean dumping has also been a popular way for coastal communities to dispose of their solid wastes in which large barges carry waste out to sea and dump it into the ocean. Most municipal and non municipal waste is sent to landfills. Landfills are popular because they are relatively easy to operate and can handle of lot of waste material. There are two types of landfills, sanitary landfills and secure landfills. Each day after garbage is dumped in the landfill, it is covered with clay or plastic to prevent redistribution by animals or the wind. In natural system, there is no such thing as waste. Everything flows in a natural cycle of use and reuse. Living organisms consume materials and eventually return them to the environment, usually in a different form, for reuse. Solid waste refers to a variety of discarded materials, not liquid or gas that is deemed useless or worthless. However, what is worthless to one person may be of value to someone else and solid wastes can be considered to be misplaced resources. Solid wastes are all the waste arising from human and animal activities that are normally solid waste and that are discarded as useless or unwanted. The term is all inclusive and it encompasses the heterogeneous mass of throwaways from the urban community as well as the homogeneous accumulations of agricultural, industrial and mineral wastes.

Electronic Waste

Electronic waste, e-waste, e-scrap or Waste Electrical and Electronic Equipment (WEEE) describe loosely discarded, surplus, outdated, broken, electrical or electronic devices. Electronic waste may be defined as all secondary computers, entertainment device electronics, mobile phones and other items such as television sets and refrigerators, whether sold, donated or discarded by their original owners. The processing of electronic waste in developing countries causes serious health and pollution problems because electronic equipment contains some very serious contaminants such as lead, cadmium, beryllium and brominates flame retardants. Electronic waste processing systems have matured in recent years, following increased regulatory, public and commercial scrutiny and a proportionate increase in entrepreneurial interest. In developed countries, electronic waste processing usually involves dismantling the equipment into various parts like metal frames, power supplies, circuit boards, plastics, by hand. The advantages of this process are the human's ability to recognize and save working and repairable parts, including chips, transistors, RAM, etc. It is a major area of concern today that the wealthy countries are dumping large quantities of e waste into the developing world. According to BBC, currently the companies export 80 per cent of the world's electronic trash to Asia. The problem of e-waste recycling in India involved the urgent need for educating consumers including the potential threat to public health and the environment posed by their products and for raising awareness for the proper waste management.

Liquid Waste

Liquid waste can be defined as such fluids as wastewater, fats, oils, grease or used oil. The disposal of such waste, such as transmission fluid, cooking oil, spent oil, fats or grease can contaminate the groundwater or negatively impact the wastewater system. The liquid waste basically the waste water discharged from the industrial and domestic area. Wastewater is water that has been used for some purpose and is deemed unfit for further use. In fact, wastewater can be used for secondary purposes in most cases. Also, efficient use of water reduces the amount of wastewater generated. Sewage is created by residences, institutions, hospitals and commercial and industrial establishments. Raw influent or sewage includes household waste liquid from toilets, baths, showers, kitchens, sinks and so forth that is disposed of via sewers. In many areas, sewage also includes liquid waste from industry and commerce. As rainfall runs over the surface of roofs and the ground, it may pick up various contaminants including soil particles and other sediment, heavy metals, organic compounds, animal waste, oil and grease. It may be originated from various sites and by different uses.

Municipal Waste

Municipal waste water is the combination of liquid or water carried wastes originating in the sanitary conveniences of dwellings, commercial or industrial facilities and institutions, in addition to any groundwater, surface water and storm water that may be present. Wastewater is the flow of used water from a community. The characteristics of the wastewater discharges vary from location to location depending upon the population and industrial sector served, land uses, groundwater levels and degree of separation between storm water and sanitary wastes. Domestic wastewater includes typical wastes from the kitchen, bathroom and laundry, as well as any other wastes that people may accidentally or intentionally pour down the drain. Sanitary waste water consists of domestic wastewater as well as those discharged from commercial, institutional and similar facilities. Industrial wastes will be as varied as the industries that generate the wastes. Municipal waste water also contains a variety of inorganic substances from domestic and industrial sources, including a number of potentially toxic elements such as arsenic, cadmium, chromium, copper, lead, mercury, zinc etc.

Industrial effluent

The effluent of the industries goes into the water system and changes the physico-chemical quality of water and also makes it unfit for drinking and other uses. Since all natural waterways contain bacteria and nutrients, almost any waste compounds introduced into such waterways will initiate biochemical reactions. These biochemical reactions are measured as BOD and COD in the laboratory. Both have been widely adopted as a measure of pollution effect. Disposal of wastewaters from an industrial plant is a difficult and costly problem. Most petroleum refineries, chemical and petrochemical plants have onsite facilities to treat their wastewaters so that the pollutant concentrations in the treated wastewater comply with the local or national regulations regarding the disposal of wastewaters into community treatment plants or into rivers, lakes or oceans. The solids can be suspended 30% as well as dissolved solids which are about 70%. The dissolved solids can be precipitated by chemical and biological processes. Organic components may consist of carbohydrates, proteins, fats and greases, surfactants, oils, pesticides, phenols etc. From a physical point of view the suspended solids can lead to the development of sludge deposits and anaerobic conditions when discharged into the receiving environment. Physically, the wastewater is usually characterized by grey colour, musty odour, 0.1% solid content and 99.9% water content.

Soil

The soil is the target of thousands of contaminants that vary in composition and in concentration. The contaminants enter the system as a result of a wide range of actions such as intentional applications, inadequate residue disposal, accidental wastes and inappropriate use. Soil pollution is defined as the buildup in soils of persistent toxic compounds, chemicals, salts, radioactive materials or disease causing agents, which have adverse effects on plant growth and animal health. Soil is the thin layer of organic and inorganic materials that covers the earth's rocky surface. The organic portion, derived from the decayed remains of plants and animals, is concentrated in the dark uppermost topsoil. The inorganic portion, made up of rock fragments, was formed over thousands of years by physical and chemical weathering of bedrock. Soil pollution is caused by the presence of manmade chemicals or other alteration in the natural soil environment. This type of contamination typically arises from the rupture of underground storage links, application of pesticides and percolation of contaminated surface water to subsurface strata, oil and fuel dumping, leaching of wastes from landfills or direct discharge of industrial wastes to the soil. The most common chemicals involved are petroleum hydrocarbons, solvents, pesticides, lead and other heavy metals. This occurrence of this phenomenon is correlated with the degree of industrialization and intensities of chemical usage. The waste contaminates the soil. The solid waste includes garbage, domestic refuse and discarded solid materials such as those from commercial, industrial and agricultural operations. They contain increasing amounts of paper, cardboards, plastics, glass, old construction material, packaging material and toxic or otherwise hazardous substances.

Human Activities

Some human activities have resulted in the accumulation of metals in the environment. Both soil and aqueous effluents have been contaminated with heavy metals as the result of numerous industrial activities, including mining, smelting, jewellery, automobile battery production, vehicle emission and land filling of industrial waste and fly ash from incineration process. This contamination of the environment poses serious health threats to humans and animals, as these heavy metals tend to persist in the environment indefinitely. This kind of contamination presents a challenge, as the presence of heavy metals in soils and aqueous effluents leads to serious problems because they cannot be biodegraded. In this case, the metal ion can only be converted to the base metal, methylated, precipitated, volatilized or complexed with an organic ligand. The more common heavy metals associated with anthropogenic activities include lead, cadmium, copper, chromium, nickel, iron, mercury and zinc. Methods of treating the contaminated effluents currently consist of chemical precipitation, solvent extraction, dialysis, electrolytic extraction, cementation, reverse osmosis, evaporative methods, ion exchange resins, carbon adsorption and dilution.

Heavy Metals

Metals play an integral role in the life processes of living organisms. Some metals like Ca, Co, Cr, Cu, Fe, K, Mg, Mn, Na, Ni and Zn are essential, serve as micronutrients and are used for redox processes, to stabilize molecules through electrostatic interactions; as components of various enzymes and regulation of osmotic pressure. The essential metals must be present in a certain concentration range. Too low concentrations of heavy metals lead to a decrease in metabolic activity and too high concentrations, it leads to toxicity. While other metals like Ag, Al, Cd, Au, Pb and Hg have no biological role and they are non essential. Non – essential metals are tolerated at very low concentrations and inhibit metabolic activity at higher concentrations. They are potentially toxic to living organism specially microorganisms. Toxicity of non essential metals occurs through the displacement of essential metals from their native binding sites or through ligand interactions. The many uses of heavy metals in several applications lead to wide distribution in soil, silt, waste and waste water. Such pollution of the environment by toxic metals and radionuclide arises as a result of many human activities, largely industrial, although such sources as agriculture and sewage disposal also contribute. Heavy metal contamination can be a consequence of industrial activities that eliminate residues in the soil that in long terms, promote their accumulation. Heavy metals in wastewater come from industries and municipal sewage and they are one of the main causes of water and soil pollution. The majority of the sources are originated by human actions like metal manufacture and mining industries with storage, disposal and transportation problems. Among the metals found more frequently there are Cd, Pb, Co, Cu, Hg, Ni, Si and Zn. For Cd, Pb, Cu and Zn, their toxicity increases as follows: Pb < Zn < Cu < Cd, depending on countless abiotic and biotic factors.

Managing Heavy Metal Pollution

In order to survive in heavy metal polluted environments, many microorganisms have developed means of resistance to toxic metal ions. These mechanisms include: metal exclusion by permeability barriers, active transport of the metal away from the cell organism, intracellular sequestration of the metal by protein binding, extracellular sequestration, enzymatic detoxification of the metal to a less toxic form and reduction in metal sensitivity of cellular targets. Most microorganisms are known to have specific genes for resistance to toxic ions of heavy metals. Mostly, the resistance genes are found on plasmids or on chromosomes. Plasmid encoded metal resistance determinants have been reported to be inducible.

The intake of heavy metal ions by microbial strains normally includes a redox reaction involving the metal. Some bacteria use heavy metals for energy and their growth. Bacteria that are resistant to heavy metals also play an important role in biogeochemical cycling of metal ions. Since, the oxidation state of a metal ion may determine its solubility, many scientists have been attempting to use microbes that are capable to oxidize or reduce metals in order to remediate metal contaminated sites. Although, some heavy metals are important and essential trace elements and others are toxic at high concentrations to microbes, some microbes have adapted to tolerate the presence of metals or even to use them to grow. In addition, a number of interactions between microbial strains and metals have important environmental and health implications. Health problem due to heavy metals pollution in human being include nausea, vomiting, bone complications, nervous system impairments and even death become a major problem throughout many countries when metal ions concentration in the environment exceeded the admissible limits. Due to that, various treatment technologies had been searched to reduce the concentration of heavy metals in the environment.

Toxic chemicals found in wastewater pass through wastewater treatment facilities that have not been designed to remove them and can interfere with their operation. In a biological treatment process toxic materials can upset a treatment process or even kill the biological community and make the process ineffective. To remove the toxic pollutants at the treatment facility can be very costly. Therefore, it is generally advantages to remove them at the source. Source control can be achieved by the use of municipal by laws limiting pollutant discharges to the sewerage system. The removal of toxic pollutants at the source can be achieved by requiring treatment prior to discharge, recycling of waste by products, manufacturing process changes and the substitution of raw material.

It is needed to remove the heavy metals from the contaminated sites/waste. Several heavy metals removal technologies including chemical precipitation, ion exchange, reverse osmosis, electrodialysis, ultra filtration and pyhtoremediation are commonly used in industries. However, these technologies are becoming uneconomical and unfavorable to remove heavy metals from industrial wastewaters. The development of new treatment method such as bioremediation to remove heavy metal ions from wastewater and solid waste which could be cost effective and more efficient has spurred to overcome the conventional method. Bioremediation technology has received much attention as it offered low cost technique and non hazardous biomaterials.

Bioremediation

The history of bioremediation is considerably shorter and it reflects many upturns and downturns as a result of political and economic forces. Interest in use of microorganisms to degrade specific hazardous organic chemicals probably dates back to Gayle (1952), who proposed the microbial infallitibility hypothesis. Gayle postulated that for any conceivable organic compound, there exists a microorganism that can degrade it under the right conditions. If not, evolution and adaptation would produce such a strain. This hypothesis cannot wrong, because failure to degrade a contaminant can be attributed to the researcher's failure to use the right strain under the right condition. In 1970s, environmental statutes of unprecedented scope passed, such as the Occupational Safety and Health Act (OSHA) of 1970, the Clean Air Act (CAA) of 1970, the Clean Water Act (CWA) of 1972, the Safe Drinking Water Act (SWA) of 1974 and the Toxic Substance Control Act (TSCA) of 1976. This regulatory pressure stimulated interest in site remediation technologies, including bioremediation. However, bioremediation failed to meet the expectations raised by many technology salespeople, who commonly advocated the addition of specialized bacteria to contaminated site *i.e.* bioaugmentation. Early proponents of this approach generally did not recognize that indigenous bacteria already present at a contaminated site where probably better predisposed physiologically and genetically to mediate the degradation of the target pollutants.

The first patent for a biological remediation agent was registered in 1974, being a strain of *Pseudomonas putida* that was able to degrade petroleum. In 1991, about 70 microbial genera were reported to degrade petroleum compounds and almost an equal number has been added to the list in the successive two decades. Bioremediation can occur naturally or through intervention processes. Natural degradation of pollutants relies on indigenous microflora that is effective against specific contaminants and it usually occurs at a slow rate. With intervention processes, the rate of biodegradation is aided by encouraging growth of microorganisms, under optimized physico-chemical conditions. Microorganisms play a vital role in heavy metal contaminated soil and wastewater by the mechanisms of biosorption. Some microorganisms possess an astonishing catabolic versatility to degrade or transform such compounds. The need for economical, effective and safe methods for removing heavy metals from wastewater has resulted in the search for unconventional materials that may be useful in reducing the levels or accumulation of heavy metals in the environment.

Bioremediation is the use of living microorganism to reduce the environmental pollution. It is a technology for removing pollution from the environment, restoring contaminated site and preventing future pollution. Bioremediation can be performed *in situ* or *ex situ*. With the onset of the Industrial Revolution, an ever increasing proportion of the earth's surface became contaminated with natural and xenobiotic toxic chemicals. The basic principle of bioremediation involves utilizing the activity of microorganisms naturally present in the soil and water or selected organisms inoculated into the environment, to biodegrade or detoxify contaminating compounds *in situ*. In the majority of cases a consortium of microorganisms will be involved in the biodegradation of the contaminant, rather than a single species. To optimize the process, promotion of the growth of indigenous microorganisms is necessary. It can be achieved by the addition of key nutrients such as nitrogen and phosphorus, which are normally present in growth limiting concentrations. This enables the natural microbial flora to develop and metabolize the contaminant.

Alternatively, known biodegraders of the contaminant that have been identified, isolated and their activities optimized can be used as an inoculants. For example, a recent addition to the growing list of microorganisms able to sequester or reduce metals is *Geobacter metallireducens*. This bacterium can remove uranium, a radioactive waste, from drainage waters in mining operations and from contaminated ground waters. However, the most radiation resistant bacterium known is *Deinococcus radiodurans*; this organism is also being developed to help clean up soil and water contaminated by solvents, heavy metals and radioactive waste. A genetically engineered strain of *D. radiodurans* has been produced which can detoxify mercury (genes derived from *Escherichia coli*) and degrade toluene (genes derived from *Pseudomonas putida*) in radioactive environments.

Bioremediation is a fairly new technology and holds the promise of becoming the solution to our polluted environment. This new technology gives us alternative routes to cleaning up contaminated sites was thought to be not possible previously. Nonetheless, the technology of bioremediation still has a long way more to go). Bioremediation faces several challenges and some of the most common ones are deficit of knowledge, lack of integrated research, lack of revenue and inadequate tool and infrastructure.

Bioremedition can be done *in situ* or *ex situ*. When bioremediation occurs on its own it is said that the process represents natural attenuation; however, when fertilizers are added it is termed biostimulation. When specific microbes are introduced to treat a pollutant, the term is referred to as bioaugmentation. The overall goal of bioremediation is to overcome the threats imposed by environmental pollution and to fight the subsequent effects on ecosystem degradation, effects that could be exacerbated in coming years by climate change, alteration of the water cycle and rain quantity, which could influence microbial diversity and the activity of microbial communities. The removal of pollutants by microbes (bioremediation) or plants (phytoremediation) are often considered independent approaches, but it is important to recall that interactions between plants and microbes can also be exploited for removal of pollutants. Bioremediation has wide applicability in the frontier area of research in environmental biotechnology. Field research is essential for evaluating the performance of full scale bioremediation processes and for conducting accelerated testing on technologies that are appropriate for scaled up application e.g., problems associated with the use of bacteria used in the laboratory include optimizing the activity of the organism under site conditions and defining the risks associated with introducing a non-native microorganisms to the site. Although bioremediation holds great promise for dealing with intractable environmental problems, it is important to reduce the cost of bioremediation. Specifically, much needs to be learned about how microorganisms interact with different hydrologic/micro environments. As these understanding increases, the efficiency and applicability of bioremediation will grow rapidly. The bioremediation technology is greener technology for cleaning the environment *i.e.*, "Nature's Way to a Cleaner Environment".

A deficit of knowledge on the different fundamental branches of sciences that are involved in the process of bioremediation hinders the progress of bioremediation. Examples of the different disciplines of sciences are such as structural and molecular biology, microbiology, genomics, geochemistry, along with hydrology and transport processes. To date, little is known on how introduced microorganisms interact with different hydrological environment. Research in each of the variety of fields is needed to further researchers' comprehension on the actual activity or rather, the chemistry that is involved and interactions between contaminants, native organisms on site and remedial organisms. There is still much to learn and gain from research as contaminated sites are complex systems, each composed of different types of contaminants, diverse organisms and dissimilar environment. Bioremediation is a multidisciplinary field and researchers from various fields need to integrate their knowledge. The success and efficiency of bioremediation requires the involvement of microbiologists, biochemists, engineers, geologists and soil scientists among others. Knowledge on the combined factors is not enough and mostly these are the rate limiting factors of the process of bioremediation. Interdisciplinary research of at the least two fields is unavoidable to advance this technology. Assimilation of scientific ideas across disciplines is most needed to optimize the potential of bioremediation.

There is no doubt that governmental and private sectors are investing on biotechnology companies but not much of the revenue goes to the improvement of bioremediation. Lack of revenue is an obstruction to advancement in bioremediation as it prevents further research and discoveries from taking place. Thereupon, progress of bioremediation is delayed as a result of material deficiency. Infrastructure and materials are needed to carry out research. Accuracy in experimental procedures is crucial to ensure successful treatment when introduced to contaminated site. However, there is inadequacy of infrastructure to analyze the conditions of contaminated sites as well as monitor the process of degradation that has been introduced to the site. Insufficiency of advanced tools specifically designed to aid research on bioremediation would also hold back development of research methodology and prevent discoveries from happening. Despite its shortcomings, its pertinence in this world is unquestionable in the light of present day environmental hazards. Bioremediation provides a technique for cleaning up pollution by enhancing the same biodegradation processes that occur in nature and potential for significant advances.